Neuropsychiatric Features of Medical Disorders

CRITICAL ISSUES IN PSYCHIATRY
An Educational Series for Residents and Clinicians

Series Editor: **Sherwyn M. Woods, M.D., Ph.D.**
University of Southern California School of Medicine
Los Angeles, California

A RESIDENT'S GUIDE TO PSYCHIATRIC EDUCATION
Edited by Michael G. G. Thompson, M.D.

STATES OF MIND: Analysis of Change in Psychotherapy
Mardi J. Horowitz, M.D.

DRUG AND ALCOHOL ABUSE: A Clinical Guide to Diagnosis and
Treatment
Marc A. Schuckit, M.D.

THE INTERFACE BETWEEN THE PSYCHODYNAMIC AND
BEHAVIORAL THERAPIES
Edited by Judd Marmor, M.D., and Sherwyn M. Woods, M.D., Ph.D.

LAW IN THE PRACTICE OF PSYCHIATRY
Seymour L. Halleck, M.D.

NEUROPSYCHIATRIC FEATURES OF MEDICAL DISORDERS
James W. Jefferson, M.D., and John R. Marshall, M.D.

ADULT DEVELOPMENT: A New Dimension in Psychodynamic
Theory and Practice
Calvin A. Colarusso, M.D., and Robert A. Nemiroff, M.D.

SCHIZOPHRENIA
John S. Strauss, M.D., and William T. Carpenter, Jr., M.D.

A Continuation Order Plan is available for this series. A continuation order will bring
delivery of each new volume immediately upon publication. Volumes are billed only upon
actual shipment. For further information please contact the publisher.

Neuropsychiatric Features of Medical Disorders

James W. Jefferson, M.D.
and
John R. Marshall, M.D.

University of Wisconsin Medical School
Madison, Wisconsin

PLENUM MEDICAL BOOK COMPANY
NEW YORK AND LONDON

Library of Congress Cataloging in Publication Data

Jefferson, James W.
  Neuropsychiatric features of medical disorders.

  (Critical issues in psychiatry)
  Bibliography: p.
  Includes index.
  1. Neuropsychiatry. 2. Neurologic manifestations of general diseases. 3.
Psychological manifestations of general diseases. I. Marshall, John R., 1939-
II. Title. III. Series. [DNLM: 1. Mental disorder—Etiology. 2. Diagnosis. 3. In-
ternal medicine. 4. Drug therapy—Adverse effects. WB 115 J453n]
  RC343.J36   616.047   81-2550
  ISBN 0-306-40674-8   AACR2

First Printing—July 1981
Second Printing—February 1983

© 1981 Plenum Publishing Corporation
233 Spring Street, New York, N.Y. 10013
Plenum Medical Book Company is an imprint of Plenum Publishing Corporation

To parents, wives, and children—*especially ours*

Foreword

When *Critical Issues in Psychiatry* was conceived, there were several subjects I considered to be of crucial importance in a series devoted to residents and clinicians in psychiatry, as well as to other mental health professionals. Of prominence was the pressing need for an in-depth and scholarly examination of the interface between medicine and psychiatry. I had been amazed to find that not a single book, to my mind, adequately addressed the psychological symptoms and manifestations of both common and rare medical illness. It seemed to me that there was a need for a work which would achieve the following goals: First, it would assist in the differential diagnosis of functional psychiatric symptoms versus symptoms secondary to recognized or unrecognized medical illness; second, it would elucidate the psychological symptoms resulting from pharmacologic and other therapeutic interventions in medical illness; and third, it would examine the use of psychopharmacological agents in the presence of medical illness and the drugs used to treat that illness.

Dr. Jefferson is Board Certified in both internal medicine and psychiatry, and both Drs. Jefferson and Marshall have extensive clinical experience from their many years of consultation/liaison work in psychiatry. Their experience and expertise have resulted in what I believe to be a monumental contribution to the literature. With both comprehensiveness and conciseness, each chapter addresses an organ system of the body and reviews those medical illnesses and disorders which can present with or be accompanied by psychiatric symptoms. In each instance, the condition's clinical features and laboratory findings are described, the psychiatric manifestations are delineated and discussed, the psychophysiological basis of the symptomatology is elucidated when the mechanisms are known, and the psychological symptoms or complications which can accompany treatment are comprehensively reviewed. Whether discussing endocrine dysfunction, ketoacidosis, or the mitral-valve-prolapse syndrome, the authors describe patients and conditions which might present in any mental health professional's office, or, for that matter, in the office of an internist or primary care physician.

It is the nightmare of every psychiatrist and nonmedical psychotherapist that despite best intentions and efforts, one will regard as functional a patient whose primary problem is an underlying medical illness. It is an unfortunate reality that there have undoubtedly been patients who have suffered (and died) because of shortsighted, unidimensional, psychological misinterpretation. Knowledge is our best insurance against such tragedies. Since it is difficult for most psychiatrists and other mental health professionals to maintain their medical expertise, the authors have done an important service to the profession by providing this first truly comprehensive resource and reference. In doing so, they have exhaustively reviewed and evaluated the existing literature, while at the same time retaining clinical relevance and readability.

As a psychiatrist and psychoanalyst, I regard this volume as essential for ready availability in my daily clinical work. It is likely that nonmedical psychotherapists and mental health professionals of all disciplines will find the book of great value. This will undoubtedly be true of internists, neurologists, family practitioners, and other primary care specialists who must address themselves daily to the differential diagnosis and management of psychological symptoms which may be related to medical illness.

Sherwyn M. Woods, M.D., Ph.D.
Series Editor

Preface

Many books have been published in recent years dealing with psychosomatic illness, liaison-consultation psychiatry, the psychological care of the medically ill, and general hospital psychiatry. Our book makes no attempt to duplicate these efforts, but rather focuses on other aspects of the medical–psychiatric interface. These include:

1. The neuropsychiatric features of medical disorders
2. The neuropsychiatric effects of medical drugs
3. Psychotropic drugs and medical disorders

It is written for clinicians in order to assist them in the difficult area of differential diagnosis, illustrating the perils of misdiagnosis and emphasizing the dictum that only accurate diagnosis can lead to specific, effective treatment. We insist that psychiatric symptoms not be automatically considered indicative of "functional" illness but that they also be recognized as integral parts (and sometimes the leading edge) of many medical disorders. This is not to deny the importance of recognizing and understanding psychological stressors, psychological responses to illness, and the psychological approaches and treatments that are a necessary aspect of dealing with these conditions. Indeed, a clinician lacking these attributes would be unidimensional and of limited affectiveness. They are simply not our subject matter.

With the exception of the introductory chapter, the book is disorder- rather than symptom-oriented and follows a general medical textbook format. While we emphasize the neuropsychiatric features of medical disorders and medical drugs, we present them in a framework that provides an overview of the disorders with regard to etiology, clinical features, diagnosis, and treatment. In this way, we stress the interrelationship between symptoms and disorder, recognizing and deploring the all too common tendency to treat them as separate, unrelated entities.

The book does not cover all medical disorders, since many do not have well defined, unique neuropsychiatric features and were, thus, excluded. We apologize for omissions that would have been appropriate inclusions and would appreciate having those brought to our attention. Neurologic disorders were intentionally excluded, in part due to the availability of texts such as *Behavioral Neurology* (Pincus and Tucker; Oxford University Press,

1978), *Psychiatric Aspects of Neurologic Disease* (Benson and Blumer; Grune and Stratton, 1975) and *Organic Psychiatry* (Lishman; Blackwell Scientific, 1978).

Although we are well aware of major controversies surrounding the use of terms such as psychological, physical, functional, organic, medical, and psychiatric, we saw little option but to use them (often within quotation marks) in the conventional sense. While recognizing that distinctions may blur and that terminology may be clumsy and subject to misinterpretation, we have attempted to use a language that, while imprecise, will be familiar to most of our readers. We recognize and value psychiatry as a medical speciality; hence the term "medical disorder" refers to a nonpsychiatric medical disorder while the term "psychiatric disorder" refers to a psychiatric medical disorder.

Readers will find it apparent that we consider unsound the common practice of assuming the presence of a psychiatric illness merely because a physical disorder seems absent. Misdiagnosis is likely if a clinician has not considered a comprehensive differential diagnosis or has not obtained the appropriate laboratory tests. It is also possible that current diagnostic techniques are not sufficiently refined to detect illnesses that will eventually fall within the nonpsychiatric medical domain. Historically, neurosyphillis was considered a psychiatric illness until the spirochete was discovered and effective treatments developed. Psychiatric diagnosis is clearly not diagnosis by elimination, and if positive support for a psychiatric diagnosis is not available, it is far better to label the disorder "of unknown etiology." This avoids stigmatizing the patient with unwarranted assumptions and allows for ongoing diagnostic considerations in both medical and psychiatric arenas.

We wish to thank the Department of Psychiatry at the University of Wisconsin and the Wisconsin Psychiatric Institute for providing an atmosphere within which writing this book was both facilitated and encouraged. We are especially grateful to our trainees who provided both tolerance and critical comment when these topics were presented in seminars. Without the secretarial assistance of Jean Thomas, Pam Miller, and *especially* Lynn DeWeese, we would have been stymied at the start. Sherwyn Woods, as Editor-in-Chief of the *Critical Issues in Psychiatry* series, provided continual encouragement, valuable suggestions, and a much appreciated tolerance for delay. Finally, Hilary Evans, Senior Medical Editor of the Plenum Publishing Company, has done all that is humanly possible to alleviate the pains of publishing.

James W. Jefferson and John R. Marshall

Madison

Contents

Chapter 3

Respiratory Disorders 51

Chapter 16

Sleep and Arousal Disorders 329

Chapter 17

Substance Abuse Disorders 341

Physical Illness and Psychiatric Symptoms

OVERVIEW

There are few, if any, psychiatric symptoms that cannot be caused or aggravated by physical illnesses. The nonspecificity of altered mood, behavior, or perception requires that clinicians continually contend with the possibility that there may be an underlying nonpsychiatric disease process accounting entirely for or contributing to an apparent "functional" disorder. Despite this ubiquitous dilemma and numerous hoary tales of misdiagnosis, studies that might delineate the validity of this concern are few and not entirely satisfactory.

While it is widely known that patients seen in medical and surgical clinics have a substantial incidence of psychiatric illness, it is less well appreciated that psychiatric patients often have undiagnosed medical disorders that sometimes account for their symptoms. Davies (1965), a general physician, examined 36 outpatients referred to a psychiatrist. Twenty-one were found to have associated physical disease, and in 15 the condition was felt to be related to the psychiatric state. The report, however, did not note whether the illness was previously known to the patient or the patient's general physician, or how obscure the clues were that led to the diagnosis.

Hall et al. (1978) studied 658 consecutive outpatients at a community mental health center. The patients underwent a detailed initial evaluation that included a thorough medical history, physical examination, and physical symptom checklist. The first 100 patients with four or more positive responses on the checklist and 100 controls (no positive responses) underwent biochemical screening. Patients with evidence of physical disease were referred for appropriate medical evaluation and treatment. A disorder was felt to be of etiologic importance in causing psychiatric symptoms if "(1) psychiatric symptoms abated significantly with medical treatment, (2) medical symptoms seemed clearly related to the onset of psychiatric symptoms, or (3) the presence of a medical disorder, even though untreatable. . . . explained the patient's symptom pattern." The authors concluded that

9.1% of the total sample had medically induced psychiatric symptoms. In addition, 46 of the 60 symptom-positive patients (77%) had previously undiagnosed medical illnesses. While the criteria used for determining a causal relationship between medical disorders and psychiatric symptoms did not take into account factors such as spontaneous remission and the placebo effect, it still seems reasonable to conclude that medical disorders produced unrecognized psychiatric symptoms in a substantial number of patients.

Koranyi (1979) found at least one major medical illness in 43% of 2090 psychiatric clinic patients, and almost half of these had been undiagnosed by the referring source. In this study "major physical illnesses" were defined as "those somatic conditions fulfilling three criteria: (1) they caused active symptoms, (2) they required medical treatment, and (3) they caused concern on medical grounds." Of the 902 patients with major medical illnesses, it was felt that the psychiatric condition was caused by the illness in 18%, aggravated by the illness in 51%, and coexisted independently with illness in 31%.

Similar studies of psychiatric inpatients have also found a substantial incidence of medical illness, much of which had not been previously diagnosed. Marshall (1949) reviewed records of 175 psychiatric inpatients and that 44% had a physical condition requiring treatment. In half of the 44%, the physical condition was felt to contribute to the development of the psychiatric illness. Herridge (1960) examined the records of 209 consecutive psychiatric admissions and found that 5% had a major physical disorder as the principal diagnosis even though they had been referred to the hospital as having only a "functional" illness.

Johnson (1968) conducted detailed physical examinations of 250 consecutive admissions to a psychiatric inpatient service and found thirty (12%) who had physical conditions that were "important etiologic factors" in the presenting psychiatric symptoms. Twenty-four of them (80%) had not been diagnosed prior to admission. Maguire and Granville-Grossman (1968), examining the records of 200 consecutive admissions to a general hospital psychiatric unit, found 67 cases (33.5%) with "significant physical morbidity." Of these patients, 47 had a physical disorder noted as severe, 33 had not been diagnosed prior to admission, and 18 required transfer to medical wards. The authors were not able to determine how causally related these disorders were to the psychiatric symptoms.

The diagnosis of conversion reaction or dissociative reaction may be inappropriately made in a substantial number of patients whose symptoms are actually due to physical disease. Watson and Buranen (1979) found that 25% of their patient sample had been misdiagnosed and, on followup, were found to have degenerative disorders "affecting skeletal, muscular, and connective tissues, the spinal cord and the peripheral nerves." When symptoms cannot be readily explained, it is in the best interest of the patient to defer the diagnosis rather than to apply a poorly substantiated diagnostic label.

Various authors have found that cardiovascular, central nervous system, endocrine, pulmonary, and infectious disorders are more likely to produce psychiatric symptoms (Davies, 1965; Johnson, 1968; Hall et al., 1978; Koranyi, 1979). Hall et al. (1978) found that endocrine and metabolic disorders were the most frequent medical cause of psychiatric symptoms in women whereas cardiovascular and pulmonary disease predominated in men. To restrict one's diagnostic evaluation to a limited set of disorders, however, would be ill advised.

In summary, there appears to be ample evidence that nonpsychiatric medical illnesses can cause psychiatric symptoms and be misdiagnosed as psychiatric disorders. Some of the conclusions reached by Hall et al. (1978) should be stressed:

1. "Medical illness often presents with psychiatric symptoms."
2. "It is difficult to distinguish physical disorders from functional psychiatric disorders on the basis of psychiatric symptoms alone."
3. "Detailed physical examination and laboratory screening are indicated as routine procedure in the initial evaluation of psychiatric patients."
4. "Most patients are unaware of the medical illness that is causative of their psychiatric symptoms."
5. "The presence of a family physician does not protect either the patient or the treating psychiatrist from unrecognized medical illness."

REPRESENTATIVE PSYCHIATRIC SYMPTOMS

Anxiety

Anxiety is an emotional state that has been experienced by everyone and under most circumstances is considered normal. Abnormal or pathological anxiety is not qualitatively different but is quantitatively characterized by being more severe, more persistent or inappropriate. A distinction is often made between "trait" anxiety, which exists as part of a long-standing personality pattern, and "state" anxiety, which is acute, episodic, and often related to easily identified environmental precipitants.

Because the word "anxiety" has different meanings to different people, an important aspect of evaluation is defining in great detail what the patient actually means. One patient, for example, complained of "nervousness" but on closer evaluation was found to be referring to a benign essential tremor and not to the subjective manifestations of anxiety. In this case, appropriate treatment involved the use of propranolol for tremor reduction.

A complaint of anxiety or nervousness should be further defined with regard to both psychic and somatic symptoms. The psychic aspects of anxiety are described by terms such as *restlessness, tension, apprehension, fearfulness, edginess, irritability,* and *hyperexcitability*. Somatic manifestations include muscle tension (shakiness, trembling, muscular aches, restlessness), autonomic hyperactivity (sweating, palpitations, dry mouth), gastrointestinal upset, cold, clammy hands, tightness in the chest or throat, difficulty in breathing, and weakness in the legs.

When initially evaluating a patient complaining of "anxiety," it is important not to be resticted by psychoanalytic assumptions such as (1) anxiety is caused by intrapsychic conflict or (2) "fear is a reaction to a real or threatened danger while anxiety is more typically a reaction to an unreal or imagined danger" (Hinsie and Campbell, 1970).

In the process of arriving at a *DSM III (Diagnostic and Statistical Manual of Mental Disorders*, 3rd edition, 1980) diagnosis of anxiety disorder, one must be careful to exclude anxiety secondary to physical or other psychiatric disorders. From the point of view of diagnosis it is important (and often difficult) to distinguish between anxiety that is an emotional response to a physical illness and anxiety symptoms that are an integral part of the illness. For example, a patient with a fractured femur may be anxious because of concern about the injury or may manifest restlessness and apprehension secondary to the respiratory and cerebral insult from fat emboli. Similar symptoms may have quite different etiologies and respond best to quite different treatments.

An extensive listing of disorders associated with symptoms of anxiety is hardly a productive approach to diagnosis. These listings are so large that they lack specificity yet at the same time can never be truly comprehensive. For example, Giannini et al. (1978) in their *Psychiatric, Psychogenic, and Somatopsychic Disorders Handbook* list 91 entities that can produce signs and symptoms of anxiety. These include such diverse disorders as barium poisoning, cabin fever, dermatitis herpetiformis, overwork syndrome, pseudocyesis, root work, and Santa Ana syndrome. A more productive approach to diagnosis, of course, is a comprehensive medical and psychiatric history. This, coupled with a background knowledge of some of the more common disorders associated with anxiety symptoms, should lead to a more definitive evaluation.

A comprehensive drug history is an essential part of such an evaluation; it should consider symptoms from both drug effect and drug withdrawal and should include both prescription and over-the-counter drugs as well as substances so much a part of our society that they are often overlooked. Caffeine intoxication (caffeinism) is listed as a "substance-induced organic mental disorder" in *DSM III* and can produce an anxiety syndrome or aggravate a preexisting anxiety state. According to Greden (1974)

> High intake of caffeine ("caffeinism") can produce symptoms which are indistinguishable from those of anxiety neurosis, such as nervousness, irritability, tremulousness, occasional muscle twitchings, insomnia, sensory disturbances, tachypnea, palpitations, flushing, arrhythmias, diuresis, and gastrointestinal disturbances.

The caffeine withdrawal syndrome and the headache associated with it may also mimic anxiety.

The total daily intake of caffeine and related xanthines from beverages and medications such as coffee, tea, cola drinks, cocoa, various analgesics, and over-the-counter stimulants may be considerable, yet not readily apparent unless a comprehensive caffeine intake history is obtained. This should be an integral part of every anxiety evaluation.

Anxiety symptoms first developing after hospitalization may be due to withdrawal from drugs that were not mentioned in the initial history. Alcohol withdrawal, of course, is the classic example and generally occurs within three days after stopping drinking. Less obvious may be withdrawal symptoms from antianxiety drugs such as diazepam and chlordiazepoxide, which often do not begin until 5–7 days after discontinuation.

Other medical disorders that might be mistaken for a primary anxiety disorder include hyperthyroidism, hyperventilation, hypoglycemia, pheochromocytoma, and hyperadrenalism. Since patients with **hyperthyroidism** have a hyperdynamic peripheral circulation they tend to have warm, moist palms as opposed to the cold and clammy palms of a patient with primary anxiety. In addition, the sleeping pulse of a hyperthyroid patient tends to remain high whereas it generally falls to normal in patients with primary anxiety. While the hyperventilation syndrome may be a manifestation of a primary anxiety disorder, it should be recognized that **hyperventilation** can occur secondary to a variety of organic disorders that produce respiratory acidosis. **Hypoglycemia** has been, in recent years, a much maligned and overused diagnosis, yet low blood sugar can certainly cause anxiety symptoms that will improve following glucose intake. An appropriately performed glucose tolerance test that correlates symptoms with blood sugar level is an important aspect of diagnosis. The anxiety-like symptoms associated with **pheochromocytoma** are almost invariably associated with a paroxysmal or sustained blood pressure elevation. Since blood pressure elevations of a labile nature may also occur in association with a primary anxiety episode, the correct diagnosis of a pheochromocytoma will require the evaluation of associated clinical findings and measurement of appropriate catecholamine levels. **Hyperadrenalism** from excessive exogenous or endogenous steroids can also cause anxiety symptoms that should not be particularly difficult to diagnose if attention is paid to a comprehensive history and physical examination.

A more extensive discussion of these entities occurs elsewhere in the book, as does a more extensive examination of anxiety as a manifestation of various nonpsychiatric illnesses (see Index). A word of caution should be added about undue efforts to categorically assign anxiety-related symptoms to either a physical or a psychological disorder. As discussed at greater length in the chapter on Cardiovascular Disorders (Chapter 2), there appears to be an association between anxiety neurosis (panic attacks) and the mitral valve prolapse syndrome that suggests some commonality between what had previously been considered two fundamentally different syndromes.

Depression

The otherwise healthy depressed patient often presents the psychiatrist with difficult diagnostic and treatment problems. When depression occurs in the nonpsychiatric medical setting these difficulties are often greatly magnified. A patient may have a depression as a reactive consequence to developing a serious medical illness. This state has been referred to as despondency and is differentiated from a more endogenous type of depression (Cassem, 1978). In addition, a patient with a particular medical illness may also have a primary affective disorder that coincidentally (or possibly causally) becomes manifest at the time of a medical illness. Another patient might have a characterological depression which is an integral part of his personality, the symptoms of which are exaggerated during times of stress (e.g., when medically ill). Still another may have depressive symptoms that represent more than a secondary response to an illness but rather appear to be part and parcel of the illness itself. The distinction between "secondary response" and "part and parcel" is often blurred, especially since successful treatment of the underlying illness is likely to resolve the depression in both situations. Nonetheless, certain medical illnesses and drugs appear able to "cause" depressive symptoms, perhaps more so in patients who are particularly predisposed. While the other types of depression are no less important, our emphasis is on those conditions that might be mistaken for and mistreated as functional or reactive depressions. An awareness of these conditions is especially important since their depressive manifestations may be the first or most prominent aspect of their presentation. Timely diagnosis of the underlying disorder is especially important since progression of the illness may result in serious and, at times, irreversible medical complications.

Just as with anxiety, to attempt to list all medical illnesses that can be associated with depressive symptoms would be futile. Giannini et al. (1978) mention 91 medical and psychiatric entities as being associated with depressive symptoms. While extensive, such a list is far from comprehensive and one wonders whether disorders listed such as appendicitis, camphor intoxication, lichen simplex chronicus, and Santa Ana syndrome need be considered in the differential diagnosis of medical disorders that might present with depressive symptoms.

Illnesses that have traditionally been associated with depressive symptoms include endocrinopathies (thyroid, parathyroid, adrenal), malignancies (especially pancreatic and other abdominal tumors), infectious illnesses (such as posthepatitis, postinfluenza, and post-infectious mononucleosis syndromes), deficiency disorders (B_{12}, folate, and others), and neurological disorders (such as tumor, multiple sclerosis). These and other disorders are discussed at length in the body of the text and are referred to in the Index.

Drug-induced and drug-withdrawal depressions should be considered in every diagnostic evaluation. This area has been reviewed at length by Whitlock and Evans (1978) who stress that drug-induced depression is more likely to occur in an individual who either is genetically predisposed, has had prior depressive illness, or is elderly. They mention also that over 200 drugs have been reputed to cause depression in certain patients but that certain drugs or classes of drugs are more likely to be implicated. These include antipsychotics, barbiturates, alcohol, antihypertensives, and oral contraceptives. Even within these classes, it is often difficult to firmly establish a cause–effect relationship. It is also important not to mistake drug-induced psychomotor slowing and sedation for a true depressive syndrome. While most drugs do not appear to cause depression, one should remain open-minded enough to suspect that any drug might be a contributing factor, especially in a predisposed individual. A trial period off medication is usually a safe and informative intervention. The role of various drugs in producing psychiatric symptoms is discussed throughout the text.

A comprehensive medical history and physical examination remains the key to diagnosing secondary depression. It is very uncommon to find depression as a truly isolated symptom of an underlying medical illness. Nonetheless, should the initial medical evaluation of a depressed patient be unrevealing, one must remain alert for the appearance of incriminating signs or symptoms as the natural course of the illness progresses. There is a tendency for a negative initial evaluation to provide an enduring false sense of security that encourages the attribution of later findings to functional causes. Since most depressions are not caused by latent medical illnesses, a clinician is faced with the need to remain alert for the unlikely yet not become a slave to repeated, extensive, costly, and futile medical evaluations. A final problem is that primary depressions (no associated medical illness) can have diagnostically misleading somatic manifestations which include weight loss, anorexia, nausea, constipation, disturbed sleep, fatigue, weakness, pain, and sexual dysfunction.

Fatigue

> There is no end to the medical disorders which may cause fatigue . . . . So wide is the reference that there is little point in extending a classification which would inevitably cover most of the conditions in medicine.
>
> F. Dudley Hart (1979)

This section will not attempt to provide an exhaustive differential diagnosis of fatigue but rather will stress the need for a comprehensive and open-minded approach to evaluating the complaint. Patients with this common medical symptom are likely to complain of being tired, weary, worn out, without ambition, or run down. If the condition exists without sufficient justification in terms of exertion, work, or energy expenditure, a search should be made for a pathological cause.

It is important, in the process of evaluation, to distinguish fatigue from weakness, the latter signifying the presence of reduced muscle power. If true generalized or focal weakness can be demonstrated, the likelihood of an organic diagnosis is greatly strengthened (myasthenia gravis, for example). The psychogenically fatigued person, on the other hand, may complain bitterly of severe weakness that cannot be verified with specific testing.

While it cannot be overstressed that one of the most common causes of fatigue is depression, a common mistake is to equate the complaint of fatigue with the diagnosis of depression. For example, of the 20% of patients initially felt to have reserpine-induced depression, only about 6% acutally had a true endogenous type of depressive illness. The remainder had what was described as "pseudodepression"—a drug-induced fatigue state with psychomotor slowing, sedation, and energy loss but lacking the affective features of a true depression (Goodwin et al., 1972). A psychiatrist who is particularly eager to uncover cases of masked or hidden depression may be especially susceptible to the misdiagnosis of fatigue. A primary care physician, on the other hand, is more likely to focus on the quest for "organic" illness and neglect to evaluate the fatigued patient carefully for associated manifestations of depression. Any fatigued patient clearly deserves close scrutiny for both "organic" and "psychological" causes of his complaint.

The nonpsychiatric causes of fatigue are legion and include both the obvious and the obscure. While severe **anemia** is unquestionably a common and rather apparent cause of fatigue, it is often difficult to assess the role of milder degrees of anemia in generating such a complaint. Fatigue is a common side effect of many drugs — a point important to recognize because adjustment of dose or drug is likely to bring prompt relief. Nonspecific fatigue and malaise, often quite severe, are the most common neuropsychiatric manifestations of **digitalis** intoxication, with some reports giving an incidence of 95–100% (Lely and Van Enter, 1972). The antihypertensive drug, **clonidine**, was reported to cause fatigue that was troublesome in 30% of patients, and to be the cause of treatment failure in 10% (Raftos et al., 1973). Tiredness and drowsiness were found in over 40% of patients receiving **methyldopa** and may have contributed to the overdiagnosis of methyldopa-induced depression.

Caffeine is an important yet underdiagnosed cause of fatigue, with symptoms appearing as part of a withdrawal syndrome in a person accustomed to a relatively high daily intake of coffee, tea, cola, or caffeine-containing drugs. Lethargy, inability to work effectively, irritability, and headache comprised a characteristic set of dysphoric symptoms in heavy users (five or more cups of coffee per day) who omitted their morning coffee (Goldstein and Kaizer, 1969). It is clear from these few examples that drugs can be a very specific cause of a nonspecific symptom.

Nonspecific constitutional symptoms such as fatigue and lethargy are associated with the **polymyalgia rheumatica-giant cell arteritis** syndrome and may predate by many months more characteristic findings. Early diagnosis is especially important for two reasons: (1) treatment with steroids often produces a dramatic response, and (2) untreated, the illness may progress to complications such as blindness.

A substantial number of patients with diagnostically puzzling complaints of fatigue and excessive daytime sleepiness are being found to have **sleep disorders** such as narcolepsy, sleep apnea, or nocturnal myoclonus. With the advent of sleep laboratories and improved diagnostic technology, certain patients previously thought to be psychoneurotic or neurasthenic have been found to have well defined and treatable disorders of sleep and wakefulness.

The possibility that **central nervous systems allergies** can cause fatigue and other nonspecific symptoms that have been previously misdiagnosed as hypochondriasis, psychophysiologic reaction, and psychoneurosis is one that deserves rigorous research evaluation. The available literature provides tantalizing yet inconclusive evidence that this might be the case (Finn and Cohen, 1978).

Like any symptom taken as an isolated finding, a complaint of fatigue has little diagnostic specificity. It is the clinician's job to tease from the patient a constellation of signs and symptoms that coupled with appropriate laboratory testing, will lead to an accurate diagnosis. The circumstances under which fatigue occurs should be examined for diagnostic clues. For example, a patient who feels better on weekends may be suffering from overwork and job stress or exposure to noxious industrial toxins or may have delayed sleep phase syndrome.

There are a number of features generally felt to be of differential value in separating "organic" from "psychological" fatigue. They will not be mentioned here because they are often more confounding and biasing than useful and because they appear to be based on hearsay than on careful scientific observation.

Hallucinations

While definitions of what constitutes a hallucination vary, a widely accepted one, given in the American Psychiatric Association publication *A Psychiatric Glossary*, is "a false sensory perception in the absence of an actual external stimulus" (Frazier et al., 1975). The phrase "absence of an actual external stimulus" tends to separate a true hallucination from an illusion (a misinterpretation of a real experience), although clinically the distinction is often somewhat arbitrary.

Fleeting hallucinatory experiences are rather ubiquitous, occurring in settings such as extended sleep loss, prolonged nighttime driving, and other forms of sensory deprivation. Hallucinations of a more persistent nature have a pathological implication and deserve careful diagnostic evaluation.

Although hallucinations occur in association with many organic disorders, it is surprising that some physicians automatically equate hallucinations with schizophrenia and refer patients with undiagnosed organic mental disorders to psychiatrists for treatment for presumed functional disorders.

On the other hand, there is a tendency to equate visual hallucinations with organic disorders and auditory hallucinations with schizophrenia and affective illness. When more closely studied, however, the phenomenological characteristics of hallucinations are less useful in differential diagnosis than is commonly believed (Goodwin et al., 1971; Lowe, 1973; Slade, 1976). For example, Goodwin et al. (1971) found visual hallucinations in 72% of patients with affective disorder and chronic schizophrenia and 89% with organic brain syndrome. Figures vary from study to study, but investigators have consistently found that a substantial number of patients with the so-called functional psychoses have visual hallucinations.

Auditory hallucinations in the presence of a clear sensorium, generally felt to be characteristic of schizophrenia, can also occur in nonschizophrenic alcoholics (alcoholic hallucinosis) and can be induced even in normal volunteers by sufficient intake of amphetamines.

The presence of hallucinations should alert the clinician to perform a comprehensive diagnostic evaluation. Associated clinical and laboratory findings will provide the information needed to arrive at a tentative diagnosis and formulate a treatment plan. The operative diagnostic criteria in the 3rd edition of *Diagnostic and Statistical Manual of Mental Disorders* (DSM-III, 1980) provides useful set of guidelines. For example, hallucinations occurring in association with a disturbance of attention, disordered memory and orientation, reduced wakefulness or insomnia, and increased or decreased psychomotor activity are suggestive of a delirium. This is especially true if there is evidence of a specific organic factor felt to be etiologically related to the disturbance. In fact, it is often the presence of the aforementioned constellation of findings that sets off an intensive search for an underlying organic etiology. Hallucinations associated with quite different constellations of findings may be found in schizophrenia, affective disorder, and hysteria, as well as other types of organic mental disorder.

It should be stressed that phenomenologically similar hallucinations may be associated with widely divergent disorders and also that the same etiologic agent (e.g., alcohol) may be associated with quite different types of hallucinations in different individuals or even in the same individual at different points in time. Finally, hallucinations occurring in a given individual may be associated with more than one disorder. For example, a paranoid schizophrenic patient with longstanding refractory auditory hallucinations developed visual hallucinations while being treated with lithium and thiothixene. Lithium-induced hypothyroidism was diagnosed and treated and the visual hallucinations promptly resolved. The diagnostic trap of automatically assuming that schizophrenic patients who hallucinate do so because they have schizophrenia was avoided.

When hallucinations develop in a patient hospitalized on a nonpsychiatric service, organic mental disorder should be the prime diagnostic consideration. This is especially important since early discovery of an organic etiology may allow specific treatment and avoid progressive medical complications with an attendant increase in morbidity and mortality. For example, visual hallucinations developing in a patient receiving intravenous atropine for complete heart block should never be assumed to represent the coincidental development of schizophrenia. Treatment with antischizophrenic drugs like chlorpromazine or thioridazine would only aggravate what is much more likely to be an atrophine-induced central anticholinergic delirium.

Visual hallucinations occurring in a cardiac patient receiving digitalis should suggest a neuropsychiatric manifestation of digitalis intoxication. If this association is not made and the patient is treated symptomatically while continuing to receive digitalis, he will be at grave risk for a fatal digitoxic arrhythmia. When Durozier (1874) first described digitalis delirium, there was an associated mortality rate of 90%.

Hallucinating patients admitted to psychiatric facilities or seen by psychiatrists as outpatients may be at a double disadvantage since the setting carries a bias toward a psychiatric (i.e., functional) diagnosis and since psychiatrists are often less astute medical diagnosticians. *DSM-III* has quite appropriately included under organic mental disorders entities such as organic hallucinosis and organic affective syndrome, which would otherwise resemble functional disorders except for "evidence from either physical examination, medical laboratory tests, or the history, of a specific organic factor that is judged to be etiologically related to the disturbance." A good example of such a condition is secondary mania as described by Krauthammer and Klerman (1978).

A truly comprehensive listing of all the possible causes of each type of hallucination (e.g., auditory, visual, olfactory, tactile) is not available. Attempts that have been made to provide such comprehensive lists are misleading because they are incomplete, contain entries that are not well substantiated, and do not provide information as to relative incidence. Consequently, lists are not provided here but readers with a need for such information are referred to Giannini et al. (1978).

In summary, hallucinations are important clinical findings. Taken in isolation, they have limited diagnostic value but should initiate a careful search for additional manifestations, which, taken together, should lead to a specific diagnosis and treatment. While a certain type of hallucination may have less diagnostic specificity than commonly believed, a thorough investigation for an underlying organic etiology is always indicated because of the potential for definitive and often curative treatment.

REFERENCES

Cassem NH: Depression, in Hackett TP, Cassen NH (eds): *Massachusetts General Hospital Handbook of General Hospital Psychiatry*. Saint Louis, CV Mosby, 1978, pp 209–225.
Davies DW: Physical illness in psychiatric out-patients. *Br J Psychiatry* 111:27–33, 1965.

Diagnostic and Statistical Manual of Mental Disorders, ed 3. Washington, American Psychiatric Association, 1980.

Duroziez P: Du délire et du coma digitaliques. *Gazette Hebdomadaire de Medecine et de Chirugie* 11:780–785, 1874.

Finn, R, Cohen HN: Food allergy: Fact or fiction? *Lancet* 1:426–428, 1978.

Frazier SH, Campbell RJ, Marshall MH, et al. (eds): *A Psychiatric Glossary.* Washington, American Psychiatric Association, 1975.

Giannini AJ, Black HR, Goettsche RL: *Psychiatric, Psychogenic, and Somatopsychic Disorders Handbook.* New York, Medical Examination Publishing, 1978.

Goldstein A, Kaizer S: Psychotropic effects of caffeine in man: III. A questionnaire survey of coffee drinking and its effects in a group of housewives. *Clin Pharmacol Ther* 10:477–488, 1969.

Goodwin DW, Alderson P, Rosenthal R: Clinical significance of hallucinations in psychiatric disorders. *Arch Gen Psychiatry* 24:76–80, 1971.

Goodwin FK, Ebert MH, Bunney WE: Mental effects of reserpine in man: A review, in Shrader RI (ed): *Psychiatric Complications of Medical Drugs.* New York, Raven Press, 1972, pp 73–101.

Greden JF: Anxiety or caffeinism: A diagnostic dilemma. *Am J Psychiatry* 131:1089–1092, 1974.

Hall RCW, Popkin MK, Devaul RA, et al: Physical illness presenting as psychiatric disease. *Arch Gen Psychiatry* 35:1315–1320, 1978.

Hart FD: Fatigue, in Hart FD (ed): *French's Index of Differential Diagnosis.* Bristol, England, John R. Wright, 1979, p 285.

Herridge CF: Physical disorders in psychiatric illness. *Lancet* 2:949–951, 1960.

Hinsie LE, Campbell RJ: *Psychiatric Dictionary.* London, Oxford University Press, 1970, p. 49.

Johnson DAW: The evaluation of routine physical examination in psychiatric cases. *Practitioner* 200:686–691, 1968.

Koranyi EK: Morbidity and rate of undiagnosed physical illnesses in a psychiatric clinic population. *Arch Gen Psychiatry* 36:414–419, 1979.

Krauthammer C, Klerman GL: Secondary mania: Manic syndromes associated with antecedent physical illness or drugs. *Arch Gen Psychiatry* 35:1333–1339, 1978.

Lely AH, Van Enter CHJ: Non-cardiac symptoms of digitalis intoxication. *Am Heart J* 83:149–152, 1972.

Lowe GR: The phenomenology of hallucinations as an aid to differential diagnosis. *Br J Psychiatry* 123:621–633, 1973.

Maguire CP, Granville-Grossman KL: Physical illness in psychiatric patients. *Br J Psychiatry* 115:1365–1369, 1968.

Marshall HES: Incidence of physical disorders among psychiatric inpatients. *Br Med J* 2:468–470, 1949.

Raftos J, Bauer GE, Lewis RG, et al: Clonidine in the treatment of severe hypertension. *Med J Aust* 1:786–793, 1973.

Slade P: Hallucinations. *Psychol Med* 6:7–13, 1976.

Watson, CG, Buranen C: The frequency and identification of false positive conversion reactions. *J Nerv Ment Dis* 167:243–247, 1979.

Whitlock FA, Evans LEJ: Drugs and depression. *Drugs* 15:53–71, 1978.

2

Cardiovascular Disorders

HEART FAILURE

General Considerations

Heart failure is a condition in which the heart is unable to pump enough blood to supply the demands of the body. Although the cardiac output is usually reduced during heart failure, it may also be normal or elevated—the critical factor being that, whatever the output, it is inadequate to meet the metabolic requirements of the body.

Schlant (1970) has divided heart failure into three categories:

1. Mechanical abnormalities
2. Myocardial (muscular) failure
3. Dysrhythmia (arrhythmias)

Examples of mechanical abnormalities include valvular stenosis with increased resistance to blood flow, valvular insufficiency, abnormal shunting, pericardial constriction, and ventricular aneurysm. Myocardial failure is characterized by impaired myocardial contractility and may be primary (cardiomyopathies and loss of muscle mass from myocardial infarction) or secondary (due to drugs, toxins, inflammation, or infection). Heart failure may also be caused by arrhythmias such as extreme bradycardias or tachycardias, conduction disturbances, asystole, or fibrillation.

Depending on the cause, heart failure may occur abruptly or gradually, with symptoms dependent on the speed of onset. For example, a ruptured papillary muscle leading to marked mitral valve insufficiency may present as fulminant pulmonary edema, while more gradually developing mitral insufficiency from rheumatic valvular disease is characterized by exertional dyspnea, fatigability, and palpitations.

Clinical Features

Symptoms commonly occurring with heart failure are described in Table 2-1. While these symptoms are often associated with heart disease they are not specific and may occur under a wide range of conditions. Depending

TABLE 2-1. Symptoms of Heart Failure

Dyspnea—Difficult or labored breathing
Exertional dyspnea—Dyspnea provoked by physical effort or exercise
Orthopnea—Difficult breathing except in the upright position
Cardiac asthma—Wheezing due to bronchospasm secondary to heart failure
Paroxsysmal nocturnal dyspnea—Sudden onset of dyspnea occurring after retiring, that wakens
    the patient and is relieved by the upright position
Cough—Tends to be nonproductive and present during recumbency
Insomnia—Difficulty sleeping that may be secondary to nocturnal dyspnea or occur in association
    with heart failure induced Cheyne–Stokes respiration
Acute pulmonary edema—Sudden left ventricular failure characterized by marked respiratory
    distress, wheezing, frothy sputum, rales
Weakness and fatigue—May be due to reduced skeletal muscle blood flow, excessive diuresis,
    electrolyte imbalance, poor appetite
Gastrointestinal symptoms—Anorexia, nausea, vomiting, diarrhea, constipation may occur sec-
    ondary to venous distention, fluid retention, drug toxicity (especially digitalis)
Cardiac cachexia—Profound state of malnutrition and general ill health related to cellular hypoxia
    associated with congestive heart failure
CNS dysfunction—May occur secondary to impaired cerebral blood flow

on the method of presentation, the presence of associated confirmatory signs and symptoms, the premorbid personality and current behavior of the patient, and the diagnostic orientation and personality of the examining physician, heart failure will be either accurately or inaccurately diagnosed.

When present as a constellation, the symptoms of heart failure should never be mistaken for psychiatric illness. A clinician may be misled, however, if they occur individually, are of minor magnitude, or develop under unusual circumstances, or if heart failure is not considered part of the differential diagnosis. It is well to remember that symptoms of heart failure will evoke emotional responses from the individual that, especially if exaggerated, may mask the underlying condition.

Shortness of breath is often a manifestation of anxiety and in the more extreme form may present as a hyperventilation syndrome. In such instances careful examination will show that associated findings of heart failure will be absent and the patient will usually respond to reassurance, carbon dioxide rebreathing, antianxiety drugs, or combinations thereof. Deliberate overbreathing will reproduce the syndrome and confirm the diagnosis.

When heart failure occurs or is exacerbated at night, a patient may complain of insomnia, restlessness, agitation, and anxiety—symptoms frequently associated with conditions such as depression, nightmares and night terrors, and anxiety neurosis. While insomnia is a cardinal manifestation of depression, heart failure symptoms such as cough, orthopnea, and nocturnal dyspnea may also impair sleep. In addition, a symptom such as paroxysmal nocturnal dyspnea (PND)—which may cause the patient repeatedly to awake suddenly and breathlessly, sit up, and even go to the window for air—can be quite distressing and evoke feelings of anxiety and agitation. It is important to look beyond such secondary manifestations if the underlying etiology is to be determined. The physical findings associated with PND may not persist beyond the duration of the symptoms, so that a negative examination done the following day can be misleading. At times, the differential diagnosis may be quite difficult, especially if symptoms occur in a patient who is anxious or depressed and also has documented heart disease.

The setting in which the symptoms develop can be misleading and one must be careful not to let biases constrict his diagnostic acumen. For example, Hurst and Logue (1970) refer to a young woman who developed acute pulmonary edema for the first time while having intercourse on her wedding night. It is not difficult to imagine symptoms of agitation, faintness, and breathlessness occurring in this setting being ascribed to situational anxiety, a panic attack, hyperventilation, or hysterical overreaction. The patient in question, however, had severe mitral stenosis, which became fulminantly symptomatic under the physiologic and emotional stress of the situation.

Weakness, fatigue, anorexia, and weight loss are nonspecific complaints that occur in association with a wide variety of medical and psychiatric illnesses. When they occur in conjunction with insomnia, a psychiatrist tends to think of the vegetative manifestations of depression. It is apparent that a similar constellation may be found in heart failure and that a more extensive diagnostic evaluation would be necessary to distinguish the two conditions.

If heart failure is sufficiently severe, cerebral blood flow and cerebral metabolism may be reduced to the point of causing central nervous system dysfunction. This is more likely in the presence of associated factors such as cerebral vascular disease, structural brain damage, or drugs that alter the central nervous system. Symptoms likely to occur under these conditions would be those found with an organic brain syndrome. Recognizing heart failure as the cause is important since this is a specifically treatable and potentially reversible brain syndrome. Hurst and Logue (1970) describe a stuperous patient who improved markedly when the arrhythmia associated with severe heart failure was corrected.

ARRHYTHMIAS

Arrhythmias (or dysrhythmias) are disturbances of cardiac rate, rhythm, and conduction and may occur in the presence or absence of intrinsic heart disease. The presence of an arrhythmia is not always associated with clinical symptoms and may be detected only by physical examination or electrocardiography. At the other extreme, a rhythm disturbance such as ventricular fibrillation or asystole is glaringly obvious since syncope resulting from cerebral hypoxia occurs within seconds, and, in the absence of effective treatment, death follows within minutes.

Symptomatic, nonfatal arrhythmias may be characterized by a subjective awareness of the abnormal rhythm or by consequences of reduced blood flow to various organs.

Palpitations

A person who complains of palpitations is said to be subjectively aware of his heart beating. Terms commonly used to describe this condition include *racing, pounding, flip-flopping, skipping, stopping,* or *fluttering in the throat.* What is felt to be a palpitation may actually originate outside the heart from causes such as respiratory irregularities, diaphragmatic flutter, or chest wall muscle contractions. Extracardiac factors that can cause a more forceful and/or rapid heartbeat include blood loss; fever; hyperthyroidism; low blood sugar; and drugs such as caffeine, alcohol, and sympathomimetic amines.

Palpitations of cardiac origin may reflect normal physiology in conditions such as a rapid forceful regular heartbeat immediately following strenuous exercise or the slow regular heartbeat that one sometimes recognizes with an ear to the pillow when falling asleep.

Many disorders of cardiac rhythm may produce palpitations, the most common being premature (ectopic) beats of supraventricular or ventricular origin. A more forceful contraction occurs following a premature beat because the increased time available for ventricular filling results in a larger end-diastolic volume. Tachyarrhythmias are another common cause of palpitations and may be regular or irregular, of sudden or gradual onset and termination, and of ventricular or supraventricular origin.

Whether a person will be aware of a rhythm disturbance and how he expresses this awareness is determined both by the characteristics of the arrhythmia, the setting in which it occurs, and the individual's personality and current perceptual set. The threshold for recognizing a rhythm alteration appears to vary both within and between individuals. Individual sensitivity may be heightened by decreased environmental stimuli, fatigue, and anxiety. The variability between individuals becomes evident when similar electrocardiograms are found in asymptomatic and symptomatic patients.

How a person who is distressed by an awareness of his heartbeat describes this sensation will greatly influence the diagnostic consideration given him. An emotionally stable, articulate person might clearly and accurately characterize an episode of paroxysmal atrial tachycardia, while a similar episode in a more emotionally labile patient might be masked by anxiety symptoms and the numbness, tingling, and lightheadedness of hyperventilation. Still more difficult to assess would be the same arrhythmia in a schizophrenic patient who might complain of being controlled by "extragalactic metronomic pulsations" reaching him through a receiver implanted in his chest. In the latter instance, a clinician would have to combine a high index of suspicion and a knack for translating schizophrenic language to arrive at an accurate diagnosis.

In appropriately predisposed individuals, palpitations may initiate a reenforcing and spiraling cycle of palpitations→ anxiety→ more palpitations→ more anxiety, with a common denominator being increased endogenous catecholamine release. Recognition of the underlying arrhythmia is important in the treatment and prevention of this syndrome since correction of the rhythm disturbance may effectively interrupt or prevent the cycle.

Arrhythmias and the Cerebral Circulation

Studies in animals and man have shown that cardiac rhythm disturbances can cause reduced blood flow to the brain (Bellet,1971;Corday and Tzu-Wang, 1970; Anonymous, 1977a). In dogs, altered cardiac rhythm caused the following reduction in internal carotid artery blood flow (Corday and Irving, 1960):

1. Premature atrial contraction—8%
2. Premature ventricular contraction—12%
3. Frequent premature systoles—25%
4. Atrial tachycardia, fibrillation, and flutter, with rapid ventricular rates—23%
5. Extremely rapid ventricular rate—40–75%

The reduction in cerebral circulation associated with a slow heartbeat (complete heart block) has been demonstrated by Shapiro and Chawla (1969) who showed a 30% increase in cerebral blood flow when electrical pacing restored a normal rate and by Sulg et al. (1969) who noted that effective pacing normalized both a reduced cerebral blood flow and a slowed electroencephalogram, and was associated with symptomatic improvement. Abdon and Malmcrona (1975) mention a patient who had been placed in a mental hospital with a diagnosis of senile psychosis. When a bradyarrhythmia was correctly diagnosed and treated, her mental status improved to the extent that she returned home.

If cerebral blood flow is sufficiently compromised, neuropsychiatric symptoms will develop. These may include syncope, seizures, focal neurological signs, visual impairment, weakness, fatigue, confusion, and even psychosis. Symptoms are more likely (1) if the arrhythmia is severe, (2) if there is preexisting compromise of the cerebral circulation, and (3) if there is preexisting central nervous system disease.

The term "cardiogenic dementia" has been used to describe the precipitation or aggravation of a dementia in the elderly by an arrhythmia-induced reduction in cerebral blood flow (Anonymous, 1977a). There is clearly a need to explore closely the possibility that a cardiac mechanism may be responsible for what, at first glance, appears to be intrinsic brain dysfunction.

Diagnosis of Arrhythmias

The first step in diagnosing an arrhythmia is to suspect it. As already noted, these disorders may have quite atypical presentations, so that exclusion by lack of a classic history is unwise. In 8 of 16 patients with transient cerebral ischemic attacks caused by cardiac arrhythmia, the correct diagnosis was not suspected at the time of initial evaluation (McAllen and Marshall, 1973). One should always ask the patient if he noted any alteration in his pulse when the symptoms were present. Though such information may be helpful, many patients have not sought such correlation, do not know how to palpate their pulse, or are unreliable data collectors. A more objective step would be to physically examine the symptomatic patient, recording cardiac rate and rhythm both peripherally and over the heart.

An electrocardiogram (ECG) is necessary to confirm or disconfirm clinical findings. While a routine 12-lead ECG (or even a rhythm strip) may suffice under certain circumstances, more extended monitoring may be necessary to detect an elusive, intermittent rhythm disturbance. The development, in recent years, of techniques for extended ambulatory monitoring has markedly reduced the need for long-term, in-hospital observations and allowed patients to record an ECG over time, in their natural environment. Through the use of three chest electrodes and a small portable recording device, records of up to 24 hours may be obtained. Patients are instructed to keep a diary of activities and also to note times at which symptoms are present so that correlation can be made with ECG. Under certain circumstances, it still may be necessary to hospitalize a patient for a more extensive evaluation, which might include provocative drug testing or all-night sleep laboratory assessment. Once an arrhythmia has been diagnosed, a causal relationship to the symptoms must still be established. Finding a close association in time is necessary, and ideally one should be able to show a remission of symptoms with suppression of the arrhythmia and recurrence of symptoms with reappearance of the arrhythmia.

BLOOD PRESSURE

Hypotension

"Low" blood pressure, like "low" blood sugar, may or may not be of pathological significance. Many people have systolic pressures which are under 100 mm of mercury in the absence of precipitating factors or clinical symptoms—a condition which represents their normal state. More difficult to evaluate is the person with a "chronically" low blood pressure who has symptoms that are compatible with those produced by low blood pressure but in whom a causal relationship has not been established. In such instances a thorough search must be made for conditions that can cause hypotension. These include adrenocortical insufficiency; malnutrition; chronic bed rest; a variety of neurological conditions such as tabes dorsalis, syringomyelia, multiple sclerosis, spinal cord section, and diabetic neuropathy; and drugs such as antihypertensives, antipsychotics, and antidepressants. If the condition can be diagnosed and treatment is accompanied by an associated increase in blood pressure and resolution of symptoms, a relationship can be reasonably well established.

The symptoms of hypotension can be varied depending on the magnitude and duration of the problem, but are invariably caused by reduced perfusion of various organs. Acute and progressive blood loss, for example, will be associated with a reduced level of consciousness, confusion, coma, and ultimately death due to cerebral hypoperfusion.

Less severe and more chronic hypotensive states have been associated with nonspecific symptoms of fatigue, weakness, dizziness, and faintness. Whether such symptoms reflect the hypotension per se or the underlying condition is often difficult to determine. For example, primary autonomic insufficiency (Shy–Drager syndrome) is characterized not only by postural hypotension and syncope but also by anhydrosis, sphincter disturbances, impotence, and extrapyramidal disturbances such as tremor, rigidity, and ataxia.

Postural hypotension is usually quite easy to recognize and diagnose since the patient becomes symptomatic when changing from recumbency to a more upright position. Recumbent and standing blood pressure measurements will confirm such a diagnosis. Under certain conditions, however, postural hypotension may not be so apparent. For example, it is less well recognized that hypotension may be absent while a person is walking, yet be quite severe when standing still. This is because contraction of the calf muscles during ambulation forces blood toward the heart and maintains an adequate venous return (Eichna et al., 1947).

Postural hypotension may also mimic sleep. This was graphically demonstrated in a report of two patients who, following antipsychotic drug administration, were able to walk to the examining room, but then became drowsy, developed slow and deep respirations and occasional snoring, and appeared to fall asleep (Jefferson, 1972). They remained sitting with their heads propped against the wall, and only when pulse and blood pressure were determined did the diagnosis become apparent. In these instances, what appeared to be a desirable sedative effect from an antipsychotic drug was actually a potentially life-threatening hypotensive side effect.

Hypertension

Symptoms of morning headaches, visual blurring, nervousness, sweating, palpitations, nose bleed, excessive fatigue, and decreasing sexual performance are commonly elicited from hypertensive patients; although they may be ameliorated during successful antihypertensive therapy, they do not really correlate very well with early hypertension. (Gill, 1975)

Boller et al. (1977) compared a group of 20 asymptomatic untreated hypertensive men (mean diastolic pressure 115 mm of mercury) with 20 normotensive controls using a neuropsychological test battery. While no differences between groups were found with tests sensitive to focal damage, the hypertensive group did show significant deficiencies in general functioning with regard to reaction time and forward digit recall. The differences were not great and the clinical implication of these findings is not clear.

Essential hypertension, unless severe, tends to be a silent disease. Attributing a causal relationship between hypertension and a multitude of bodily symptoms is generally not warranted, since such an association is usually coincidental.

If untreated, however, hypertension may proceed through its silent or latent period and produce symptomatic complications consequent to damage to the myocardium and blood vessels. Differential diagnosis is rarely a problem, since blood pressure measurement is an integral part of evaluating renal and cardiac failure, angina pectoris, myocardial infarction, and cerebrovascular accidents.

Hypertensive Encephalopathy

Hypertensive encephalopathy tends to develop acutely or subacutely, and is characterized by headache, visual impairment, impaired consciousness, confusion, delirium, nausea, vomiting, and convulsions, usually occurring in the absence of focal neurological findings. Altered state of consciousness and severe headache are the most consistent findings. The presence of focal neurological findings during an episode portends a focal neurological residual following treatment (Chester et al., 1978). The syndrome is associated with (1) increased arterial blood pressure, usually extreme, (2) decreased cerebral blood flow, (3) cerebral arteriolar constriction, and (4) cerebral edema (Finnerty, 1968). More recently, it has been suggested that the encephalopathy results from a decompensation of cerebral vascular tone with increased cerebral blood flow leading to cerebral edema (Chester et al., 1978; Ram, 1978). Regardless of the underlying mechanism, aggressive treatment of hypertensive encephalopathy is indicated, since lowering of the blood pressure is generally associated with neurological improvement and minimization of renal and cardiac complications.

Two conditions may mimic hypertensive encephalopathy and require exclusion before antihypertensive drug treatment is started. The extremely high blood pressure that may accompany pulmonary edema secondary to hypertensive heart disease responds well to treatment of the pulmonary edema, whereas aggressive antihypertensive drug therapy in this situation may precipitate serious hypotension. Secondly, an acute anxiety episode in a patient with labile hypertension may cause marked blood pressure elevation. In this instance, the retinal blood vessels and the heart size tend to be normal, as does the electrocardiogram. Treatment should be directed at anxiety reduction through verbal interventions and/or the use of antianxiety drugs.

Neuropsychiatric symptoms occurring in the presence of systemic hypertension may be more closely associated with the underlying disease process and not directly related to the elevated blood pressure.

Pheochromocytoma

Pheochromocytomas are chromaffin tumors arising in the adrenal gland or in extramedullary chromaffin tissue. About 90% are found in the adrenal gland and 10% of these are bilateral. Symptoms caused by these tumors are attributed to the release of dopamine, norepinephrine, and epinephrine. The ratio of these catecholamines varies from tumor to tumor and may account for the variability in symptoms. The hypertension associated with pheochromocytoma may be either paroxysmal or sustained, although rare cases have occurred in the absence of any blood pressure elevation.

In a series of 100 patients with pheochromocytoma, the most common paroxysmal symptoms were headache (characteristically of rapid onset, severe intensity, throbbing quality, and short duration), perspiration (often drenching the patient in sweat), and palpitations (with or without tachycardia) (Thomas et al., 1966). Subjective complaints, listed in order of frequency, are shown in Table 2-2. Another report mentioned that mental symptoms occurred in 40% of cases with paroxysmal hypertension (Magee, 1975).

Of particular interest to the psychiatrist is the high incidence of neuropsychiatric symptoms which could be mistaken for psychoneurotic anxiety or panic attacks. Drake and Ebaugh (1956) describe a 34-year-old woman with a 5-year history of depression and weak spells who was diagnosed as having "an anxiety reaction with depressive features, associated with psycholepsy." Electroshock therapy was initiated but after the first treatment she experienced a cardiorespiratory arrest and died. At autopsy, a 128-gram pheochromocytoma of the adrenal gland was found. Manger and Gifford (1977) mention depressive psychosis occurring in association with pheochromocytoma and resolving with removal of the tumor.

To further complicate the clinical picture, paroxysmal episodes due to pheochromocytomas have been precipitated by such misleading factors as hyperventilation, emotional stress, laughing, sleeping, sexual intercourse, shaving, gargling, straining at the stool, and sneezing (Green, 1960).

The presence of a normal blood pressure between episodes should not impart a false sense of security, and once a pheochromocytoma is considered as part of the differential diagnosis, appropriate screening should be done by measuring urinary excretion of catecholamines and their metabolites.

TABLE 2-2. Symptoms in 100 Patients with Pheochromocytoma[a]

Symptom	Patients (Number or %)	Symptom	Patients (Number or %)
Headache	80	Tightness in throat	8
Perspiration	71	Dizziness or faintness	8
Palpitation (with or without tachycardia)	64	Convulsions	5
		Neck–shoulder pain	5
Pallor	42	Extremity pain	4
Nausea (with or without vomiting)	42	Flank pain	4
		Tinnitus	3
Tremor or trembling	31	Dysarthria	3
Weakness or exhaustion	28	Gagging	3
Nervousness or anxiety	22	Bradycardia (noted by patient)	3
Epigastric pain	22	Back pain	3
Chest pain	19	Coughing	1
Dyspnea	19	Yawning	1
Flushing or warmth	18	Syncope	1
Numbness or paresthesia	11	Unsteadiness	1
Blurring of vision	11	Hunger	1

[a] From Thomas et al. (1966) with permission. Copyright American Medical Association.

Primary Aldosteronism

Primary aldosteronism is associated with hypertension as well as hypokalemia. Symptoms from reduced potassium levels include muscle weakness, which may be episodic or sustained and tends to be most prominent in the legs, as well as headache, paresthesias, and fatigue. Although such neuropsychiatric manifestations are common, they appear to be secondary to the underlying disease rather than to the hypertension itself.

ATHEROSCLEROTIC HEART DISEASE

Angina Pectoris

Angina refers to a spasmodic, choking, suffocative pain, and the term angina pectoris has come to represent a syndrome characterized by episodic pain or discomfort secondary to myocardial ischemia, the commonest cause of which is coronary atherosclerosis.

Most commonly, the pain of angina pectoris is located in the substernal region and may remain localized or radiate to the neck, jaws, shoulder, back, abdomen, or arms. Atypical locations are all too frequent, however, and pain has been described as occurring *only* in the neck, jaws, shoulder, back, abdomen, or arms. Misdiagnosed angina localized to the jaw may result in unnecessary dental procedures and ultimate edentulism. All in all, location alone should not be too heavily relied upon in diagnosing angina pectoris.

The symptoms of myocardial ischemia have been described in many ways, often in terms that do not include actual pain. Patients might speak of pressure, constriction, heaviness, burning, tingling, stabbing, choking, and indigestion, so that merely questioning them about chest pain may result in a false negative history. Disregarding such complaints or relegating them to a category of nonsignificant or psychosomatic can be a grave disservice to the patient.

The constricting character of the anginal distress may be spontaneously demonstrated by the patient holding his clenched fist over his sternum (Levine's sign). Such a display, however, is by no means diagnostic, for similar findings have been reported in the psychiatric literature as characteristic of "functional" illness. For example, Lindberg (1965) described the "depressive gesture" in which the depressed patient points to his chest as the location of his distress.

The circumstances under which angina occurs are an important aspect of making a correct diagnosis. Physical exertion and emotional upset are classic precipitants, with symptom relief occurring rapidly after removal of the precipitating factor. Angina, however, can occur at rest, can occur during activities which are usually well tolerated, and may actually disappear even though the precipitating activity is continued.

The duration of angina pectoris tends to be brief (3–5 min) if the precipitating factor is removed, and sublingual nitroglycerine usually produces prompt relief in 1–2 min. Pain lasting for considerably longer periods may be due to noncardiac causes or may represent an intermediate stage between stable angina pectoris and myocardial infarction known as preinfarction angina, acute coronary insufficiency, or crescendo angina.

It should now be apparent that the diagnosis of myocardial ischemia may not be readily made from clinical description alone, although a thorough and comprehensive history does remain the cornerstone of proper diagnosis. The electrocardiogram (ECG) is often thought to be the key to definitive diagnosis, and frequently it is. The resting ECG, however, may be normal (50–70% of patients with effort angina and no prior infarction have normal resting ECGs) (Logue and Hurst, 1970), and such a finding is, therefore, of little or no diagnostic value.

Exercise electrocardiography (stress testing) is a valuable source of diagnostic information especially if symptoms can be reproduced during the procedure. At times it may be necessary to deviate from standard testing procedures and allow the patient to recreate the situation that precipitates the symptoms. Extended ambulatory electrocardiogrphy may be quite useful if testing in the laboratory is unproductive. The use of coronary arteriography may be helpful in resolving diagnostically confusing situations, although it is important to realize that anatomy and physiology are not necessarily synonymous.

Neurotic, psychotic, psychosomatic, hysterical, and hypochondriacal patients are not immune from the ravages of atherosclerotic heart disease.

This is unfortunate not only for the patient but also for the clinician whose diagnostic task would be greatly simplified were the conditions mutually exclusive. Such patients may sorely tax the abilities of the physician to recognize potentially life-threatening conditions and the frequent cry of "wolf" has, no doubt, resulted in the untimely demise of a good number of these folks. Also, the inability of patients with certain disorders such as schizophrenia or mental retardation to communicate effectively with the physician will greatly impair proper diagnosis and treatment. In such situations, it is especially important to "listen" to the patient since a change or alteration in their usual behavioral pattern, however atypical, may signify an emerging medical problem.

Chest pain that is not due to angina may be due to a wide variety of other conditions, some of which fall under the rubric of "emotional disorders." These include:

1. Anxiety neurosis (also known as neurocirculatory asthenia, cardiac neurosis, cardiophobia, etc.)
2. Hyperventilation syndrome
3. Depression
4. Musculoskeletal conditions such as xyphoidalgia, costochondritis, and painful shoulder syndrome
5. Briquet's syndrome (hysteria)—A 72% incidence of chest pain was noted in hysteria by Perley and Guze (1962)
6. Drug addiction—The addict may quite effectively mimic angina in an attempt to obtain narcotics

Nonangina chest pain associated with emotional disorders tends to be either sharp, stabbing, intermittent, and of brief duration or dull, aching, and lasting hours to days. Such pain also tends not to have the same relationship to exercise as does angina, and a distinction can usually be made without difficulty. Growing awareness of an association between the "functional cardiac disorders," mitral valve prolapse syndrome, and the improvement of the atypical chest pain often associated with these conditions with propranolol treatment, is discussed below.

Evans and Lum (1977) emphasize that hyperventilation can be an important cause of "pseudoangina." They describe a group of 50 patients referred to them for chest pain evaluation who were hyperventilators. Organic heart disease was also present in 13. With treatment that involved explanation and respiratory physiotherapy, 76% of them remained symptom free over an 11- to 68-month followup period.

Myocardial Infarction

The symptoms of myocardial infarction are usually quite graphic, with pain being the most common complaint. The pain tends to be more severe and of longer duration than anginal pain, but may have a similar location and pattern of radiation. The pain, usually substernal, has been described as "crushing," "vise-like," "squeezing," or "like someone sitting on my chest." Associated symptoms may include weakness, sweating, nausea, and vomiting, and in more extreme situations there may be cardiovascular collapse with syncope and shock.

On the other hand, myocardial infarction may be quite atypical, with about 15% of episodes occurring *without* any symptoms. Often, pain may be absent, with a patient presenting with an arrhythmia, acute pulmonary edema, vascular collapse, or syncope. The elderly are a group in which appropriate diagnosis may be especially difficult. In one study, only 19% of the patients had the classic symptom of substernal or epigastric distress. The other 81% presented with findings such as stroke, peripheral gangrene, renal failure, pulmonary embolism, syncope, dyspnea, giddiness, palpitations, recurrent vomiting, sweating, weakness, and restlessness (Logue and Hurst, 1970). Many of these symptoms, especially appearing in a person with some degree of senile impairment, could all too easily be mistaken for emotional upset. Similar diagnostic problems will occur in patients with functional psychiatric disorders that interfere with their ability to effectively communicate their distress.

If a myocardial infarction is suspected from the patient's history, laboratory confirmation should be attempted by serial determinations of serum enzymes and by serial electrocardiograms. It is essential to realize that in the early phase of myocardial infarction, both enzymes and electrocardiograms may be normal. Therefore, if clinical suspicion so warrants, a patient should be hospitalized for observation.

According to Logue and Hurst (1970), anxiety attacks and especially hyperventilation episodes may be misdiagnosed as myocardial infarction leading to prompt administration of narcotics and oxygen, which then further confuses the picture. Differentiating these conditions may be especially difficult, since anxiety is the characteristic emotional response of people who are experiencing a myocardial infarction. A correct diagnosis may be possible only with more extended observation and appropriate laboratory testing, and it is wise to assume that an infarction is present until it can be clearly proven otherwise.

SYNCOPE

Syncope or fainting is often of circulatory origin and under such circumstances occurs due to cerebral hypoxia from inadequate blood flow to the brain (see section on Hypotension). Adams and Braunwald (1974) divided circulatory causes of syncope into:

1. Inadequate vasoconstriction mechanisms—vasovagal or vasodepressor syncope, postural hypotension, carotid sinus syncope of the vasodepressor type, primary autonomic insufficiency
2. Hypovolemia

3. Mechanical reduction of venous return—e.g., Valsalva's maneuver, cough, micturition, atrial myxoma
4. Reduced cardiac ouput—e.g., obstructed left ventricular outflow, obstructed pulmonary flow, cardiac tamponade
5. Arrhythmias

These possible etiologies must be explored when evaluating a patient having syncopal episodes and must be definitively excluded before a diagnosis of hysterical syncope can be strongly entertained. The classic presentation of the latter condition is that of an emotionally labile young female who gracefully and without injury swoons to the floor or a chair, where she remains unresponsive to voice for minutes or even hours in the presence of normal blood pressure, pulse, and skin color. A traditional confirmatory finding is that when the patient's arm is held over her face and dropped, it invariably falls to the side without striking the face. Such a finding was noted in a 55-year-old woman who had been diagnosed as having psychogenic convulsions (conversion hysteria). Some, but not all of her symptoms, were later found to be due to Adams–Stokes attacks secondary to paroxysmal heart block, and these were prevented by implantation of a cardiac pacemaker (Spudis and Griffin, 1974).

Hypersensitivity of the carotid sinus is an uncommon cause of syncope. Normally, stimulation of the carotid sinus results in a transient slowing of heart rate and a mild fall in blood pressure, but in sensitive individuals these changes may be extreme, leading to episodes of dizziness, faintness, and, at times, unconsciousness. There are two types of carotid sinus hypersensitivity—cardioinhibitory and vasodepressor—which can coexist in the same patient (Walter et al., 1978). Spontaneous episodes may occur or an attack may be associated with shaving, a tight collar, or movement of the head. In a most unusual case, the patient often fainted when he swallowed a bolus of food (Weiss and Ferris, 1934). The attacks could be reproduced by distension of the esophagus with a rubber balloon in the area of a traction diverticulum and prevented by vagal blockade, suggesting that they were of vasovagal origin.

To properly screen a patient for circulatory causes of syncope, efforts should be made to obtain pulse, blood pressure, and ECG during an episode. If these measurements are normal, attention should then be directed towards metabolic, cerebrovascular, and emotional causes. Infrequency and unpredictability of epidoses may make such a diagnostic evaluation quite difficult. At times, it may be possible to reproduce the circumstances under which the episode occurred and obtain a more definitive diagnosis (e.g., deliberate hyperventilation or carotid sinus massage).

CARDIAC TUMORS

Tumors that involve the heart may be primary or secondary, benign or malignant, mural or intracavitary (Harvey, 1968). Of particular interest with regard to diagnostic puzzles and neuropsychiatric manifestations is the myxoma—a primary, benign, intracavitary tumor. Most myxomas are atrial in origin, with 75% located in the left atrium. Although benign, their precarious location makes them a tumor of high potential lethality (Greenwood, 1968).

Their clinical presentations may be quite varied and include manifestations such as "syncope, epileptiform seizures, coma, shock, acute pulmonary edema, cyanosis, gangrene of the nose and toes, or episodic bizarre behavior" (Wenger, 1970). These tumors may produce widespread embolization of tumor fragments or thrombi from the tumor surface. Systemic emboli can cause a wide variety of neurological signs and symptoms, the distribution and often transient nature of which can be suggestive of a functional illness.

In addition, myxomas often obstruct blood flow resulting in heart failure, pulmonary hypertension, or valvular stenosis or insufficiency. If the tumor is on a pedicle, it may move from atrium to ventricle and back causing intermittent symptoms such as syncope due to a ball–valve effect.

Finally, myxomas may be associated with constitutional manifestations such as fever, weight loss, weakness, anemia, elevated sedimentation rate, and hyperglobulinemia.

The diagnostic and therapeutic confusion that can be caused by an atrial myxoma is graphically illustrated in a report by Wharton (1977). A middle-aged woman had an episode of sweating, nausea, and transient blurred vision. Three months later there was a transient episode of tremor, dizziness, and left-sided weakness but no physical abnormalities were found. After 7 more months, she was hospitalized with weight loss and a transient episode of tremor, dizziness, and right-sided weakness. Examination by a neurologist and internist were unrevealing. Later, she underwent psychiatric evaluation and treatment and was seen "twice weekly at first and then biweekly for 40 sessions over the next 15 months before the diagnosis of atrial myxoma was finally made." Despite repeated reassurance by her internist that she did not have significant cerebral, vascular, or cardiac/disease, she had another transient neurological episode following which an echocardiogram led to a definitive diagnosis which was promptly followed by surgical excision of the tumor. Recognition of the tumor in this case was made more difficult by the presence of non-tumor-related psychiatric issues which did respond favorably to psychotherapy.

INFECTIVE (BACTERIAL) ENDOCARDITIS

Infective endocarditis refers to a microbial infection that involves the heart valves, endocardium, or endothelium of adjacent blood vessels. Symptoms result from local cardiac damage, embolization, immunologic host response, and systemic infection.

Acute bacterial endocarditis is caused by organisms having a high pathogenicity, often occurs in a previously normal heart, usually has an abrupt onset, and may run a rapid, fulminant course. On the other hand, **subacute bacterial endocarditis** is caused by a pathogen of low virulence, in a heart with preexisting structural damage of an acquired or congenital nature. The onset and clinical course tend to be insidious, although without treatment serious and often lethal complications will occur.

Common complaints early in the course of subacute bacterial endocarditis include weakness, malaise, loss of appetite, sweating, and low-grade fever—symptoms suggestive of a mild viral infection. One third of the time, initial presenting manifestations are related to emboli involving sites such as brain, kidney, gastrointestinal tract, lung, and extremities.

Neuropsychiatric manifestations of subacute bacterial endocarditis may be predominant and, as a result, delay diagnosis. More obvious neurological findings include seizures, coma, hemiplegia, sudden blindness, and meningitis. On reviewing 218 patients with bacterial endocarditis, 84 (39%) with neurological lesions were found (Pruitt et al., 1978). In 36 the neurological symptoms were the first evidence of endocarditis, in 24 the findings were important in making the correct diagnosis and in 5 there were no other suggestions of the underlying endocarditis. Specific neurologic complications included cerebral embolism (37 patients), cerebral myeotic aneurysm (10 patients), brain abscess (9 patients) and seizures (24 patients).

Initial psychiatric symptoms may be those of an organic brain syndrome or occasionally of a schizophreniform psychosis. Antel et al. (1955) described a 55-year-old man ultimately diagnosed as having subacute bacterial endocarditis whose initial symptoms were neuropsychiatric. These included forgetfulness, insomnia, religious preoccupation, bizarre behavior, suspicion, visual and auditory hallucinations, and disorientation.

In a report by Fetterman and Ashe (1938) almost 50% of their cases presented with a neuropsychiatric complaint. Four of their 42 patients had psychoses, two of which were schizophreniform. One patient had "forgetfulness, negligence of the amenities, morosity, lethargy, negativism, and incoherent speech." Later, auditory hallucinations and delusions developed in the absence of physical symptoms and it was not until several weeks later that marked pallor led to the correct diagnosis.

In recent years, the diagnosis of subacute bacterial endocarditis has been complicated by a shift in mean age of onset to the mid-50's and to the excessive and often careless use of antibiotic drugs. A high index of suspicion is essential for early detection, and diagnosis should always be entertained in someone with a fever and a heart murmur. Finding positive blood cultures will help confirm the diagnosis, but there are times when even blood cultures will be negative and treatment must be instituted on clinical grounds alone.

FUNCTIONAL CARDIAC DISORDERS

Occupying the "gray zone" between cardiology and psychiatry is a condition (or set of conditions) that has been known by many names and clinical descriptions. These include:

DaCosta syndrome   Cardiac neurasthenia
Neurovegetative tachycardia   Cardiasthenia
Cardiophobia   Autonomic imbalance with tachy-
                                      cardia
Nervous heart syndrome   Irritable heart syndrome
Effort syndrome   Hyperkinetic heart syndrome
Disorder action of the heart   Vasoregulatory asthenia
Cardiac neurosis   Cardiac muscular exhaustion
Hyperkinetic circulatory state   Essential circulatory hyperkinesis
Soldiers heart   Hyperdynamic beta-adrenergic cir-
                                      culatory state
Neurocirculatory asthenia

Whether this represents a single disorder or is a heterogeneous group of conditions, and whether this should be considered a "functional psychiatric" illness or an "organic medical" illness remains to be determined (see section on Mitral Valve Prolapse Syndrome). While the lethality is low (essentially none in the absence of mitral valve prolapse), these conditions produce a high degree of subjective distress, often of a chronic nature. Symptoms are such that differentiating them from the more potentially hazardous cardiovascular diseases may be quite difficult.

Patients are likely to complain of:

1. Increased cardiac awareness
2. Palpitations—usually increased awareness of normal beats
3. Breathing difficulties—both with exertion and at rest, often sighing, sometimes smothering feelings
4. Chest pain—sticking, stabbing, or dull and prolonged
5. Decreased exercise tolerance
6. Fatigue, exhaustion, lack of energy
7. Excessive sweating
8. Tremor
9. Dizziness, lightheadedness, faintness
10. Anxiety

While these complaints are usually episodic in nature, the illness overall may become a chronic debilitating problem. Generally these symptoms occur in the absence of diagnosable underlying cardiovascular disease but they may also be superimposed on more traditionally "organic" disease and consequently present difficult diagnostic and management issues.

Although the etiology of these disorders has not been established, there are some data that implicate overactivity of the sympathetic nervous system. Frohlich et al. (1969) described an exaggerated responsiveness to the infusion of the beta receptor agonist, isoproterenol, in a group of such patients, some of whom also responded with an almost uncontrollable hysterical outburst which was promptly reversed by the beta receptor antagonist, propranolol. The use of beta-receptor-blocking drugs to treat these disorders has met with some success suggesting that either sympathetic overactivity or beta receptor hypersensitivity plays a role in the disorders (Jefferson, 1976).

The natural history of these disorders tends to be chronic and characterized by remissions and exacerbations. A small percent of patients will recover completely, others will have symptoms without disability, some will have symptoms with intermittent disability, and finally some will become permanently disabled. The effectiveness of treatments, including drugs, reassurance, and supportive and uncovering psychotherapy has been quite variable, and there is a need for well designed studies if there is to be better understanding of these disorders.

MITRAL VALVE PROLAPSE SYNDROME (MVPS)

Once thought to be rare and of extracardiac origin, nonejection systolic clicks and the often associated apical systolic murmurs are actually quite common and are caused by an abnormality of the mitral valve mechanism. It has been suggested that as high as 6–20% of otherwise healthy people have prolapse of a mitral valve leaflet (usually posterior) which is responsible for the characteristic auscultatory findings (Anonymous, 1978). More conservatively, Rizzon et al. (1973) found that 0.33% of 1009 female students had these findings. The prevalence in the general population is probably somewhere between these extremes.

MVPS has been referred to by a variety of terms which include "systolic click–late systolic murmur syndrome," "mitral valve prolapse-click syndrome," "Reid–Barlow syndrome," "Barlow's syndrome," "billowing posterior mitral leaflet syndrome," and "billowing mitral leaflet syndrome." Barlow and Pocock (1975) suggest that the presence of one or more of the following principal features should be helpful in suspecting or detecting the syndrome.

1. A non-ejection click or clicks most often late systolic but at times confined to early systole. An associated murmur of mild mitral regurgitation may or may not be present.
2. Electrocardiographic evidence of abnormal T waves, conduction defects or arrhythmias.
3. Intermittent chest pain, usually of short duration and atypical for angina pectoris.
4. Anxiety and palpitations.
5. Greater prevalence in females and the likelihood of familial occurrence.

The chest pain associated with the MVPS is characteristically precordial in location, sharp in character, short in duration, and unrelated to exercise or emotion. At times it may more closely resemble the pain of coronary artery disease, creating troublesome diagnostic issues. It has been suggested that the syndrome is the commonest cause of non-coronary artery disease chest pain but that the diagnosis is often missed due to lack of suspicion or incomplete examination (Barlow and Pocock, 1975). Indeed, 21% of the 380 MVPS patients described by Naggar (1979) had normal auscultatory findings. Suggestive clinical history, ECG abnormalities, or arrhythmias led to correct diagnosis by echocardiography. The mechanism by which the pain is produced is unclear, one speculation being that it is due to abnormal tension on the papillary muscles.

In addition to chest pain, palpitations and exertional dyspnea are common symptoms. Other manifestations include hyperventilation syndromes, psychotic symptoms, and psychoneuroses. In a group of 230 MVPS patients, migraine was present in 28%, as compared to an expected prevalence of 10%. The authors suggest that all patients with migraine be carefully evaluated for MVPS (Litman and Friedman, 1978).

There are many similarities between the neuropsychiatric symptoms associated with MVPS and those reported for the functional cardiac disorders, anxiety neuroses, and panic states, suggesting that the syndromes may well be related (Wooley, 1976; Pariser et al., 1978) (see section on Functional Cardiac Disorders). The patient reported by Pariser et al. (1978) fulfilled diagnostic criteria for anxiety neurosis (Washingtion University Criteria) and panic disorder (Research Diagnostic Criteria) and had auscultatory and echocardiographic findings of MVPS. When 21 patients with anxiety neurosis were evaluated by Venkatesh et al. (1978), eight were found to have mitral valve prolapse. Finally when exercise tolerance was studied in anxiety neurotics, impaired tolerance was present in the group with MVPS, while those without mitral valve abnormalities did not differ from controls (Crowe et al., 1979).

How these disorder interrelate requires further definition. Barlow and Pocock (1975) suggest that, in some instances, the "psychoneurotic" manifestations may be iatrogenic. For example, a patient with atypical chest pain due to undiagnosed MVPS may be subjected to bias and labeling from his physician once coronary artery disease has been ruled out. By exclusion, his illness therefore becomes "functional," "hypochondriacal," "all in his head," and the mitral valve pathology may remain undiagnosed.

Psychiatrists must also institute a careful search for MVPS when a patient presents with anxiety neurosis or panic attacks. While the syndrome has a good overall prognosis, the patient with MVPS is at risk for developing bacterial endocarditis and should receive antibiotic prophylaxis for procedures such as dental surgery. In addition, there have been rare reports of sudden death and of progression of the valvular lesion to severe mitral regurgitation.

Treatment of MVPS includes general measures such as patient education and support and reassurance in addition to specific drug therapies for arrhythmias, palpitations, and chest pain. At present, propranolol appears to be the most useful agent, although there is a need for well-designed and controlled studies in order assess treatment outcome more accurately.

IMPOTENCE

Impotence (more specifically, erectile dysfunction) is classically found with progressive atherosclerotic obstruction of the aorta and iliac arteries, in association with exercise-induced muscular pain in the lower back, buttocks, and lower extremities (LeRiche's syndrome). Characteristically, the femoral pulses are absent or greatly reduced and abdominal bruits are present.

Impotence, however, may also be caused by vascular obstruction in the *absence* of LeRiche's syndrome and in the *absence* of signs of diminished femoral artery pulses, because of more localized involvement of the hypogastric or internal pudendal arteries or their more distal branches. Techniques are available to measure penile pulses and blood pressure (Abelson, 1975; Gaskell, 1971) and there has been some success reported in restoring erectile function by revascularization procedures (Anonymous, 1976, 1977b). Also of interest is a recent report of impotence of $2\frac{1}{2}$ years' duration that was responsive to the vasodilating drugs, glyceryl trinitrate (nitroglycerine) and pentaerythritol tetranitrate (Mudd, 1977).

These findings suggest that impotence secondary to vascular causes may be substantially underdiagnosed, especially in the absence of supportive findings such as diminished or absent lower extremity pulses or intermittent claudication. A major concern, of course, is that such cases would be relegated, by default, to the category of psychogenic impotence and treated inappropriately and with great frustration by the "new sex therapies." It should be reemphasized that the diagnosis of "psychogenic" impotence should never be made solely by exclusion of "organic" causes.

THORACIC OUTLET SYNDROME

Neurovascular compression syndromes in the neck and shoulder girdle regions result from pressure or tension on the subclavian or axillary artery and the brachial plexus. Based on the anatomical location of the compression, these syndromes have been divided into the:

1. Cervical rib and anomalous first thoracic rib syndrome
2. Scalenus anticus syndrome
3. Costoclavicular syndrome
4. Hyperabduction syndrome

Symptoms may be unilateral or bilateral, and consist of pain, paresthesias, numbness, and weakness in the upper extremities which tend to be intermittent in nature and positionally related. Inconsistent paresthesias in the absence of positive neurological findings is a common presentation. In more severe cases, venous or arterial thrombosis, ulceration and gangrene of the fingers, and rupture of the subclavian artery may occur (such events being quite rare).

It is the milder, intermittent cases that may be attributed to functional causes unless one is aware of the syndromes and can perform the necessary diagnostic maneuvers. These manuevers are described in detail by Fairbairn and Clagett (1972) and, when positive, will cause a diminution or obliteration of the radial pulse. Since similar pulse changes may also occur in asymptomatic individuals, it is necessary to correlate the symptoms carefully with vascular compression. Once diagnosed, patients may improve with a program of shoulder girdle exercises, although surgical intervention may be necessary in severe or refractory situations.

CAROTIDYNIA

The term "carotidynia" refers to a syndrome of vascular neck pain arising from one or both carotid arteries. Symptoms include a dull or deep seated neck pain that is aggravated by swallowing or positional changes, the direct location of which is often difficult to pinpoint. Radiation over the neck, side of the face, and scalp is common. The pain may persist for several weeks and be compounded by secondary apprehension and worry. Physical findings are restricted to tenderness and sometimes swelling over the involved carotid artery, which is usually most pronounced at the bifurcation.

Misdiagnoses are common, and include infection, tonsillitis, thyroid disease, and aneurysm. Unless the condition is suspected, medical evaluation may be negative (over half the patients reported by Lovshin (1977) had had prior medical evaluation but none had been correctly diagnosed), and negative medical evaluations of chronic pain syndromes are likely to result in a misdiagnosis of "functional" pain. Anxiety and depression may be secondary complications if the disorder is not correctly diagnosed (Bank, 1978). Since carotidynia appears to be quite responsive to drugs that aie effective in the treatment and prophylaxis of migraine, correct diagnosis is quite important (Murray, 1979). Some feel that the disorder is actually a migraine variant occurring in the carotid artery.

GIANT CELL ARTERITIS, TEMPORAL ARTERITIS, POLYMYALGIA RHEUMATICA

Although not firmly resolved, polymyalgia rheumatica (PMR) is likely to occupy part of the clinical spectrum of giant cell arteritis (also called temporal arteritis or cranial arteritis) (Ettlinger et al., 1978 Mumenthaler, 1978). Biopsies of medium-sized arteries in patients with PMR show a high incidence of giant cell arteritis, even in the absence of palpable tenderness of the vessels (Hamilton et al., 1971).

It is uncommon for PMR to develop in people under the age of 60. Onset may be either insidious or abrupt, and symptoms may consist of pain, aching, and stiffness of proximal muscles involving shoulders, upper arms, back, buttocks, and thighs. Discomfort may be worse after inactivity or with exertion. In contrast to the prominent symptoms, physical findings in PMR are scant or absent. Muscles may be tender, but weakness or atrophy is generally absent.

The clinical findings in giant cell arteritis (GCA) are determined by the vessels involved. Commonly affected are branches of the internal and external carotids, resulting in headache (classically temporal in location), scalp tenderness, masticatory claudication, and a variety of visual symptoms including sudden blindness. Involvement of the appropriate vessels can result in cerebrovascular accident, myocardial infarction, myocarditis, peripheral neuropathy, and claudication in the extremities. Although the classic physical finding in giant cell arteritis is a tender, nodular, and easily palpable temporal artery, there have been positive biopsies of this vessel despite a negative physical examination.

Nonspecific constitutional manifestations associated with PMR-GCA are common and may predate more definitive findings by *many months*. These include fatigue, lethargy, apathy, depression, anorexia, weight loss, sweats, fever, malaise, and myalgia. Even when more advanced, PMR in the absence of obvious arteritis may be characterized only by vague nonspecific complaints. The potential for misdiagnosis is well stated by Anderson and Bayles (1974):

> Faced with nonspecific complaints and a negative examination, and often also with apathy or depression, the physician may feel quite comfortable attributing these vague symptoms to "functional" or situational complaints in a senior citizen.

While these poorly defined symptoms are the most likely manifestations to confront the psychiatrist, more advanced mental disturbances have been reported. Hart (1967) described two patients with cranial arteritis who had formed visual hallucinations (e.g., "The patient experienced images of menacing people and flapping, brightly coloured curtains which promptly disappeared as soon as systemic corticosteroid therapy was begun.") Depression is a not uncommon prodromal manifestation and depressive symptomatology may obscure other more subtle yet more specific findings. At least one patient was admitted to a mental hospital before the correct diagnosis was made (Vereker, 1952). Other findings may include confusion, disorientation, impaired memory, aggressive behavior, altered level of consciousness, and focal neurological signs (Paulley and Hughes, 1960). Focal intellectual impairment, as manifested by impaired visual nonverbal memory in the presence of otherwise good cognitive function, has been described (Cochran et al., 1978).

Given the complex and often confusing symptoms associated with PMR-GCA, it is well to remember that the erythrocyte sedimentation rate (ESR) is usually markedly elevated and may be the only abnormal laboratory finding. According to Anderson and Bayles (1974), the ESR by the Westergren method is usually over 50 and often greater than 100. As important as this diagnostic clue might be, it is important to be aware that the ESR is occasionally normal in the presence of active giant cell arteritis (Hamilton et al., 1971).

A diagnosis of PMR should be entertained in an elderly patient with proximal muscle discomfort, a lack of physical findings, and an elevated ESR. Arteritis should be suspected in an elderly patient with the initial onset of "tension headache" or other head or facial pain. In addition to "functional" illness, diseases such as infection, malignancy, systemic lupus erythematosus, rheumatoid arthritis, scleroderma, and polymyositis must also be excluded.

The proper diagnosis of PMR-GCA can be established by characteristic findings on temporal artery biopsy, although a negative biopsy by no means excludes the diagnosis. At times, treatment must be initiated on clinical findings alone with response to treatment, in turn, helping to confirm the diagnosis.

The treatment of choice for PMR-GCA is corticosteroids. Response tends to be rapid and dramatic, with symptomatic improvement sometimes beginning within hours. Initial treatment of PMR with as low as 10 mg/day of prednisone may be effective, while higher doses (40–80 mg/day) are commonly used in the treatment of temporal arteritis.

Once the clinical manifestations and ESR elevations have been supressed, low dose therapy is maintained until the disease runs its course. Both PMR and GCA appear to be self-limiting processes, lasting on the average of two years. Steroid therapy is intended to relieve symptoms and prevent complications such as blindness. The lowest possible maintenance dose should be used to minimize the likelihood of drug side effects, and the dose should be tapered periodically until eventually the drug can be discontinued without exacerbation of the disease.

Correctly diagnosing PMR-GCA requires a high index of clinical suspicion. The fact that it occurs in the geriatric age group further increases the likelihood of misdiagnosis, which is especially tragic since specific and highly effective treatment is available. It would be well for every physician working with this age group to periodically review the subject (Hamilton et al., 1971; Anderson and Bayles, 1974; Ettlinger et al., 1978; Mumenthaler, 1978).

NEUROPSYCHIATRIC EFFECTS OF CARDIOVASCULAR DRUGS

Digitalis

Digitalis intoxication is characterized primarily by gastrointestinal and cardiovascular manifestations. While less common, neuropsychiatric toxicity is not rare and, unfortunately, does not produce a characteristic clinical picture. Greenblatt and Shader (1972) have comprehensively reviewed the subject and include a listing of symptoms that have been *attributed* to digitalis (Table 2-3). The authors do point out that such findings often occur in complex clinical settings, and to attribute their cause to a single etiology (i.e., digitalis) may be unwarranted. A wide variety of visual symptoms may also occur in conjunction with digitalis toxicity, such as blurred vision, scotomata, color disturbances including yellow or green vision, flickering lights and even more vivid distortions. Trigeminal neuralgia has been reported in association with digitalis intoxication (Bernat and Sullivan, 1979).

Neuropsychiatric symptoms may, on occasion, be the presenting manifestations of digitalis toxicity (Shear and Sacks, 1978) at which time prompt recognition will not only allow reversal of the delirium but will also prevent progression to potentially life-threatening cardiac arrhythmias. A high index of suspicion coupled with determination of serum digitalis levels are integral steps in making the correct diagnosis but, at times, a clinical trial period of drug discontinuation may be necessary.

TABLE 2-3.   Neuropsychiatric Symptoms Attributed to Digitalis[a]

Headache
Weakness, lassitude, fatigue
Somnolence, drowsiness
Apathy
Depression
Changes in affect or personality
Memory loss
Dizziness, vertigo, ataxia

Confusion, disorientation
Aphasia
Irritability, nervousness, restlessness
Euphoria, giddiness
Excitement, agitation, combativeness
Belligerence, violence
Delusions
Hallucinations

Psychosis
Delirium
Mania
Insomnia, nightmares
Neuralgias

Paresthesias
Muscle pain and weakness
Syncope
Seizures
Stupor, coma

[a] From Greenblatt (1972) with permission of author and publisher.

Antiarrhythmic Drugs

Quinidine

Rarely, even small doses of quinidine may cause symptoms such as visual disturbance, tinnitus, headache, and confusion. Large doses can cause a syndrome known as cinchonism, the neuropsychiatric symptoms of which include headache, apprehension, excitement, confusion, delirium, and syncope (Moe and Abildskov, 1975).

Of interest is a report of a 72-year-old woman with a dementia of *several years' duration* who improved dramatically when quinidine (which she had taken for 14 years) was discontinued (Gilbert, 1977). While on the drug she was described as "severely confused and disoriented and had vivid nocturnal hallucinations." A month after stopping quinidine "her memory had greatly improved. She was perfectly oriented to time and place, her power of concentration was markedly improved and she has resumed her hobbies of reading and embroidery."

Procainamide

Moe and Abildskov (1975) mention that weakness, depression, giddiness, and psychosis with hallucinations have been ascribed to procainamide. A reasonably well documented case of procainamide-induced psychosis was reported by McCrum and Guidry (1978). In addition, the drug may induce a systemic lupus erythematosus-like syndrome which can have associated central nervous system manifestations.

Lidocaine

Lidocaine is usually given intravenously for the control of ventricular arrhythmias and is commonly used in cardiac intensive care units. With increasingly higher doses, symptoms may include drowsiness, lightheadedness, numbness, confusion, disorientation, convulsions, central nervous system depression, and death.

Phenytoin (Diphenylhydantoin)

Although primarily an anticonvulsant, phenytoin also has an established role as an antiarrhythmic agent. Intoxication with this drug produces a characteristic picture, which includes nystagmus, ataxia, dysarthria, and lethargy, and may also include confusion, hyperactivity, and hallucinations. Although there have been reports of phenytoin-induced conversion symptoms, tactile and visual hallucinatory states with somatic delusions, and schizophrenic psychoses, a causal relationship has not been well established (Stores, 1975).

Propranolol

Propranolol is now widely used in the treatment of arrhythmias, hypertension, and angina pectoris. A wide range of neuropsychiatric side effects have been attributed to this drug (Jefferson, 1974). These include:

Toxic psychosis	Fatigue
Hallucinations (often hypnogogic and almost always visual)	Weakness
Vivid dreams and nightmares	Lethargy
Insomnia	Headache
Ataxia	Paresthesia
Lightheadedness	Depression

The overall incidence of these side effects is quite low with a greater tendency to occur at higher doses.

Although it seems prudent to consider depression as a potential adverse reaction to propranolol, the true incidence is difficult to determine with reports varying from 0.02% to 50% of patients evaluated. The drug does not appear to have the "depressogenic" potential of reserpine or even methyldopa.

In addition to possibly exacerbating angina or precipitating myocardial infarction, abrupt discontinuation of a beta-receptor-blocking drug can also cause anxiety, palpitations, and tachycardia (Williams et al., 1979).

Disopyramide

Disopyramide, while not chemically related to other antiarrhythmic drugs, has a mechanism of action similar to that of procainamide and quinidine. The use of this drug has been associated with the onset of acute psychosis, but reports are few and a causal relationship has not been established (Falk et al., 1977; Padfield et al., 1977). These psychotic episodes may have been related to the anticholinergic action of the drug. Additional side effects include headache, fatigue, malaise, nervousness, insomnia, impotence, and depression, but, again, the incidence is quite low and the symptoms may well have been coincidental with, rather than secondary to, use of the drug.

Antihypertensives

Hydralazine

This drug can cause a systemic lupus erythematosus syndrome. In addition, there have been reports of paresthesias, tingling, dizziness, tremors, depression, disorientation, and anxiety. With the exception of headache, neuropsychiatric symptoms are not major side effects of hydralazine.

Methyldopa

Sedation is a common side effect of methyldopa, and patients may experience a persistent lassitude and drowsiness. Additional problems have included weakness, nightmares, impaired mental activity, hallucinations, paranoia, forgetfulness, sexual dysfunction, and depression (Adler, 1974; Kurtz, 1976; Endo et al., 1978). The incidence of methyldopa-induced depression is difficult to establish. References in the literature appear to be based on anecdotal reports, and what constitutes depression is often loosely defined (Pariente, 1973). For example, in an article titled "Methyldopa and Depression" the two cases described contained no mention of depression, but rather described psychomotor retardation and increased sleepiness (Dubach, 1963). Many do feel that of the antihypertensive agents, methyldopa is second only to reserpine in aggravating, unmasking, or causing depression (Whitlock and Evans, 1978).

Reserpine

In recent years, reserpine has played a more limited role in the treatment of hypertension. It tends to be used in fixed-dose drug combinations in doses considerably lower than once employed. There has been a corresponding decrease in the incidence of reserpine-induced neuropsychiatric reactions.

Reserpine-induced depression is a well defined clinical entity which has been thoroughly reviewed by Goodwin et al. (1972). The average incidence of depression based on 16 reports was 20% although only 6% developed "a syndrome analogous to naturalistic endogenous depression." The likelihood of developing depression was greater if a patient had a past history of depression or was on greater than 0.5 mg of reserpine per day. The severity of symptoms ranged from mild to full blown psychotic depression that required treatment with electroconvulsive therapy.

In addition to depression, other side effects associated with reserpine use include nightmares, vague somatic complaints, anxiety attacks, restlessness, organic brain syndrome with vivid visual hallucinations, and sexual dysfunction.

Clonidine

Sedation is a common side effect of clonidine. Depression is also a possible side effect with a reported incidence ranging from as high as 10% to no different from placebo (Whitlock and Evans, 1978). Dementia of five months duration in an elderly patient was reversed when clonidine was discontinued (Lavin and Alexander, 1975). Abrupt withdrawal of the drug has been associated with a rapid rise in blood pressure to pretreatment levels and symptoms of insomnia, headache, flushing, sweating, and apprehension (Reid et al., 1977).

Propranolol

See Antiarrhythmic Drug Section.

Guanethidine

Depression has been reported in patients treated with guanethidine, despite the limited ability of the drug to pass the blood—brain barrier (Whitlock and Evans, 1978). Reports have been few, however, and incidence and causality are difficult to determine. Additional side effects of guanethidine include dizziness, weakness, lassitude, and inhibition of ejaculation.

Pargyline

It is well to remember that pargyline is a monoamine oxidase inhibitor, and that patients receiving this drug are at risk for hypertensive crises if they ingest foods with a high tyramine content or sympathomimetic drugs. A depressed patient taking pargyline for hypertension should not be treated with a tricyclic antidepressant unless the pargyline has been discontinued for two weeks.

Sodium Nitroprusside

Although quite effective in treating acute hypertensive crises, sodium nitroprusside can cause toxic psychoses if the serum concentration gets too high (as reflected in serum thiocyanate level).

Vasopressors

Side effects from vasopressors are related to sympathetic stimulation, and can include anxiety, restlessness, palpitations, and insomnia.

Anticoagulants

Neurological complications from anticoagulant therapy are produced by bleeding involving the brain (intracerebral and subarachroid hemorrhage, subdural hematoma), spinal cord (epidural and subdural hematoma), and peripheral nerves (especially femoral nerve compression from bleeding into the iliacus muscle) (Silverstein, 1979). Mental status changes in the elderly due to anticoagulant-induced subdural hematoma may be incorrectly attributed to the aging process.

Comment

The cardiovascular drugs discussed above should not be considered an inclusive listing of those causing neuropsychiatric side effects. In the presence of an unexplained reaction, any drug should be considered suspect and subject to temporary discontinuation to attempt to relieve symptoms and establish a causal relationship.

CARDIOVASCULAR DRUG-INDUCED SEXUAL DYSFUNCTION

With a few exceptions, the role of cardiovascular drugs in causing sexual dysfunction is not clear. Often erectile or ejaculatory difficulties or a decrease in libido are mentioned as possible side effects without careful documentation of a cause and effect relationship. Unfortunately, questions about sexual dysfunction are all too often omitted at the time of both initial and ongoing evaluation, leading to considerable problems with diagnosis and treatment. A comprehensive review of the effect of antihypertensive drugs on ejaculation and erectile function has been done by Segraves (1977).

Several drugs have been implicated more often than others. The antihypertensive **guanethidine** is said to cause reduced emission and delay or failure of ejaculation without loss of erectile ability in as high as 60% of patients receiving large doses (Mills, 1975). **Methyldopa** has been implicated in causing decreased libido, erectile dysfunction, reduced emission, and delayed ejaculation 2–33% of patients (Newman and Salerno, 1974). It has been stated that impotence and constipation occur in 10–20% of patients on chronic **clonidine** therapy (Nickerson and Ruedy, 1975).

Two case reports suggest that **propranolol** may cause impotence (erectile dysfunction) since the difficulty began shortly after the drug was started, resolved on discontinuation, and reappeared when the patient was rechallenged with the drug (Knarr, 1976; Miller, 1976). Erectile dysfunction with intact libido has been reported with the antiarrhythmic agent **disopyramide** and has been attributed to its anticholinergic activity (McHaffie et al., 1977). Even a class of drugs as "sexually innocuous" as the **thiazides** have fallen under suspicion. Freis (1978) has stated: "Nevertheless, the clinical experience of many physicians indicated that in some middle-aged to older hypertensive patients, continuous treatment with thiazide diuretics may result in the appearance of impotence." An earlier survey found erectile difficulties in 33% of a group of middle aged hypertensives who were receiving only diuretics (Bulpitt and Dollery, 1973).

In evaluating sexual dysfunction, there is no substitute for a comprehensive medical and psychosocial history. Otherwise medication may be "blamed" for what is actually an interpersonal problem or, conversely, marital discord may arise secondary to drug-induced dysfunction. Also, a preexisting problem may be first uncovered during treatment with a cardiovascular drug because more attention is paid to the possibility of adverse reactions. The preexisting problem may then be falsely assumed to be a drug side effect. Finally, it may be quite difficult to separate pharmacological and psychological drug side effects, as suggested by the Veterans Administration Cooperative Study Group on Antihypertensive Agents (1972), which found that the incidence of impotence during a double-blind trial was as high on placebo as it was on a combination of thiazides, reserpine, and hydralazine.

If drug side effect is suspected as the cause of sexual dysfunction, perhaps the most practical clinical approach would be a trial period off the medication to try to establish a causal relationship. Prior to beginning drug treatment, a thorough sexual history should be taken and the possibility of sexual side effects clearly explained to the patient. Such an approach should help prevent the development of complicated and confusing situations in which multiple medications, psychosocial factors, and iatrogenic distortions have become needlessly fused.

PSYCHOTROPIC DRUGS AND CARDIOVASCULAR DISORDERS

In general, patients with cardiovascular disease are at higher risk for developing cardiovascular toxicity from psychotropic drugs—the more severe the disease, the greater the risk. These patients also tend to be on a greater number of medications, which increases the possibility of adverse drug–drug interactions. A number of reviews have been written dealing with the cardiovascular effects and toxicity of the various classes of psychotropic drugs and will provide the reader with a more complete appreciation of the subject (Ebert and Shader, 1970; Ayd, 1970; Greenblatt and Shader, 1974; Jefferson, 1975; Fowler et al., 1976; Bigger et al., 1978; Jefferson and Greist, 1979).

Antipsychotic Drugs

The more potent antipsychotic drugs such as haloperidol, trifluoperazine, and thiothixene have a lower incidence of cardiovascular side effects than do less potent drugs such as chlorpromazine and thioridazine and, thus, are favored for use in patients with cardiovascular disease. No antipsychotic drug, however, is without the potential for causing hypotension and arrhythmias, and all should be used with greater than usual caution in the high risk patient.

Blood Pressure

Hypotensive changes caused by antipsychotic drugs are most likely to occur early in the course of therapy, often resolve spontaneously over several days, and tend to be of a postural nature. Both recumbent and standing blood pressure measurements should be made with the standing pressure being the most sensitive indicator of a hypotensive effect. Patients who are taking antihypertensive medications or who are in a state of fluid–electrolyte imbalance can be expected to be especially susceptible to these changes. Cigarette smoking has been shown to be inversely related to the likelihood that chlorpromazine will cause hypotension (Swett et al., 1977).

Electrocardiogram

Repolarization changes in the form of T wave alterations are common, benign, and reversible cardiac effects of antipsychotic drugs. It is important that these drug-induced changes not be mistaken for serious cardiac pathology.

Arrhythmias and Sudden Death

Both serious arrhythmias and sudden death have been attributed to the use of antipsychotic drugs, but such occurrences are quite rare, appear to be idiosyncratic, and often occur in a setting in which it is difficult to isolate a specific etiologic agent. Although chlorpromazine and thioridazine have been most often associated with sudden death, it has not been fully resolved if thses two drugs are truly more hazardous. Given the extremely low incidence of these serious side effects, a definitive answer will probably not be forthcoming. Nonetheless, since the higher milligram potency drugs are clearly less likely to cause hypotension and may be less likely to cause arrhythmias, their use is preferred in patients with cardiovascular disease.

Drug Interactions

Antipsychotic drugs can reverse the antihypertensive action of **guanethidine**, probably by blocking neuronal uptake of the latter drug. This has been most clearly demonstrated with chlorpromazine, and it also occurs with haloperidol and thiothixene (Hussar, 1973) but does not occur with molindone. In general, however, because of their ability to cause hypotension, it is more common for the antipsychotics to potentiate the effects of antihypertensive agents.

Two patients on a constant dose of **methyldopa** developed organic brain syndrome symptoms when placed on haloperidol and which cleared when the latter was discontinued, suggesting a possible interaction between the two drugs (Thornton, 1976).

Antipsychotic drug-induced liver microsomal enzyme induction has not been shown to be of clinical importance with regard to decreasing the effect of oral anticoagulents (Hartshorn, 1975), but should be considered a possibility.

Antianxiety Drugs

Benzodiazepines are very well tolerated clinically, even in patients with advanced cardiovascular disease. The cardiovascular effects of these drugs have been thoroughly reviewed by Greenblatt and Shader (1974).

Barbiturates are potent inducers of liver microsomal enzymes and can substantially decrease the effect of oral anticoagulants (Hussar, 1973). These drugs, fortunately, have been largely replaced by the benzodiazepines both as hypnotics and anxiolytics.

Antidepressants—Tricyclics

The tricyclic antidepressants have potent cardiovascular effects and toxicity (Jefferson, 1975; Spiker et al., 1975; Bigger et al., 1978). Patients with cardiovascular disease are more susceptible to these adverse reactions, and while the tricyclics are not contraindicated in such situations, appropriate caution must be exercised. Tricyclic overdose can cause profound alterations in blood pressure, cardiac rhythm, and cardiac contractility even in the presence of an otherwise normal cardiovascular system.

Blood Pressure

Postural hypotension is a common side effect of the tricyclics, especially early in the course of therapy. Recent work (Glassman et al., 1979) suggests that substantial postural hypotension persists for weeks during therapy and should be considered the most serious cardiovascular complication of the tricyclics. On rare occasions, a hypertensive response can occur.

Electrocardiogram

Benign, reversible T-wave changes are the most common ECG alterations that occur with therapeutic doses of the tricyclic antidepressants. With intoxication, a wide variety of arrhythmias, at times life-threatening or fatal, can occur. In some situations, the tricyclics may actually have an antiarrhythmic effect. Recently it has been shown that imipramine can suppress atrial and ventricular ectopic beats. On the other hand, preexisting conduction disturbances were either unchanged or aggravated (Glassman et al., 1978).

Sudden Death

An increased incidence of sudden death in patients with cardiovascular disease has been associated with the use of tricyclic antidepressants. Whether patients are at greater risk on certain tricyclics has not been resolved, and studies in both animal and man have been contradictory (Jefferson, 1975).

Drug Interactions

All tricyclics interfere with the antihypertensive effect of **guanethidine** by blocking its uptake into the adrenergic neuron. **Clonidine** may also be less effective when used in conjunction with tricyclics, although the mechanism of this interaction is not clear. The antihypertensive **pargyline** is a monoamine oxidase inhibitor and should not be used in conjunction with tricyclic antidepressants. Since it also has antidepressive activity, some feel it would be a useful drug for the depressed, hypertensive patient.

The tricyclics are inhibitors of liver microsomal drug metabolizing enzymes and have been shown to substantially increase the half-life of the oral anticoagulant, **dicumarol**. **Propranolol** metabolism is also inhibited but whether this is of clinical importance has not been established.

Antidepressants—Monoamine Oxidase Inhibitors

Postural hypotension is a common side effect of monoamine oxidase inhibitors and, consequently, these drugs may potentiate the action of antihypertensive drugs. In addition, the interaction of monoamine oxidase inhibitors with **sympathomimetic amines** and certain antihypertensives such as **reserpine** and **methyldopa** may lead to hypertensive crises.

Lithium

The use of lithium in patients with cardiovascular disease, while not contraindicated, is not without hazard. Factors which include unstable fluid–electrolyte balance, diuretic drug use, and sodium restriction can greatly complicate treatment. The cardiovascular effects and toxicity of lithium have been recently reviewed in depth (Jefferson and Greist, 1979).

Blood Pressure

Lithium does not cause major alterations in blood pressure.

Electrocardiogram

The most common effect of lithium on the electrocardiogram is benign and reversible alterations in T-wave morphology.

Lithium-induced arrhythmias are rare although there have been several reports of sinus node dysfunction associated with its use.

Drug Interactions

The use of **thiazide** and possibly **potassium sparing diuretics** with lithium causes increased serum lithium levels and can lead to lithium toxicity. There have been several case reports of an adverse interaction between lithium and **methyldopa** (Byrd, 1977), but the two drugs have also been used together without difficulty in many patients.

REFERENCES

Abdon N-J, Malmcrona R: High pacemaker implantation rate following "Cardiogenic Neurology." *Acta Med Scand* 198:455–461, 1975.

Abelson D: Diagnostic value of the penile pulse and blood pressure: A Doppler study of impotence in diabetes. *J. Urology* 113:636–639, 1975.

Adams RD, Braunwald E: Faintness, syncope, and episodic weakness, in Wintrobe MW, Thorn GW, Adams RD, et al (eds): Harrison's Principles of Internal Medicine, ed. New York, McGraw–Hill, 1974, pp 72–78.

Adler S: Methyldopa-induced decrease in mental activity. *JAMA* 230:1428–1429, 1974.

Anderson, LG, Bayles TB: Polymyalgia rheumatica and giant cell arteritis. *Disease-a-Month*, pp 1–36, Jan 1974.

Anonymous: Bypass to raise penile blood said to correct impotence. *Med Tribune* Mar 10, 1976.

Anonymous: Cardiogenic dementia. *Lancet* 1:27–28, 1977(a).

Anonymous: New surgical treatment for impotence: Revascularization. *Med World News* Jan 10, 1977(b), p 26.

Anonymous: Prolapsed mitral leaflet could be most common valve disorder. *JAMA* 239:687–688, 1978.

Antel JJ, Rome HP, Geraci JE, et al: Toxic-organic psychosis as a presenting feature in bacterial endocarditis. *Mayo Clin Proc* 30:45–50, 1955.

Ayd FJ: Cardiovascular effect of phenothiazines. *Int Drug Ther Newsl* 5:1–8, 1970.

Bank H: Idiopathic carotiditis. *Lancet* 1:726, 1978.

Barlow JB, Pocock WA: The problem of nonejection systolic clicks and associated mitral systolic murmurs: Emphasis on the billowing mitral leaflet syndrome. *Am Heart J* 90:636–655, 1975.

Bellet S: *Clinical Disorders of the Heart Beat*. Philadelphia, Lea & Febiger, 1971, p 658.

Bernat JL, Sullivan JK: Trigeminal neuralgia from digitalis intoxication. *Jama* 241:164–165, 1979.

Bigger JT, Kantor SJ, Glassman AH, et al: Cardiovascular effects of tricyclic antidepressant drugs, in Lipton MA, DiMascio A, Killam KF (eds): *Psychopharmacology: A Generation of Progress*. New York, Raven, 1978, pp 1033–1046.

Boller F, Vrtunski PB, Mack JL, et al: Neuropsychological correlates of hypertension. *Arch Neurol* 34:701–705, 1977.

Bulpitt CJ, Dollery CT: Side effects of hypotensive agents evaluated by a self-administered questionnaire. *Br Med J* 3:485–490, 1973.

Byrd GJ: Lithium carbonate and methyldopa: Apparent interaction in man. *Clin Toxicol* 11:1–4, 1977.

Chester EM, Agamanolis DP, Banker BQ et al: Hypertensive encephalopathy: A clinical pathologic study of 20 cases. *Neurology* 28:928–939, 1978.

Cochran JW, Fox JH, Kelly MP: Reversible mental symptoms in temporal arteritis. *J Nerv Ment Dis* 166:446–447, 1978.

Corday E, Irving DW: Effect of cardiac arrhythmias on the cerebral circulation. *Am J Cardiol* 6:803–808, 1960.

Corday E, Tzu-Wang L: Hemodynamic consequences of cardiac arrhythmias, in Hurst JW, Logue RB (eds): *The Heart*. New York, McGraw–Hill, 1970, pp 484–489.

Crowe RR, Pauls DL, Venkatesh A, et al: Exercise and anxiety neurosis: Comparison of patients with and without mitral valve prolapse. *Arch Gen Psychiatry* 36:652–653, 1979.

Drake FR, Ebaugh FG: Pheochromocytoma and electroconvulsive therapy. *Am J Psychiatry* 113:295–301, 1956.

Dubach UC: Methyldopa and depression. *Br Med J* 1:261–262, 1963.

Ebert MH, Shader RI: Cardiovascular effects, in Shader RI, DiMascio A (eds): *Psychotropic Drug Side Effects*. Baltimore, Williams & Wilkins, 1970, pp 149–163.

Eichna LW, Horvath SM, Bean WB: Postexertional orthostatic hypotension. *Am J Med Sci* 213:641–654, 1947.

Endo M, Hirai K, O'Hara M: Paranoid-hallucinatory state induced in a depressive patient by methyldopa: A case report. *Psychoneuroendocrinology* 3:211–215, 1978.

Ettlinger RE, Hunder GG, Ward LE: Polymyalgia rheumatica and giant cell arteritis. *Ann Rev Med* 29:15–22, 1978.

Evans, DW, Lum LC: Hyperventilation: An important cause of pseudoangina. *Lancet* 1:155–157, 1977.

Fairbairn JF, Clagett OT: Neurovascular compression syndromes of the thoracic outlet, in Fairbairn JF, Juergens JL, Spittell JA (eds) *Peripheral Vascular Diseases*. Philadelphia, WB Saunders, 1972, pp 459–475.

Falk RH, Nisbet PA, Gray TJ: Mental distress in patient on disopyramide. *Lancet* 1:858–859, 1977.

Fetterman JL, Ashe WF: Cerebral debut of certain cases of cardiac disease. *Ohio State Med J* 34:1354–1358, 1938.

Finnerty FA: Hypertensive encephalopathy. *Am Heart J* 75:559–563, 1968.

Fowler NO, McCall D, Chou T-C: Electrocardiographic changes and cardiac arrhythmias in patients receiving psychotropic drugs. *Am J Cardiol* 37:223–230, 1976.

Freis ED: Thiazides and impotence. *Drug Ther* 8:161, 1978.

Frohlich ED, Tarazi RC, Dustan HP: Hyperdynamic beta-adrenergic circulatory state. *Arch Int Med* 123:1–7, 1969.

Gaskell P: The importance of penile blood pressure in cases of impotence. *Can Med Assoc J* 105:1047–1051, 1971.

Gilbert GJ: Quinidine dementia. *JAMA* 237:2093–2094, 1977.

Gill RJ: Essential hypertension (hypertensive vascular disease, hypertensive cardiovascular disease, primary hypertension), in Horwitz D. Magee JH (eds): *Index of Suspicion in Treatable Diseases*. Philadelphia, Lea & Febiger, 1975, pp 439–447.

Glassman, AH, Bigger JT, Kantor SJ, et al: Cardiovascular effects of imipramine. *NCDEU Intercom* 7:8–12, 1978.

Glassman AH, Bigger JT, Giardina EV, et al: Clinical characteristics of imipramine-induced orthostatic hypotension. *Lancet* 1:468–472, 1979.

Goodwin FK, Ebert MH, Bunney WE: Mental effects of reserpine in man: A review, in Shader RI (eds): *Psychiatric Complications of Medical Drugs*. New York, Raven Press, 1972, pp 73–101.

Green HL: Pheochromocytoma—a survey of current concepts. *Henry Ford Hosp Med Bull* 8:103–115, 1960.

Greenblatt DJ, Shader RI: Digitalis toxicity, in Shader RI (ed): *Psychiatric Complications of Medical Drugs*. New York, Raven Press, 1972, pp 25–47.

Greenblatt DJ, Shader RI: *Benzodiazepines in Clinical Practice*. New York, Raven Press, 1974, pp 141–171.

Greenwood WF: Profile of atrial myxoma. *Am J Cardiol* 21:367–375, 1968.

Hamilton CR, Shelley WN, Tumulty PA: Giant cell arteritis: Including temporal arteritis and polymyalgia rheumatica. *Medicine* 50:1–27, 1971.

Hart, CT: Formed visual hallucinations: A symptom of cranial arteritis. *Br Med J* 3:643–644, 1967.

Hartshorn EA: Interactions of CNS drugs: Psychotherapeutic agents—The antipsychotic drugs. *Drug Intell and Clin Pharm* 9:536–550, 1975.

Harvey WP- Clinical aspects of cardiac tumors. *Am J Cardiol* 21:328–343, 1968.

Hurst JW, Logue RB: Etiology and clinical recognition of heart failure, in Hurst JW, Logue RB (eds): *The Heart*. New York, McGraw–Hill, 1970, pp 434–454.

Hussar DA: Drug interactions. *Am J Pharm* 145:65–116, 1973.

Jefferson JW: Atypical manifestations of postural hypotension. *Arch Gen Psychiatry* 27:250–251, 1972.

Jefferson JW: Beta-adrenergic receptor blocking drugs in psychiatry. *Arch Gen Psychiatry* 31:681–691, 1974.

Jefferson JW: A review of the cardiovascular effects and toxicity of tricyclic antidepressants. *Psychosom Med* 37:160–179, 1975.

Jefferson JW: Use of beta-adrenergic blocking drugs in psychiatry, in Saxena PR. Forsyth RP (eds):*Beta-Adrenoceptor Blocking Agents*. Amsterdam, North–Holland Pub Co, 1976, pp 239–271.

Jefferson JW, Greist JH: The cardiovascular effects and toxicity of lithium, in Davis JM. Greenblatt D (eds): *Psychopharmacology Update: New and Neglected Areas*. New York, Grune & Stratton, 1979, pp 65–79.

Knarr JW: Impotence from propranolol? *Ann Int Med* 85:259, 1976.

Kurtz JB: Methyldopa and forgetfulness. *Lancet* 1:202–203, 1976.

Lavin P, Alexander CP: Dementia associated with clonidine therapy. *Br Med J* 1:628, 1975.

Lindberg BJ: Somatic complaints in the depressive symptomatology. *Acta Psychiatr Scand* 41:419–427, 1965.

Litman GI, Friedman HM: Migraine and the mitral valve prolapse syndrome. *Am Heart J* 96:610–614, 1978.

Logue RB, Hurst JW: Clinical recognition of coronary atherosclerotic heart disease and its complications, in Hurst JW, Logue RB (eds): *The Heart*. New York, McGraw–Hill, 1970, pp 946–984.

Lovshin LL: Carotidynia. *Headache* 17:192–195, 1977.

McAllen PM, Marshall J: Cardiac dysrhythmia and transient cerebral ischemic attacks. *Lancet* 1:1212–1214, 1973.

McCrum ID, Guidry JR: Procainamide-induced psychosis. *JAMA* 240:1265–1266, 1978.

McHaffie DJ, Guz A, Johnston A: Impotence in patient on disopyramide. *Lancet* 1:859, 1977.

Magee JH: Vascular crises: Pheochromocytoma, in Horwitz O, Magee JH (eds): *Index of Suspicion in Treatable Diseases*. Philadelphia, Lea & Febiger, 1975, pp 458–459.

Manger WM, Gifford RW: *Pheochromocytoma*. New York, Springer–Verlag, 1977, pp 141–142.

Miller RA: Propranolol and impotence. *Ann Int Med* 85:682–683, 1976.

Mills LC: Drug-induced impotence. *Am Fam Physician* 12:104–106, 1975.

Moe GK, Abildskov JA: Antiarrhythmic drugs, in Goodman LS, Gilman A (eds): *The Pharmacological Basis of Therapeutics*. New York, MacMillan Publishing Co, 1975, pp 683–704.

Mudd JW: Impotence responsive to glyceryl trinitrate. *Am J Psychiatry* 134:922–925, 1977.

Mumenthaler M: Giant cell arteritis (cranial arteritis, polymyalgia rheumatica). *J Neurol* 218:219–236, 1978.

Murray TJ: Carotidynia: A cause of neck and face pain. *Can Med Assoc J* 120:441–443, 1979.

Naggar CZ: The mitral valve prolapse syndrome, spectrum and therapy. *Med Clin North Am* 63:337–353, 1979.

Newman RJ, Salerno HR: Sexual dysfunction due to methyldopa. *Br Med J* 4:106, 1974.

Nickerson M, Ruedy J: Antihypertensive agents and the drug therapy of hypertension, in Goodman LS, Gilman A (eds): *The Pharmacological Basis of Therapeutics*. New York, MacMillan, 1975, pp 705–726.

Padfield PL, Smith DA, Fitzsimons EJ, et al: Disopyramide and acute psychosis. *Lancet* 1:1152, 1977.

Pariente D: Methyldopa and depression. *Br Med J* 4:110–111, 1973.

Pariser SF, Pinta ER, Jones BA: Mitral valve prolapse syndrome and anxiety neurosis/panic disorder. *Am J Psychiatry* 135:246–247, 1978.

Paulley JW, Hughes JP: Giant-cell arteritis or arteritis of the aged. *Br Med J* 2:1562–1566, 1960.

Perley MJ,Guze SB: Hysteria—the stability and usefulness of clinical criteria. N Eng J Med 266: 421–426, 1962.

Pruitt AA, Rubin RH, Karchmer AW: Neurologic complications of bacterial endocarditis. Medicine 57:329–343, 1978.

Ram CVS: Hypertensive encephalopathy, recognition and management. Arch Int Med 138:1851–1853, 1978.

Reid JL, Dargie HJ, Davies DS, et al: Clonidine withdrawal in hypertension. Lancet 1:1171–1174, 1977.

Rizzon P, Biasco G, Brindicci, G, et al: Familial syndrome of midsystolic click and late systolic murmur. Br Heart J 35:245–259, 1973.

Schlant RC: Altered physiology of the cardiovascular system in heart failure, in Hurst JW, Logue RB (eds): The Heart. New York, McGraw–Hill, 1970, pp 405–423.

Segraves RT: Pharmacological agents causing sexual dysfunction. J Sex Marital Ther 3:157–176, 1977.

Shapiro W, Chawla N: Effects of pacing on cerebral blood flow and cardiac dynamics. Circulation (suppl 3 to Nos. 39–40): 184, 1969.

Shear MK, Sacks MH: Digitalis delirium: Report of two cases. Am J Psychiatry 135:109–110, 1978.

Silverstein A: Neurological complications of anticoagulation therapy. Arch Int Med 139:217–220, 1979.

Spiker DG, Weiss An, Chang SS, et al: Tricyclic antidepressant overdose: Clinical presentation and plasma levels. Clin Pharmacol Ther 18:539–546, 1975.

Spudis EV, Griffin A: Adams-Stokes attacks associated with hysteria. JAMA 229:1636, 1974.

Stores G: Behavioral effects of anti-epileptic drugs. Dev Med Clin Neurol 17:647–658, 1975.

Sulg IA, Cronqvist S, Schuller H, et al: The effect of intracardial pacemaker therapy on cerebral blood flow and electroencephalogram in patients with complete atrioventricular block. Circulation 39:487–494, 1969.

Swett, C, Cole JO, Hartz SC: Hypotension due to chlorpromazine. Arch Gen Psychiatry 34:661–663, 1977.

Thomas JE, Rooke ED, Kvale WF: The neurologists experience with pheochromocytoma. JAMA 197:754–758, 1966.

Thornton WE: Dementia induced by methyldopa with haloperidol. N Eng J Med 294:1222, 1976.

Venkatesh A, Pauls DL, Crowe R, et al: Mitral valve prolapse in anxiety neurosis. Clin Res 26:656A, 1978.

Vereker R: The psychiatric aspects of temporal arteritis. J Ment Sci 98:280–286, 1952.

Veterans Administration Cooperative Study Group on Antihypertensive Agents: Effects of treatment on mortality in hypertension: III. Influence of age, diastolic pressure, and prior cardiovascular disease; further analysis of side effects. Circulation 45:991–1004, 1972.

Walter PF, Crawley IS, Dorney ER: Carotid sinus hypersensitivity and syncope. Am J Cardiol 42:396–402, 1978.

Weiss S, Ferris EB: Adams-Stokes syndrome with transient complete heart block of vasovagal reflex origin. Arch Int Med 54:931–951, 1934.

Wenger NK: Tumors of the heart, in Hurst JW, Logue RB (eds): The Heart. New York, McGraw–Hill, 1970, pp 1275–1290.

Wharton RN: Atrial myxoma masquerade. Am J Psychiatry 134:1441–1442, 1977.

Whitlock FA, Evans LEJ: Drugs and depression. Drugs 15:53–71, 1978.

Williams LC, Turney JH, Parsons V: Beta-blocker withdrawal syndrome. Lancet 1:494–495, 1979.

Wooley CF: Where are the diseases of yesteryear? Circulation 53:749–751, 1976.

3

Respiratory Disorders

RESPIRATORY FAILURE

General Considerations

Respiratory insufficiency or failure exists when the lungs are unable to perform their function of adequate gas exchange. Confirmation of the diagnosis is made by measurement of arterial blood gases. Useful guidelines (under resting conditions at sea level) for diagnosing arterial hypoxemia is a partial pressure of oxygen (pO_2) of less than 60 mm Hg, while arterial hypercapnia would be diagnosed if the partial pressure of CO_2 (pCO_2) is greater than 49 mm Hg. Respiratory failure may be acute and fully reversible, chronic and unremitting, or chronic with superimposed acute exacerbations. Abnormal arterial blood gases are not invariably due to lung disease, as demonstrated by the low pO_2 seen in association with those forms of congenital heart disease having a substantial right to left intracardiac shunt.

Mild respiratory insufficiency may be detectable only during exercise, while at the same time more advanced blood gas abnormalities will also be present at rest. While a complaint of dyspnea or breathlessness often accompanies respiratory failure, the association is not inevitable. For example, a patient with primary alveolar hypoventilation and blood gases consistent with respiratory failure may not complain of dyspnea. On the other hand, if by increasing pulmonary work a patient can maintain normal blood gases, he may complain of marked dyspnea without meeting the requirements for a diagnosis of respiratory failure.

Depending on the characteristics of the arterial blood gas abnormality, there are two types of acute respiratory failure. The first is **hypoxemic respiratory failure**, a condition in which the lungs are unable to deliver sufficient oxygen to the blood, resulting in arterial hypoxemia (low pO_2). At the same time, CO_2 transfer is not impaired and pCO_2 is either normal or low. Conditions in which hypoxemic acute respiratory failure occur include: (1) diffuse pulmonary infection, (2) aspiration pneumonia, (3) interstitial pneumonia, (4) inhalation of irritant gases, (5) oxygen toxicity, (6) fat embolism, (7) "shock lung," (8) immunologic disorders, (9) alveolar filling diseases, and (10) inhalation burns (Moser, 1974).

The second type, **hypercapnic respiratory failure**, is also characterized by arterial hypoxemia (low pO_2), but is further defined by the presence of hypercapnia (high pCO_2). Impaired elimination of CO_2 can occur owing to hypoventilation in the presence of normal lungs in conditions which depress the respiratory center. Such conditions include: (1) the use of drugs such as opiates and barbiturates; (2) encephalitis; (3) bulbar poliomyelitis; (4) neuromuscular disorders affecting respiratory muscles such as Guillain–Barre syndrome, myasthenia gravis, and muscular dystrophies; (5) metabolic alkalosis; (6) thoracic cage abnormalities, as with trauma and kyphoscoliosis; (7) upper airway obstruction; and (8) idiopathic hypoventilation (West, 1974). Because lung disease is absent in these patients, the presence of hypercapnic respiratory failure may be overlooked.

Hypercapnic respiratory insufficiency associated with intrinsic pulmonary disease occurs with conditions such as emphysema, bronchitis, and asthma. Impaired CO_2 elimination is secondary to altered characteristics of the lung itself, although these disorders may be secondarily compounded by the administration of respiratory depressants.

Clinical Features

Hypoxia

The brain is acutely sensitive to oxygen lack, and within seconds hypoxia can cause electroencephalographic abnormalities. Restlessness and apprehension often characterize mild hypoxia, while more severe acute hypoxia may cause CNS irritability and an agitated delirium. If oxygen deprivation is chronic, there may be associated impairment of judgement and cognitive function and neuromuscular irritability. More profound hypoxia may be associated with depressed CNS function, visual disturbances, incoordination, dysarthria, coma, and ultimately death.

Perhaps the greatest diagnostic pitfall lies in mistaking the restlessness and apprehension of an early hypoxic delirium for psychologically-based anxiety. Misdiagnosis at this juncture can have perilous consequences, since the use of a sedative–anxiolytic drug to relieve the "anxiety" can, in fact, suppress respiration and further aggravate the hypoxia.

Hypercapnia

Since hypercapnia is usually associated with both hypoxia and respiratory acidosis, it is difficult to assess the relative contributions of each.

High concentrations of CO_2 have a depressant effect on the CNS. In fact, in 1937 Waters successfully anesthetized three patients with 30% CO_2 (but one had a convulsion and the technique was quickly discarded) (from Westlake et al., 1955). If normal people breathe increased concentrations of CO_2, they may develop depression, irritability, anxiety, somnolence, confusion, and delirium (Sieker and Hickam, 1956).

A rise in arterial CO_2 level will cause dilatation of cerebral blood vessels, an increase in cerebral blood flow, and an increase in intracranial pressure. This probably accounts for the papilledema which may occur in the presence of marked hypercapnia.

Kilburn (1965) studied 24 patients in respiratory failure and found that the neuropsychiatric manifestations correlated closely with increased arterial blood pCO_2 and acidosis but not with the degree of arterial hypoxemia. As hypercapnia and acidosis became more severe, there was a higher incidence of disorientation, somnolence, coma, asterixis, tremor, seizure, headache, and death.

The severity of symptoms is also correlated with the rate at which CO_2 retention develops. Patients with chronic respiratory acidosis may be quite resistant to neuropsychiatric impairment despite high levels of arterial CO_2. Indeed, as Gross and Hamilton (1963) point out, symptoms correlate best with the degree to which CO_2 has increased above the *usual* level for the patient.

The need for physicians to be aware of the manifestations of hypercapnia has been stressed by Kilburn (1965) who states:

> However, patients have been described as forgetful, drowsy, somnolent, confused, anxious, disoriented, irritable, irrational, obstreperous, paranoid, psychotic, and psychopathic. Because of abrupt or gradual personality deterioration patients have been admitted to psychiatric as well as neurologic wards.

Correct diagnosis is especially important since reduction of CO_2 levels towards normal will result in dramatic neuropsychiatric improvement.

Treatment

Oxygen is an important factor in the treatment of hypercapnic respiratory failure, but too much oxygen can actually aggravate CO_2 retention and cause clinical deterioration.

Acute CO_2 retention stimulates respiration through a decrease in cerebrospinal fluid (CSF) pH, a decrease in arterial pH, and a decrease in arterial pO_2. With persistent hypercapnia, however, bicarbonate retention normalizes CSF pH within 24 hr and blood pH within 3 to 5 days so that hypercapnia is no longer a major respiratory stimulus. Ventilation is then maintained, to a large extent, by the effect of reduced arterial oxygen tension on peripheral chemoreceptors. If excessive oxygen is administered to the hypercapnic patients, this ventilatory drive is removed, alveolar ventilation will decrease, and further CO_2 retention will occur (Moser, 1974). The previously described symptoms of CO_2 intoxication may then develop (Westlake et al., 1955; Sieker and Hickam, 1956).

For example, Westlake et al. (1955) described a patient with moderate cyanosis, mild CO_2 retention (pCO_2 = 52 mm Hg), and a normal blood pH (7.38), who was placed in an oxygen tent and then developed euphoria and disorientation which progressed to stupor, coma, and death. Arterial pCO_2 had risen to 129 mm Hg and pH dropped to 7.13. Another patient, in the presence of ample oxygenation, developed progressive CO_2 retention and became restless, confused, and disoriented, and eventually sank into semi-coma.

Treatment of the hypercapnic, hypoxemic patient requires the judicious administration of oxygen, and *gradual* lowering of the pCO_2, with frequent monitoring of arterial blood gases. If in the presence of chronic hypercapnia, CO_2 levels are lowered too rapidly by mechanical ventilation, neuropsychiatric complications can develop (Rotheram et al., 1964; Kilburn, 1966; Faden, 1976). Because CO_2 freely diffuses across the blood–brain barrier while bicarbonate crosses more slowly, rapid removal of CO_2 can result in CSF alkalosis. This, in turn, may cause cerebral hypoxia through cerebral vasoconstriction and by adversely shifting the oxyhemoglobin dissociation curve. The use of aminophylline to treat respiratory failure may further aggravate the situation, since this drug can also cause cerebral vasoconstriction and reduce cerebral blood flow.

Symptoms associated with the overzealous correction of hypercapnia include hypotension, tachypnea, arrhythmias, multifocal and generalized seizures, tremor, asterixis, and myoclonic jerks. Kilburn (1966) described anxiety and hyperactivity as early signs, which, if unheeded, could progress to confusion, disorientation, and ultimately coma. Recognizing and correcting the alkalosis is imperative if the condition is to be effectively treated. If the initial manifestations were mistaken for functional (neurotic) anxiety, inappropriate treatment would only further clinical deterioration.

Acute (Adult) Respiratory Distress Syndrome

The acute respiratory distress syndrome (ARDS), is a form of respiratory failure precipitated

> by an acute illness or injury which directly or indirectly affects the lung, including direct chest trauma, prolonged or profound shock, fat embolism, massive blood transfusion, cardiopulmonary bypass, oxygen toxicity, sepsis, acute hemorrhagic pancreatitis, aspiration or viral pneumonia, near-drowning, drug overdose, or inhaled irritants (Anonymous, 1977).

Since the survival rate with prompt treatment is 60–70% and without treatment only 10–20%, early diagnosis is quite important.

The syndrome tends to develop several days after the initiation of treatment for an injury or illness and may interrupt what appears to have been an uneventful recovery. Initial manifestations are not unique and include dyspnea, rapid and labored respiration, anxiety, apprehension, hypoxemia, and variable cyanosis. In the early phases, these findings, coupled with the setting in which they occur, may be suggestive of situational anxiety or of an evolving delirium. Consequently, the consulting psychiatrist may be called upon to assist with diagnosis and treatment, and it is important that he be aware of the possibility of ARDS.

HYPERVENTILATION (RESPIRATORY ALKALOSIS)

General Considerations

Hyperventilation has been defined as "ventilation in excess of that required to maintain normal arterial blood pO_2 and pCO_2" (Missri and Alexander, 1978). Under acute conditions an increase in rate and/or depth of respiration increases CO_2 loss leading to a fall in pCO_2 and a consequent increase in blood pH (acute respiratory alkalosis). If hyperventilation is maintained, compensatory changes occur which reduce plasma bicarbonate concentration (renal bicarbonate reabsorption decreases and bicarbonate may be transfered into the cells) and restore arterial blood pH to normal. Under conditions of chronic hyperventilation pCO_2 remains low, rendering the patient susceptible to symptoms from relatively small further reductions in CO_2.

Causes

While hyperventilation is often considered synonymous with "the hyperventilation syndrome," overbreathing may occur in association with a wide variety of conditions (Levinsky, 1977). These include:

Arterial hypoxemia

Arterial hypercapnia

Metabolic acidosis (e.g., diabetic ketoacidosis)
Muscular exercise
Fever

Hypermetabolism
Systemic hypotension

Drug poisoning (especially with salicylates)
Excessive mechanical ventilation
Cerebral disease
Pregnancy
Chronic hepatic insufficiency
Anxiety

Pathophysiology

By overbreathing, large quantities of CO_2 are blown off, producing hypocapnia. Abrupt reduction in arterial blood pCO_2 causes intense vasoconstriction of cerebral blood vessels and a decreased cerebral blood flow. In addition, the alkalosis produced causes a shift to the left of the oxyhemoglobin dissociation curve (Bohr effect), causing hemoglobin to bind oxygen more tightly, making it less available to the tissues. The combination of reduced cerebral blood flow and the Bohr effect may explain the CNS symptoms associated with hyperventilation.

Other physiologic changes occurring with hyperventilation include constriction of arterioles in the skin, intestines, and kidneys, increased coronary artery resistence, and a decrease in cardiac output and stroke volume. Serum levels of sodium, potassium, magnesium, and total calcium remain unchanged, while organic phosphate levels are reduced and ionized calcium levels may decrease (possibly accounting for the appearance of tetany) (Missri and Alexander, 1978; Waites, 1978).

Clinical Features

Because of factors such as severity and rate of onset, underlying illness, premorbid personality, and coexisting anxiety, the signs and symptoms associated with hyperventilation can be quite varied.

Despite one hour of hyperventilation, which lowered arterial blood pCO$_2$ to almost half normal and produced a rather severe respiratory alkalosis (pH = 7.58), normal volunteers experienced relatively few symptoms (Saltzman et al., 1963). Those that did appear included altered awareness, lightheadedness, a sensation of unreality, tingling and numbness of the hands, feet, and circumoral region, distal extremity cramps, and a feeling of abdominal warmth. Despite these symptoms and the appearance of Chvostek's sign and carpal spasm, none of the subjects complained of anxiety or apprehension.

The **hyperventilation syndrome** (sustained or recurrent episodes of hyperventilation with no apparent organic cause) is a common yet frequently unrecognized occurrence in medical and psychiatric practices. Rice (1950) found a 10.7% incidence in 1000 consecutive office patients; McKell and Sullivan (1947) noted that 5.8% of patients with gastrointestinal complaints had symptoms attributable to hyperventilation; and Tucker (1963) observed that hyperventilation was a clinical factor in symptom production in 60% of patients with a diagnosis of anxiety neurosis or anxiety hysteria.

The signs and symptoms that may be associated with the hyperventilation syndrome are many (Table 3-1). On rare occasions, hyperventilation has resulted in both visual and auditory hallucinations (Allen and Agus, 1968). Not well appreciated is the observation that *unilateral* neurovascular findings may result from hyperventilation (Tavel, 1964). For a more complete appreciation of the varied manifestations of the hyperventilation syndrome, the reader is referred to several reviews (Rice, 1950; Singer, 1958; Stead, 1960; Tucker, 1963; Lum, 1975).

TABLE 3-1.   Signs and Symptoms of Hyperventilation Syndrome[a]

General—Chronic and/or easy fatigability, general weakness with no specific muscle group involved, sleep disturbances, history of low-grade fever

Cardiovascular—atypical chest pains, tachycardia, palpitations, exaggerated sensation of heartbeat in the ears

Neurological—faintness, dizziness, impairment of concentration and memory, feeling of emptiness in head, sensation that the vision is defective although all of the visual field is clear, peripheral paresthesias

Gastrointestinal—Globus hystericus, aerophagia, belching, bloating and flatulence, mucosal dryness

Respiratory—inability to get a deep enough breath, tightness in or on the chest, excess yawning or sighing, nonproductive cough secondary to throat "tickle"

Musculoskeletal—Generalized tetany and carpopedal spasm with acute episodes; myalgias and arthralgias; generalized areas of spasm

Psychic—Variable anxiety, tension, and apprehension; reports of inability to slow down or relax; if hysterical, inappropriate pseudocalmness

[a] From Waites (1978) with permission. Copyright 1978, American Medical Association.

Diagnosis

Although hyperventilation is often clinically quite obvious, some patients, especially between episodes, may exhibit apparently normal breathing patterns. By definition, arterial blood pCO_2 will be reduced, and, depending on the chronicity of the condition, pH may be increased or normal and bicarbonate may be normal or decreased.

Diagnosing the hyperventilation syndrome is especially important, since the syndrome is often misdiagnosed and mistreated as "organic" disease of the neurologic, cardiovascular, respiratory, gastrointestinal, or endocrine systems. For example, the chest pain associated with hyperventilation must be distinguished from that of angina pectoris (Wheatley, 1975; Evans and Lum, 1977).

Once the syndrome is suspected, the diagnosis can be confirmed by the hyperventilation test. The patient is encouraged to breath deeply and rapidly for at least 90 seconds. A positive test occurs when the procedure reproduces the majority of signs and symptoms (since sufficient hyperventilation will produce some symptoms in anyone, it is important that a correlation be made between the patients' complaints and the symptoms produced by the test).

Treatment

Hyperventilation and respiratory alkalosis produced by organic causes are corrected by treating the underlying disorder.

Treatment of the hyperventilation syndrome begins with the supervised reproduction of the syndrome and explanation of its pathophysiology. Missri and Alexander (1978) suggest that a friend or relative be present during the test, as they find that patients need frequent reminding of the cause of the symptoms. An acute episode of hyperventilation may respond to reassurance, rebreathing of CO_2 (paper bag technique), slow breathing through the nose, or antianxiety medication. Over a longer term, physical therapy to modify breathing technique and psychotherapy or behavior therapy to treat underlying emotional difficulties may be of value (Missri and Alexander, 1978; Walker, 1978; Waites, 1978).

DYSPNEA

General Considerations

For the purpose of this discussion, the term "dyspnea" will be used to describe the sensation of difficult, labored, uncomfortable, or unpleasant breathing. In this sense it is a *subjective* term and should not be confused with the more objective descriptions of breathing abnormalities such as tachypnea (shallow, rapid breathing), hyperpnea (increased depth of respiration), and oligopnea (hypoventilation) (Olsen, 1963).

Causes

Because of its subjective nature, dyspnea, like pain, may be strongly influenced by emotional factors and it may be quite difficult at times to place the "organic" and "psychological" aspects in their proper perspective. Since appropriate treatment depends, to a large extent on accurate diagnosis, understanding and recognizing the many causes of dyspnea is quite important.

According to Fritts and Thomas (1974), a chief complaint of dyspnea is usually associated with one of the following:

1. Heart disease
2. Pulmonary emboli
3. Obstructive lung disease
4. Interstitial or alveolar lung disease
5. Disorders of the chest wall or respiratory muscles
6. Anxiety neurosis

Other conditions that may result in respiratory discomfort include fever, exercise, hyperthyroidism, systemic acidosis, carbon monoxide poisoning, cerebral disease, and acute hypotension. A more comprehensive listing of disorders associated with dyspnea is beyond the scope of this book.

Pathophysiology

Although much attention has been devoted to the topic of dyspnea, defining the disordered physiology responsible for the subjective state of breathlessness has been difficult. Various theories involve respiratory muscle fatigue, stimulation of stretch receptors in the lungs, and respiratory center–cortical relationships (Howell and Campbell, 1966).

Clinical Features

The type of respiration associated with the complaint of dyspnea may be of diagnostic value (Rabin, 1963). Rapid, shallow breathing is characteristic of diseases that increase lung rigidity or interfere with lung expansion by pleural or chest wall involvement. Pulmonary emboli may also present with this respiratory pattern.

Deep respirations may be found with obstructive disease such as asthma and emphysema, and with fever, toxic conditions, and metabolic disturbances that result in increased respiratory center stimulation.

So called "purse-string" respiration is characteristic of emphysema and involves expiring through puckered lips. By increasing expiratory pressure, narrowing and collapse of the smaller air passages is prevented and respiratory efficiency is improved.

Wheezing is characteristic of obstruction to air flow and may occur during inspiration, expiration, or both. Inspiratory wheezing or stridor occurs with partial obstruction of the larynx or trachea, while wheezing associated with bronchospasm, as in asthma, is predominantly expiratory.

Orthopnea, or difficult breathing when recumbent, is usually associated with heart disease, although it may also occur in the presence of severe pulmonary disease. Patients with advanced emphysema tend not only to prefer to be upright but often lean forward in order to facilitate breathing. Trepopnea refers to a condition in which breathing is more comfortable in a particular recumbent position, usually on one side or the other. It may occur in patients with tension pneumothorax, pleural effusion, or marked left atrial enlargement.

Respiratory distress secondary to psychogenic causes is often characterized by periodic deep sighing expiration. There tends not to be an association between exercise and increased distress, and the disturbance disappears during sleep. Other factors which would point to a psychogenic etiology include a clear association with emotional stress and a discrepancy between symptoms, physical signs, blood gases, and pulmonary function tests (Sparer and Davis, 1963).

When dealing with a dyspneic patient it is important to realize that the degree of distress is determined by a combination of physical and emotional factors. Emotionally overresponsive patients (sometimes pejoratively referred to as hysterical) are at an immediate disadvantage, since a serious, even life-threatening, disorder may be hidden by secondary signs and symptoms of anxiety. Treatment of the secondary anxiety without dealing with the underlying disorder can have grave consequences. For example, sedation of an agitated asthmatic patient may cause further respiratory decompensation and even death.

One must also avoid making unwarranted etiological assumptions based on coincidental rather than causal relationships. For example, a young military recruit was brought to the emergency room with symptoms of anxiety and hyperventilation that developed at the airport when he was returning to base after Christmas vacation. When first evaluated, he was diagnosed as having separation anxiety and was treated unsuccessfully with diazepam. A more detailed history revealed, however, that the soldier actually enjoyed the military and was looking forward to returning to camp. When a psychological explanation for his symptoms became less tenable, a more extensive medical evaluation was pursued, with the subsequent detection and treatment of a spontaneous pneumopericardium and pneumomediastinum.

ASTHMA

General Considerations

Asthma (bronchial asthma) is characterized by recurrent episodes of generalized airway obstruction caused by a combination of bronchospasm (contraction of bronchial muscle), mucosal edema, and intraluminal secretions. Between attacks, a person is likely to be symptom free and have normal or near normal pulmonary function tests.

Factors which may be associated with the precipitation of asthmatic attacks include: (1) allergy, (2) respiratory infection, (3) psychosocial stresses, (4) atmospheric pollution, and (5) exercise. Multiple factors may play a role in any particular case. Williams et al. (1958) reviewed 487 cases and found that single factor was present in only 15.5% (infection, 11%; allergy, 3.3%; psychological, 1.2%) while infection was involved to some extent in 88%, psychological factors in 70%, and allergy in 64%.

Pathophysiology

The airway obstruction in asthma is unevenly distributed throughout the lungs. Continued perfusion of poorly ventilated areas results in hypoxemia, with compensatory hyperventilation following early in the course of an episode. If the attack is severe, progressive airway obstruction coupled with muscle fatigue will not only aggravate the hypoxemia but will cause CO_2 retention and respiratory acidosis.

Clinical Features

The predominant manifestations of asthma are dyspnea and wheezing. Although wheezing is present in both inspiration and expiration, obstruction in the latter phase of respiration tends to be more severe. Crofton and Douglas (1975) emphasize this point by quoting an asthmatic as saying "that if he could once get the air out of his lungs he would take good care never to let it in again!"

If an attack is especially severe, however, wheezing may be markedly reduced or absent owing to a reduction in air flow from mucus plugging and fatigue. In the asthmatic with a "quiet chest," anxiety, agitation, and breathlessness may be mistakenly attributed to emotional factors. Such an error could be fatal if aggressive treatment of the obstruction is delayed and if respiration is further suppressed by the use of antianxiety medications. Determination of arterial blood gases will quickly allow the severity of the episode to be accurately assessed.

Other symptoms associated with an asthmatic attack include cough, fatigue, weakness, anxiety, and restlessness. Should respiratory failure intervene, CNS manifestations such as confusion, disorientation, and depressed consciousness are likely to occur.

Assessment

For the most part, the diagnosis of bronchial asthma is not difficult, given the accompanying constellation of signs and symptoms. Greater clinical acumen is needed, however, to place in proper perspective the neuropsychiatric aspects of the illness. A distinction must be made between emotional precipitants of an attack and the emotional response to an attack. Respiratory distress is universally anxiety provoking. Although the anxiety may further compound the breathing difficulty, treatment is generally best directed at relieving the bronchospasm and normalizing blood gas abnormalities. This, in turn, will almost certainly have a beneficial effect on the anxiety. In certain circumstances, the judicious use of a benzodiazepine anxiolytic is appropriate in conjunction with treatment of the bronchospasm.

PULMONARY EMBOLISM

General Considerations

Emboli to the lungs most often originate in the pelvic veins or deep veins of the legs while other sites of origin include the right heart chambers and upper extremity veins. Nonthrombotic emboli consisting of amniotic fluid, fat, air, or tumor are much less common.

Pulmonary embolization is a common event and is a major cause of morbidity and mortality. On routine autopsy, evidence of pulmonary embolus is found in 20–30% of all patients, and if special postmortem diagnostic techniques are utilized, the figure increases to 60% (Moser, 1974). With regard to premortem diagnosis, however, Horwitz (1975) states that pulmonary embolism "may be more common, more lethal, more satisfactorily treatable, and more frequently undiagnosed than any other disease."

Pathophysiology

The consequences of pulmonary embolism depend on the size and number of emboli as well as the patient's prior cardiorespiratory status. A large embolus can cause immediate death, while a small one may go unnoticed. The immediate effect of an embolus is to partially or completely obstruct a portion of arterial blood flow to the distal lung. This results in a portion of lung that is ventilated but not perfused resulting in "wasted ventilation." In addition, increased lung resistance, decreased compliance, loss of alveolar surfactant, and atelectasis are likely to occur. The arterial obstruction results in an increase in pulmonary vascular resistance leading to pulmonary hypertension, which, if of sufficient magnitude, will cause right ventricular failure and shock. Arterial blood gases may show hypoxemia (from right to left shunting) and hypocapnia (from hyperventilation), with an associated respiratory alkalosis.

Pulmonary infarct (death of lung tissue) is an infrequent (10%) consequence of pulmonary embolism. Apparently, an intact bronchial circulation provides enough collateral blood flow to protect the lung tissue when pulmonary artery flow is obstructed.

Clinical Features

A massive pulmonary embolus may result in sudden death or, if not fatal, will cause severe cardiorespiratory distress, chest pain, dyspnea, cyanosis, tachycardia, sweating, and collapse. While the diagnosis may not be straightforward, it is unlikely that this clinical presentation will be confused with that of a functional illness.

If the embolization is less severe, however, establishing a diagnosis may be quite difficult. Breathlessness may be the only symptom; consequently, sudden unexplained dyspnea should always suggest the possibility of pulmonary embolus. The breathlessness associated with pulmonary embolism tends to be characterized by rapid, shallow respiration, as contrasted to the deep, sighing respiration often seen in the hyperventilation syndrome. Other associated and nonspecific findings may include anxiety, apprehension, restlessness, and tachypnea. Such a constellation, of course, brings to mind conditions such as anxiety neurosis, panic attacks, hyperventilation syndrome, and hysterical overbreathing. A diagnosis of functional illness may be further supported by a paucity of abnormal findings on physical examination. Other confusing presentations may include syncope, seizures, and neurological deficits, which are suggestive of a primary neurological disorder but are actually due to reduce cardiac output and secondary cerebral ischemia.

Diagnosis

In view of such varied and deceptive presentations, the diagnosis of pulmonary embolus often requires a high index of suspicion coupled with the appropriate ultilization of laboratory tests such as chest x-ray, electrocardiogram, serum enzymes and bilirubin, arterial blood gases, lung scan, and pulmonary angiography. Since pulmonary embolism is a disorder which is potentially lethal yet at the same time amenable to treatment, prompt and accurate diagnosis is imperative.

Fat Embolism

Fat emboli occur in association with long bone fractures and other types of tissue trauma. It is unclear whether they form from disruption of fat-containing extravascular tissues and are released into the circulation or whether they are formed within the vessels from physiochemical alteration of circulating lipids. The end result is obstruction of pulmonary and systemic vasculature. Fat emboli cause pulmonary symptoms similar to those found with thromboemboli, but, in addition, cause systemic vascular obstruction and may produce petechial skin hemorrhage, deposit in retinal vessels, and occlude cerebral blood vessels. Central nervous system manifestations include altered levels of consciousness, restlessness, confusion, disorientation, seizures, and delirium. The psychiatrist is often called upon to evaluate and treat an acute brain syndrome (delirium) in a critically ill patient, and fat embolism should be part of the differential diagnosis. A definitive diagnosis can usually be made given a characteristic clinical course and chest x-ray, and finding fat globules in the blood and urine (Evarts, 1970).

HICCUP

General Considerations

Almost everyone has experienced hiccup. An episode is usually brief and, if it does not resolve spontaneously, can be terminated by any number of simple maneuvers such as breath holding, rapid swallowing, or a sudden loud noise. Rarely, episodes may be more refractory and can lead to complications such as insomnia, weight loss, fatigue, exhaustion, dehydration, severe mental stress, and death (Souadjian and Cain, 1968). In the postoperative patient, hiccup can cause wound dehiscence. Some episodes have lasted weeks, months, and even years.

Pathophysiology

When hiccup was studied with electromyography (EMG) and air flow measurements, the following was found:

> Each hiccup consisted of one or several discrete bursts of activity in inspiratory muscles occurring synchronously in diaphragm and external (inspiratory) intercostal muscles. It is associated with a coincident inhibition of expiratory intercostal muscle activity. Glottal closure occurs about 35 msec after the onset of the diaphragmatic discharge and persists until this discharge has virtually ceased, so that the direct ventilatory effect of the hiccup is negligible (Davis, 1970).

If glottal closure is bypassed, as it would be with a tracheostomy, hiccup can cause marked hyperventilation, as was demonstrated in a patient who developed an arterial blood pH of 7.58 and a minute ventilation of over 20 liters (Davis, 1970).

Fluoroscopic examinations of people during episodes of hiccup have shown that the entire diaphragm, one hemidiaphragm, or parts of a hemidiaphragm may be involved and that each contraction may be single or may involve several spasms in quick succession (Samuels, 1952).

The neural pathways involved in hiccup have not been fully elaborated. Afferent pathways are felt to include the vagus and phrenic nerves and the sympathetic chain from T_{6-12}. The main efferent pathway is the phrenic nerve but also involved are efferents to the glottis and other respiratory muscles. In addition, there appears to be a central neural mechanism for hiccup distinct from the respiratory center with an interaction between respiratory rhythm and hiccup discharge occurring at the spinal level (Salem et al., 1967; Davis, 1970).

Etiology

It is felt that there are many causes of hiccup (Table 3-2). A clear cause and effect relationship has not been demonstrated for many of these disorders, and it seems likely that in some of these conditions the association with hiccup has only been coincidental (and this seems equally true for both "organic" and "functional" etiologies). Rather than presuming etiology, the approach of Souadjian and Cain (1968) in listing "diseases seen in patients with hiccup" seems preferable. It is certainly true that for every patient with

TABLE 3-2.   Possible Causes of Hiccup[a]

Central causes	—Toxic conditions such as uremia, gout, and malaria
	—Organic lesions such as meningitis, encephalitis, syphilis, and brain and spinal cord tumors
	—Psychogenic causes
	—Traumatic conditions such as skull fracture and brain injury
Peripheral causes	—Swallowing irritant substances such as hot or cold food or drink
	—Gastrointestinal disorders such as esophagospasm, gastritis, gastric dilatation, intestinal obstruction, ileus, subphrenic abscess, pancreatitis, peritonitis, enteritis, diaphragmatic or hiatal hernia, hepatitis, metastatic cancer, gall bladder disease, and ulcer
	—Thoracic disorders such as pneumonia, pleurisy, mediastinal and lung tumors, and coronary occlusion
	—Neck disorders such as tumor, branchial cyst, diverticulum, and scalenus antecus syndrome
Surgical and anesthetic causes	—Inadequate ventilation, anesthetic drugs, weaning from anesthesia, traction in abdominal and thoracic viscera, and traction on phrenic or sciatic nerves

[a] Adapted from Samuels (1952) and Salem et al. (1967).

one of these disorders and hiccup, there are hundreds or thousands with the disorder who do not have hiccup.

In the past, the diagnosis of psychogenic hiccup has often been made in the absence of any credible substantiation. Samuels (1952), for example, stated that the majority of cases of prolonged hiccup are psychogenic, and within this classification he included malingerers, publicity seekers, postpartum women, borderline mental cases, and patients with conditions such as mental shock, prolonged nervous strain, cardiospasm, and pylorospasm. He listed two main psychogenic classes as "(1) Nervous debilitated persons who have received a recent acute mental shock . . . and (2) patients of neurotic tendencies who have long complained of minor stomach or other digestive disturbances, for which no organic basis has been found." His example of a man who began to hiccup two weeks after receiving a sterile semen report hardly establishes causality.

Souadjian and Cain (1968), in a report of 220 cases of intractable hiccup, stated that 92% of women (31/39) and 7% of men (12/181) had a diagnosis of psychogenic hiccup, but no supporting data were presented. One is faced with the statement that these patients "had enough psychiatric manifestations to warrant a diagnosis of psychogenic hiccup" which was apparently based on associated psychiatric diagnoses of addiction, conversion hysteria, grief reaction, anorexia nervosa, mental deficiency, anxiety, psychoneurosis, enuresis, and malingering.

Theohar and McKegney (1970) reviewed the literature on psychogenic hiccup and presented a case of two weeks duration which was cured by hypnosis. They felt that the hiccups were "best characterized as a conversion reaction, respresenting repressed hostility and guilt over sexual conflicts in the patient and her family constellation" but they were unable to explain why hiccup was the "chosen symptom."

The literature does not provide firm support from the existence of a well-defined entity known as "psychogenic hiccup." It appears that this diagnosis is usually arrived at by a process of elimination; i.e., if an organic etiology is not apparent, the cause must be functional. It would seem more reasonable to apply the honest, unbiased diagnosis of "hiccup of unknown etiology" to such cases if a more specific diagnosis cannot be substantiated. It is possible that secondary gains can become associated with prolonged or intractable hiccup just as with any other illness, but such secondary psychiatric consequences should not be confused with underlying etiology. In addition, there is the danger that "secondary gains" exist more in the mind of the clinician as a way of explaining a confusing situation than in reality. It is often gratifying to discover how rapidly a patient will give up such "secondary gains" once the underlying disorder is corrected.

Treatment

The usual episode of hiccup does not require medical attention. It will either remit spontaneously or respond to one of a variety of "folk remedies" which include swallowing bread or crushed ice, breath holding, hyperventilation, expiration against a closed glottis, a sudden stimulation such as a loud noise, or rapid drinking of water (at least 10 consecutive swallows).

By definition, prolonged or intractable hiccup does not respond to conventional measures and causes the patient to seek medical assistance. Ideally, evaluation should be directed toward defining the underlying etiology so that treatment can be specifically directed to eliminating the cause. In those situations in which etiology remains unknown or is known but cannot be eliminated, treatment must be directed at the hiccup itself. In such situations a wide variety of measures have been employed with varied degrees of success (Samuels, 1952; Salem et al., 1967). These include:

Carotid massage
Eyeball pressure (not recommended)
Carbon dioxide inhalation
Drugs such as short-acting muscle
    relaxants, amyl nitrite, ether inhalation, intravenous atropine, barbiturates, narcotics, chlorpromazine, methamphetamines, quinidine, procaine, edrophonium, phenytoin, diazepam
Anesthesia
Pharyngeal stimulation
Blockade of the vagus nerve in the neck or beneath the diaphragm

Paravertebral block of the C_{3-5} nerves or epidural block below C_5
Crushing or interruption of one or both phrenic nerves
Hypnosis

Salem et al. (1967) found that pharyngeal stimulation with a nasal catheter immediately inhibited hiccup in 84 of 85 patients. The duration of hiccup in these cases ranged from 1 hour to 5 days. This benign and easily performed intervention should be one of the first considered in an obstinate case of hiccup.

Very little has been written about treating hiccups by psychiatric techniques, and the lack of a reliable approach further detracts from defining psychogenic hiccup as a specific diagnostic entity. In a review of the literature, Theohar and McKegney (1970) found four cases (including their own) of hiccups that were successfully treated by hypnosis. This treatment approach should be considered in all cases of prolonged hiccup without preselecting patients on the basis of presumed organic or functional etiology.

DIAPHRAGMATIC FLUTTER (RESPIRATORY MYOCLONUS, LEEUWENHOEK DISEASE)

General Considerations

Unlike the familiar hiccup, the entity known as diaphragmatic flutter is relatively unknown and often misdiagnosed. Initial erroneous diagnoses have included angina pectoris; myocardial infarction; pericarditis; arrhythmias such as atrial fibrillation, ventricular tachycardia, and paroxsysmal supraventricular tachycardia; abdominal aortic aneurysm; and psychogenic causes such as conversion reaction, hyperventilation syndrome, and hysterical disorder of breathing. In one particular case the psychiatric consultant diagnosed "chronic anxiety reaction" and advised 50 insulin subshock treatments and chlordiazepoxide (Graber and Sinclair-Smith, 1965). Diaphragmatic flutter was first described in 1723 by Anton van Leeuwenhoek, the father of microscopy, who diagnosed the disorder in himself.

In this disorder, there are paroxysms of irregular diaphragmatic contractions (at a rate ranging from 35–480 contractions per minute) superimposed upon normal diaphragmatic movement (Rigatto and DeMedeiros, 1962). Generally, both hemidiaphragms are involved, although unilateral involvement is not rare. The paroxysms of flutter usually last seconds or minutes, yet can continue for days, weeks, or months. There is also a wide variation in the interval between episodes.

Electromyographic (EMG) studies of one patient showed "intermittent bursts of EMG activity interposed with frequent total interruption of activity." These findings were present in all respiratory muscles tested (scalene and intercostal), and the authors felt that the condition was a form of myoclonus (Phillips and Eldridge, 1973).

Clinical Features

The clinical presentation of diaphragmatic flutter may include respiratory distress, muscular fatigue or pain in the epigastrium or lower chest, or a jumping, jerking, or quivering in the upper abdomen. One patient described being awakened at night with clonic jerking of the abdomen (Graber and Sinclair-Smith, 1965), and another mentioned an upper abdominal sensation "like a balloon inflating and deflating" and felt that between episodes his breathing was "out of rhythm" (Phillips and Eldridge, 1973). Usually the respiratory rate is unaltered in the presence of diaphragmatic flutter, although tachypnea may be present.

On physical examination, there may be visible pulsations in the lower intercostal spaces or over the upper abdomen that are not synchronous with the heart beat. A variety of auscultatory findings have been reported, some of which are clearly different from the heart beat in terms of rhythm, loudness, and location, while others may be mistaken for atrial fibrillation or a pericardial rub. In some cases, a splashing sound was heard over the epigastrium, which was felt to be caused by shaking of the stomach contents.

The electrocardiogram tends to be normal although ST segment and T wave changes have been reported during paroxysms. The fluttering of the adjacent diaphragm can also produce a confusing electrocardiographic artifact.

Diagnosis

Diagnosis is best established by fluoroscopy done during an episode. EMG studies of the respiratory muscles are also of value.

Etiology

Causes of diaphragmatic flutter may be either central or peripheral. Phillips and Eldridge (1973) feel that the disorder is caused by an abnormality of the central neural respiratory system, and a number of cases have occurred in close association with viral encephalitis. Further causes include irritation of the phrenic nerve from a variety of sources or direct irritation of the diaphragmatic muscle. Although a clear-cut etiology may not be apparent, there is no evidence to support a "functional" etiology for this disorder. To assume so would be a disservice to the patient. Phillips and Eldridge (1973) note that:

> This disorder has been an example of how a lack of understanding of the cause and pathophysiology of a condition has been used as license to label it as psychogenic. This stigma usually leads to delayed effective evaluation and misguided handling of the patients.

Treatment

Since there have been less than 50 cases of diaphragmatic flutter reported and since presumed etiologies have been many, there is no standardized treatment protocol. At times it may be possible to direct specific corrective surgical or medical treatment at a specific etiology. A more drastic approach, which does not address etiology, involves blockade or surgical interruption of the phrenic nerve. Finally, a variety of drug treatments have been directed at suppressing the flutter. These have included quinidine, cortisone, sedatives, carbon dioxide, and phenytoin. In one patient, the response to phenytoin was quite definitive, with the disorder recurring each of three times that the drug was discontinued (Phillips and Eldridge, 1973).

PSYCHOTROPIC DRUGS AND RESPIRATORY DISORDERS

The respiratory effects and toxicity of psychotropic drugs is a subject which has received little attention. Most clinicians follow the rule that drugs with sedative activity are likely to have adverse effects on previously compromised respiratory function. For the most part, this is a reliable guideline. To assume, however, that these drugs are absolutely contraindicated in such patients may actually deprive them of an appropriate and relatively safe treatment. For readers wishing a more complete overview of the area, the review by Steen (1976) is recommended.

Antipsychotic Drugs

Unexplained sudden death is a rare occurrence in patients receiving antipsychotic drugs. Although it is generally held that these deaths are due to drug-induced cardiac arrhythmias or hypotensive episodes, asphyxia due to respiratory depression has been offered as an alternative explanation. There has been little firm support for this hypothesis, although asphyxia may occur indirectly consequent to aspiration during a drug-induced seizure. We recently saw a patient who, during the course of rapid tranquilization with haloperidol, developed cardiorespiratory arrest that was initiated by marked respiratory depression *followed* by a severe cardiac arrhythmia. Hypoxia from respiratory depression appeared to be the initiating factor.

Although uncommon, the extrapyramidal reactions to antipsychotic drugs may result in disordered respiration. Ayd (1979) described respiratory dyskinesias associated with early onset extrapyramidal reactions as consisting of "(1) episodes of respiratory spasms or tics associated with grunting, snorting, or puffing; (2) disturbed respiratory rate and depth; and (3) disturbed respiratory rhythm." Patients with these symptoms were also restless and hyperkinetic and responded well to either dose reduction or addition of an antiparkinson drug. When respiratory dysfunction was associated with tardive dyskinesia, it consisted of "primarily irregular respiration, usually dyspnea, along with orofacial, limb, and truncal dyskinetic movements."

Weiner et al. (1978) reported four patients with acute dyspnea and chest pain in the absence of cardiac or pulmonary disorders which were part of a more generalized choreiform movement disorder. Three patients had antipsychotic drug-induced tardive dyskinesia and one had levodopa-induced dyskinesia.

Finally, Casey and Rabins (1978) described a patient with orofacial dyskinesia and irregular respirations who developed "potentially life-threatening ventilatory and gastrointestinal disturbances" following antipsychotic drug discontinuation which required treatment with haloperidol to restore a normal breathing pattern and blood gases.

It has been suggested that antipsychotic drug-induced respiratory dyskinesias are far more common than heretofore recognized and that with accurate diagnosis these conditions will often be responsive to appropriate therapeutic intervention.

The effect of antipsychotic drugs (especially those in common use in the United States) in patients with impaired respiratory function has not been well studied. Tandon (1976) examined the effects on respiration of single intramuscular doses of diazepam (10 mg), chlorpromazine (50 mg), and haloperidol (5 mg) in patients with severe chronic obstructive lung disease. Significant respiratory depression occurred in five of ten patients given diazepam and three of eight patients given chlorpromazine while no respiratory depression was noted in any of the ten patients given haloperidol.

Keeping in mind the limitation of a single dose study, it nonetheless seems reasonable to recommend the use of one of the relatively nonsedating, high milligram potency drugs (haloperidol, thiothixene, fluphenazine, etc.) when antipsychotic treatment is needed in a patient with compromised respiratory function.

There are several reports (Steen, 1976) suggesting that phenothiazines may prolong the respiratory depressant effect of narcotic analgesics and, consequently, these drugs should be combined with caution, especially in patients with pulmonary disease.

Antidepressants—Tricyclics

Several reports (summarized in Steen, 1976) have shown that there are beneficial effects of imipramine and amitriptyline on the clinical course of asthma. Meares et al. (1971) found, in a series of 12 asthmatics, a significant increase in forced expiratory volume in one second (FEV_1) following an intramuscular injection of 25 mg of amitriptyline. They also found in guinea pigs that the bronchoconstrictor effect of histamine, 5-hydroxytryptamine, and acetylcholine was counteracted by amitriptyline. They felt that the beneficial effect of amitriptyline on the course of asthma was not due to its antidepressant activity, but rather to its effect on bronchoconstrictor substances. These studies are of sufficient promise to warrant better controlled and larger scale investigations, but these have not, as yet, been done.

There do not appear to be studies, single dose or long term, on the effect of tricyclics on respiration in patients with severe lung disease. Given the availability of a number of tricyclics, it would seem reasonable to avoid using the more sedating (amitriptyline, doxepin) in favor of the less sedating (desipramine, protriptyline) in patients with compromised respiratory function. Even in patients with normal pulmonary function, an overdose of any tricyclic antidepressant can produce severe respiratory depression.

Antidepressants—Monoamine Oxidase Inhibitors

In a placebo controlled study of patients with bronchial asthma, Mathov (1963) found that 37% of patients tested became worse while taking a monoamine oxidase inhibitor. The drugs tested included both phenelzine and nialamide. Based on this single report, monoamine oxidase inhibitors should be used with caution, if at all, in patients with asthma.

Antianxiety Drugs

Barbiturates

In general, these drugs are potent respiratory depressants affecting both respiratory drive and rhythm. The extent of depression depends both on dose and predrug respiratory status. Given the ready availability and relative safety of the benzodiazepines, the barbiturates are approaching obsolesence as antianxiety–sedative–hypnotics and their use is not advised, especially in patients with already compromised respiratory function.

Benzodiazepines

Conflicting reports of the effect of these drugs on respiration appear to be the result of patient selection, choice of drug, dose, rate and duration of administration, and length of study (Steen, 1976). In short, the benzodiazepines must be considered potential respiratory depressants, yet, even in the presence of severe lung disease, they may be used with relative safety and therapeutic benefit. The following two studies attest to the difficulty in reaching uniform treatment recommendations: Model and Berry (1974), in a randomized, double-blind placebo controlled crossover study of seven patients with respiratory failure due to chronic bronchitis, found that chlordiazepoxide (10 mg t.i.d. for three days) caused a significant increase in

pCO_2 and a significant fall in FEV_1. They suggested that the use of chlordiazepoxide is contraindicated in such a patient population.

On the other hand, Kronenberg et al. (1975) gave diazepam (10 mg q.i.d. for five days) to six patients with severe but stable chronic obstructive lung disease, CO_2 retention and hypoxia and found no significant change in arterial blood gases or FEV_1. Most of their patients also reported reduced anxiety while on the drug.

Rather than impose an absolute contraindication to the use of benzodiazepines in patients with severe lung disease, it seems reasonable that each patient with severe lung disease be assessed on an individual basis, and that treatment be initiated with a conservative dose of drug, which would then be adjusted according to clinical response and tests of pulmonary function.

Despite several reports of respiratory arrest following intravenous diazepam (Steen, 1976), the drug has been given extensively by this route with a very low overall incidence of adverse reactions. Factors involved in the respiratory arrests may have included hypersensitivity, reaction to solvent vehicle, and rapid rate of administration.

Lithium

There is no evidence to suggest that lithium is a respiratory depressant. Aminophylline does increase lithium clearance and it is conceivable, though not established, that a patient taking aminophylline would require more lithium to reach a desired serum level. On the other hand, there have been anecdotal reports of respiratory improvement in asthmatic patients receiving lithium for other indications (Nasr and Atkins, 1977; Putnam, 1978). Finally, reports (summarized in Jefferson and Greist, 1977) have shown that lithium prolongs the duration of action of certain neuromuscular blocking agents (including pancuronium and succinylcholine) in both animal and man.

NEUROPSYCHIATRIC EFFECTS OF RESPIRATORY DRUGS

Beta-Adrenergic Stimulants—Isoproterenol, Ephedrine, Metaproterenol, Terbutaline, and Salbutamol

Nervousness, tremor, and palpitations are common side effects of these drugs. Toxic psychoses which resemble amphetamine psychoses have been reported with ephedrine (Kane and Florenzano, 1971; Roxanas and Spalding, 1977), and an atypical psychosis with salbutamol (Gluckman, 1974). A preliminary report (Simon et al., 1979) suggests that salbutamol, a selective beta-2 receptor stimulant, may have antidepressant activity.

Xanthine Bronchodilators—Theophylline, Aminophylline

Central nervous system symptoms of lightheadedness, nervousness, insomnia, agitation, dizziness, headache, and seizures can occur with these drugs. Aminophylline has been shown to cause a decrease in renal blood flow and may play a role in the toxic psychosis often seen in patients being treated for respiratory failure (Faden, 1976).

Cromolyn—Disodium Cromoglycate

This drug appears to cause little central nervous system toxicity.

Steroids

The neuropsychiatric side effects of steroids are many. These are discussed elsewhere.

REFERENCES

Allen TE, Agus B: Hyperventilation leading to hallucinations. *Am J Psychiatry* 125:632–637, 1968.

Anonymous: Acute respiratory distress syndrome, in Berkow R (ed): *The Merck Manual*, ed 13. Rahway, Merck & Co., 1977, pp 571–573.

Ayd FJ: Respiratory dyskinesias in patients with neuroleptic-induced extrapyramidal reactions. In *Drug Ther Newsl* 14:1–3, 1979.

Casey DE, Rabins P: Tardive dyskinesia as a life-threatening illness. *Am J Psychiatry* 135:486–488, 1978.

Crofton J, Douglas A: *Respiratory Diseases*, ed 2. Oxford, Blackwell Scientific, 1975, p 439.

Davis JN: An experimenal study of hiccup. *Brain* 93:851–872, 1970.

Evans DW, Lum LC: Hyperventilation: An important cause of pseudoangina. *Lancet* 1:155–157, 1977.

Evarts CM: Fat embolism syndrome. *Am Fam Physician/GP* 1:78–86, 1970.

Faden A: Encephalopathy following treatment of chronic pulmonary failure. *Neurology* 26:337–339, 1976.

Fritts HW, Thomas HM: Dyspnea, in Wintrobe MM, Thorn GW, Adams RD, et al (eds): *Harrison's Principle of Internal Medicine*, ed 7. New York, McGraw–Hill, 1974, pp 166–170.

Gluckman L: Ventolin psychosis. *N Z Med J* 80:411, 1974.

Graber AL, Sinclair-Smith BC: Paroxysmal flutter of the diaphragm, a report of five cases. *Am J Cardiol* 15:252–258, 1965.

Gross NJ, Hamilton JD: Correlation between the physical signs of hypercapnia and the mixed venous pCO_2. *Br Med J* 4:1096–1097, 1963.

Horwitz O: Venous thrombosis—pulmonary embolus complex, in Horwitz O, Magee HJ (eds): *Index of Suspicion in Treatable Disease*. Philadelphia, Lea & Febiger, 1975, pp 494–500.

Howell FBL, Campbell EJM (eds): *Breathlessness*. Oxford, Blackwell Scientific, 1966.

Jefferson JW, Greist JH: *Primer of Lithium Therapy*. Baltimore, Williams and Wilkins, 1977, p 115.

Kane FJ, Florenzano R: Psychosis accompanying use of bronchodilator compound. *JAMA* 215:2116, 1971.

Kilburn KH: Neurologic manifestations of respiratory failure. *Arch Int Med* 116:409–415, 1965.

Kilburn KH: Shock, seizures, and coma with alkalosis during mechanical ventilation. *Ann Int Med* 65:977–984, 1966.

Kronenberg RS, Cosio MG, Stevenson JE, et al: The use of oral diazepam in patients with obstructive lung disease and hypercapnia. *Ann Int Med* 83:83–84, 1975.

Levinsky NG: *Acidosis and alkalosis*, in Thorn GW, Adams RD, Braunwald E, et al (eds): *Harrison's Principles of Internal Medicine*, ed 8. New York, McGraw–Hill, 1977, pp 375–382.

Lum LC: Hyperventilation: The tip and the iceberg. *J Psychosom Res* 19:375–383, 1975.

McKell TE, Sullivan AJ: Hyperventilation syndrome in gastroenterology. *Gastroenterology* 9:6–16, 1947.

Mathov E: The risks of monoamine oxidase inhibitors in the treatment of bronchial asthma. *J Allergy* 34:483–488, 1963.

Meares RA, Mills JE, Horvath TB: Amitriptyline and asthma. *Med J Aust* 2:25–28, 1971.

Missri JC, Alexander S: Hyperventilation syndrome, a brief review. *JAMA* 240:2093–2096, 1978.

Model DG and Berry DJ: Effects of chlordiazepoxide in respiratory failure due to chronic bronchitis. *Lancet* 2:869, 1974.

Moser KM: Pulmonary thromboembolism, in Wintrobe MM, Thorn GW, Adams RD, et al (eds): *Harrison's Principles of Internal Medicine*, ed 7. New York, McGraw–Hill, 1974, 1974, pp 1303–1307.

Moser KM: Management of acute respiratory failure, in Wintrobe MM, Thorn GW, Adams RD, et al (eds): *Harrison's Principles of Internal Medicine*, New York, McGraw–Hill, 1974, pp 1338–1343.

Nasr SJ, Atkins RW: Coincidental improvement in asthma during lithium treatment. *Am J Psychiatry* 134:1042–1043, 1977.

Olsen AM: What is dyspnea?, in Banyai L, Levine Er (eds): *Dyspnea: Diagnosis and Treatment.* Philadelphia, FA Davis, 1963, pp 2–5.

Phillips JR, Eldridge FL: Respiratory myoclonus (Leeuwenhoek's disease). *N Eng J Med* 289:1390–1395, 1973.

Putnam PL: Possible positive "side effects" of lithium. *Am J Psychiatry* 135:388, 1978.

Rabin CB: Diagnosis of conditions causing dyspnea, in Banyai AL, Levine ER (eds): *Dyspnea: Diagnosis and Treatment.* Philadelphia, FA Davis, 1963, pp 17–25.

Rice RL: Symptom patterns of the hyperventilation syndrome. *Am J Med* 8:691–700, 1950.

Rigatto M, DeMedeiros NP: Diaphragmatic flutter, report of a case and review of literature. *Am J Med* 32:103–109, 1962.

Rotheram EB, Safar P, Robin ED: CNS disorder during mechanical ventilation in chronic pulmonary disease. *JAMA* 189:993–996, 1964.

Roxanas MG, Spalding J: Ephedrine abuse psychosis. *Med J Aust* 2:639–640, 1977.

Salem MR, Baraka A, Rattenborg CC, et al: Treatment of hiccups by pharyngeal stimulation in anesthetized and conscious subjects. *JAMA* 202:126–130, 1967.

Saltzman HA, Heyman A, Sieker HO: Correlation of clinical and physiologic manifestations of sustained hyperventilation. *N Eng J Med* 268:1431–1436, 1963.

Samuels L: Hiccup, a ten year review of anatomy, etiology, and treatment. *Can Med Assoc J* 67: 315–322, 1952.

Sieker HO, Hickam JB: Carbon dioxide intoxication: The clinical syndrome, its etiology and management with particular reference to the use of mechanical respirators. *Medicine* 35:389–423, 1956.

Simon P, Lecrubier Y, Binouk F, et al: A report from France. *Psychopharmacol Bull* 15:1–2, 1979.

Singer EP: The hyperventilation syndrome of clinical medicine. *N Y State J Med* 58:1494–1500, 1958.

Souadjian JV, Cain JC: Intractable hiccup, etiologic factors in 220 cases. *Postgrad Med* 43:72–77, 1968.

Sparer PJ, Davis HL: Psychogenic dyspnea, in Banyai AL, Levine ER (eds): *Dyspnea: Diagnosis and Treatment*. Philadelphia, F. A. Davis, 1963, pp 334–348.

Stead EA: Hyperventilation. *Disease-a-Month*. Chicago, Year Book Publishers, February, 1960, pp 5–31.

Steen SN: The effects of psychotropic drugs on respiration. *Pharmacol Ther Bull* 2:717–741, 1976.

Tandon MK: Effect of respiration of diazepam, chloropromazine and haloperidol in patients with chronic airways obstruction. *Aust N Z J Med* 6:561–565, 1976.

Tavel ME: Hyperventilation syndrome with unilateral somatic symptoms. *JAMA* 187:147–149, 1964.

Theohar C, McKegney FP: Hiccups of psychogenic origin: A case report and review of the literature. *Comp Psychiatry* 11:377–384, 1970.

Tucker WI: Hyperventilation in differential diagnosis. *Med Clin North Am* 47:491–497, 1963.

Waites TF: Hyperventilation—chronic and acute. *Arch Int Med* 138:1700–1701, 1978.

Walker HE: How to manage the hyperventilation syndrome. *Behav Med* 5:30–37, 1978.

Weiner WJ, Goetz CG, Nausieda PA, et al: Respiratory dyskinesias: Extrapyramidal dysfunction and dyspnea. *Ann Int Med* 88:327–331, 1978.

West JB: Disorders of regulation of respiration, in Wintrobe MM, Thorn GW, Adams RD, et al (eds): *Harrison's Principles of Internal Medicine*, ed 7. New York, McGraw–Hill, 1974, pp 1298–1302.

Westlake EK, Simpson T, Kaye M: Carbon dioxide narcosis in emphysema. *Quart J Med* 24:155–173, 1955.

Wheatley CE: Hyperventilation syndrome: A frequent cause of chest pain. *Chest* 68:195–199, 1975.

Williams DA, Lewis-Faning E, Rees L, et al: Assessment of the relative importance of the allergic, infective and psychological factors in asthma. *Acta Allergol* 12:376–395, 1958.

Renal Disorders

RENAL FAILURE

The multiple causes of renal disease result in a plethora of early signs and symptoms. If the illness progresses, the final common clinical picture is renal failure. A basic understanding of this syndrome is important for an appreciation of neuropsychiatric disturbances associated with renal disorders.

Renal failure is defined as the reduction in function to a point at which the kidneys are no longer able to maintain chemical homeostasis in the organism. An accepted definition is that level at which reduction of function is severe enough to cause a 24 hr urine volume of less than 400 ml and/or a 24-hour endogenous creatinine clearance of less than 5 ml/min. (The normal range is approximately 85–140 ml/min.)

Failure may occur acutely in hours or days or chronically over a periods of weeks to months. Typical causes of failure with acute tubular necrosis include sudden injury or illness associated with shock or intense renal vasoconstriction. Common are crushing injuries, transfusion reactions, bacteremic shock, burns, heat stroke, and surgical or obstetrical conditions resulting in vascular collapse or renal ischemia. Tubular necrosis and resulting failure may also follow ingestion, absorption, or inhalation of a large number of chemical or biologic products that are toxic to the kidney. Though most of these conditions are medically or surgically related, acute renal failure may also occur in patients with excessive sweating, vomiting, malnutrition, and general dehydration secondary to psychiatric disorders.

The early period is characterized initially by oliguria, a marked decrease in urine output (50–400 ml/24 hr) followed by increasing clinical and chemical evidence of renal failure. During the first stage of oliguria, the clinical picture is dominated by the underlying illness. If the condition is not soon recognized, edema and/or hyponatremia may result from the unrestricted intake of fluids. Prominent early signs and symptoms are secondary to the hyperkalemia and pulmonary edema. Following this initial period, if the critical point of tubular damage has not been exceeded and if proper treatment has been instituted, diuresis will occur. Water and metabolites which have accumulated during the oliguric phase are excreted and the patient begins to recover.

Uremia

When the diuretic phase is delayed or does not occur, the clinical picture becomes the uremic syndrome. It is at this point that mental status changes become prominent. Uremia is essentially a symptom-complex or syndrome accompanying an accumulation in the body fluids of the end products of metabolism through accelerated catabolism and/or decreased excretion. Its chief biochemical sign is an extreme degree of azotemia, an elevated concentration of serum nonprotein nitrogen. (Normal blood urea nitrogen is 10–20 mg/100 ml.) Azotemia and the uremic syndrome are not synonymous. Nonprotein nitrogen concentration is only a brief way to describe renal dysfunction, and urea is quantitatively the largest component of the nonprotein nitrogen which accumulates in azotemia.

It is still unclear which of the end products of metabolism accumulating in body fluids are responsible for neuropsychiatric changes. Urea alone does not appear to be causal, since patients may be dialyzed against a bath containing a urea concentration equal to their blood level and still demonstrate marked clinical improvement (Merrill et al., 1953). Urea has also been administered intravenously in large amounts without obvious toxic effects (Javid and Settlage, 1956).

There are many theories. As in most forms of metabolic encephalopathy, there is a decrease in cerebral oxygen consumption, and this may cause an increased vulnerability of the brain to uremic toxins (Scheinberg, 1954; Heyman et al., 1951). Some workers have suggested that a deficiency status exists or that abnormally widespread or excessive effects from hormones or other substances produce adaptational responses to the bodily changes of renal dysfunction (examples include increased production of parathyroid hormone, natriuretic hormone, or sodium transport inhibitor) (Bricker, 1972; Avram et al., 1978). The nervous system might well be a vulnerable target for such effects. Present evidence speaks for a dialyzable, probably endogenous, neurotoxin as the most likely cause (Massey and Sellers, 1976).

Clinical Features

The clinical picture of uremia is highly variable because it is influenced by so many factors, including the age and nutritional state of the patient, the underlying disease, the presence or absence of hypertensive vascular disease, the rate of development of renal failure, and the particular combination of biochemical disorders associated with the azotemia. The symptomatic responses to a given degree of renal failure also have wide individual differences. Signs and symptoms occur in multiple systems. Cardiovascular manifestations include peripheral edema, pulmonary edema, heart failure, pericarditis, and hypertension. Gastrointestinal disturbances include mouth ulcers, anorexia, hiccups, nausea, and vomiting. Normocytic normochronic anemia and bleeding tendencies are hematologic findings, and the skin acquires accumulations of carotene-like pigments resulting in a sallow, yellow cast. Infections are common.

Neuropsychiatric Features

Clinical findings due to nervous system dysfunction are prominent in the uremic syndrome. As with all life-threatening illness, the question remains, what represents toxic encephalopathy (organic impairment) and what is due to psychological responses to the pervasive actuality and symbolic meaning of the condition? In this discussion we avoid dwelling on this complex dichotomy and focus upon symptoms. The thrust of the literature suggests that most of the behaviors to be described are primarily due to interference with the functioning of nervous system tissue. One such line of evidence is the reversibility of the phenomena upon dialysis.

The patient with beginning renal failure "just doesn't feel well." Early complaints are of fatigue and drowsiness. Relatives note apathy, general lethargy, and withdrawal. Personality changes range from constriction of affect, giving a picture of emotional dullness, to lability with impatience, petulance, demanding behavior, and occasional angry outburst. The ability to cooperate declines except for brief procedures.

Early intellectual impairment is marked by inability to concentrate and a diminished attention span. This is initially episodic, with functioning intact for short periods, but deteriorates rapidly if sustained activity is required. Clinically, administration of serial sevens or other rapid single series of calculations will highlight this deficit. Schreiner describes an engineer who finished a difficult mathematical assignment by working in 15-minute intervals during the "good days" that were interspersed with entire days of ineffectiveness (Schreiner, 1959). Psychological testing also shows diminished abilities for visual and motor coordination and for nonverbal abstraction. Ginn et al. (1975) have demonstrated deficits in uremic patients by using or developing performance measurements that test cognitive integrity by ipsitive or serial comparisons of patient performance over time. Deficiencies were found on the Trail Making Test (from the Reitan battery), in auditory short-term memory, and in answer recognition. These tests primarily measure sustained attention, alertness, short-term recall, and reaction time.

Long-term memory is also erratic during this period, ranging from forgetting small details to experiencing days and even weeks of amnesia. When combined with the common psychological mechanism of denial, patients may be unable to care for themselves, "forgetting" that they are ill or the instructions they were to follow. This may occur in persons who have previously demonstrated a good understanding of their illness. All of these phenomena might be interpreted as defenses against the knowledge and threat of serious illness, except that they are commonly noted by the patient and family prior to initial contact with a physician and, of course, before receiving the diagnosis and understanding the serious implications of their illness.

A slowing and general restriction of activities is also usually noted. Speech may be slurred. Patients often describe a need to keep moving and are irritable and complain of restlessness. Muscle fatigue occurs quickly after exercise, with postural muscles showing the first signs of weakness. This may coincide with generalized fibrillary muscle twitching, increased tendon reflexes, and cramps, particularly of the extensor muscle groups. One writer described a patient who was psychoanalyzed for several months in an attempt to remove a tic which took the form of a kicking movement at the knee (Schreiner, 1959). Subsequent medical investigation revealed azotemia secondary to chronic pyelonephritis. These muscle movements often intensify at night, just before sleep, and contribute to the common complaint of insomnia despite daytime drowsiness. Restless-leg syndrome may be seen, though it is not clear whether this represents subclinical neuropathy (Callaghan, 1966). Patients may also pick at their bedclothes or engage in other purposeless movements.

As uremia continues, sexual interests and performance diminish. (See section on Sexual Disturbance.) Appetite decreases, often secondary to the nausea, with resulting weight loss. Other kinds of symptoms secondary to neuropathies of the autonomic tracts may occur. The patient's condition is also quite dependent upon the state of the disease process, such as whether there is dehydration or a fluid overload. Wise (1974), writing on the pitfalls of diagnosing depression in patients with renal disease, pointed out that many of the above signs and symptoms are those of depression, particularly of the agitated type, and that extreme caution must be used in differentiating them. This is particularly important when a judgment is needed about suitability for dialysis or other kinds of treatment programs. Psychological testing is only of limited value in this determination. Occasionally only time and adequate medical treatment will differentiate these syndromes.

Uremic Delirium

With the progression of the uremic syndrome, neuropsychiatric symptoms become more pronounced and lead to obvious delirium. In this transitional phase, depending on underlying personality factors, a patient may become more withdrawn, demanding, angry, or paranoid. One study noted a significant number of patients with "negativistic, aggressive attitudes" towards their therapy and the medical personnel (Stenbäck and Haapanen, 1967). When clinical improvement of the renal failure occurred, this negativism disappeared. They reported patients urinating and defecating in bed, and that the nurses tended to interpret this behavior as being willful. Such behavior may fluctuate dramatically, with interspersed reasonable, lucid periods seemingly unrelated to known chemical changes.

As with other deliria (toxic psychoses), uremic delirium varies in intensity and symptomatology. Attention span is further shortened and memory deficits are more global. Faulty or diminished orientation, delusions, and hallucinations may be present. A specific description of a uremic delirium is probably not valid, though a particular type of organic psychosis characterized by bizarre behavior, confusion, seeing vivid colors, other sensory hallucinations, and muttering speech has been described (Schreiner, 1959). Earlier descriptions describe many forms of delirium such as asthenic, schizophrenic, manic, depressed, and paranoid. However, the causal association to uremia is unclear, and it is suspect whether appropriate diagnosis was made (Balser and Knutson, 1946).

It would be helpful if these neuropsychiatric symptoms could be precisely correlated with serum chemistries, yet such efforts have generally revealed wide individual variation among patients with similar laboratory values. In one attempt, Stenbäck and Haapanen (1967) divided 90 patients into a high urea group, with serum concentrations of 250 mg/100 ml or over (n = 51), and a low group, with concentrations of 50 to 199 mg/100 ml (n = 39). Psychiatric disturbances were found significantly more frequently in the high urea group. When only patients with delirium were considered, Stenbäck and Haapanen (1967) found that five patients with serum urea concentrations below 250 mg/100 ml were so affected, whereas the corresponding figure in the high serum urea group was 28. They found no differences in psychiatric symptoms when comparing acute versus chronic cases.

Occasionally, patients will pass on to stupor and coma without obvious delirium. In others, subsequent to the delirium, neurologic signs begin to become prominent. Slurred speech progresses to incoherency and mumbling. Meningeal irritation, cerebellar signs of unsteadiness, changes in gait, and nystagmus may occur. Muscle twitching may lead to convulsions that may manifest themselves as focal, Jacksonian, or grand mal type. Transient monoplegia, hemiplegia, aphasia, apraxia, amaurosis, deafness, and severe vertigo often occur prior to coma and death (Tyler, 1965).

Electroencephalographic Findings

Disturbances in the patient's electroencephalogram usually parallel the severity of his or her clinical disorder. Abnormal recordings are seen in most patients with blood urea nitrogen levels of about 60 mg/100 ml (Tyler, 1965). Conversely, those with less than 42 mg/100 ml appear normal. In mild states of uremia, the recordings are usually normal or of low voltage type. There is a slight tendency for loss of well-recognized alpha activity. When the illness is more severe, the pattern is characterized by progressive slowing, disorganization, and by intermittent slower activity. Eventually diffuse slowing with spiking is seen. Experienced encephalographers have attempted to delineate characteristic patterns. The most common abnormality described by Ginn et al. (1975) takes the form of diffuse slowing with a tendency for paroxysmal bursts of slow waves. These arise bilaterally from the frontal–parietal–parasagittal areas. These paroxysmal slow waves frequently occur without clinical evidence of seizures. This type of record suggests diffuse disturbance of central nervous system functioning. Kiley and Hines (1965) note that the wave frequency becomes slower prior to seriously deranged electrolyte imbalances, but attempts have not been successful to correlate encephalography changes with any single electrolyte abnormality.

Chronic Failure and Hemodialysis

The development and widespread use of dialysis now permits interruption and, at least, temporary reversal of the uremic syndrome and, with it, many of the mental status changes thus far described. The two most common techniques used at present are peritoneal dialysis and hemodialysis with an artificial kidney. Both have drawbacks. Peritoneal dialysis, while often used only as a holding action, has a reported increased risk of both toxic psychosis and seizures (Tyler, 1968). Tyler (1968) places this incidence at 1–2%, noting that, in his opinion, the psychosis occurs in patients with preexisting unstable personalities.

Long-term hemodialysis presents its own unique problems. The severe effects of the required dependency of the patient on both the machine and on the medical personnel, as well as other related psychological stresses, have been extensively described (Levy, 1974; Wright, Sand and Livingston, 1966; Shea et al., 1965; Abram, 1968; Abram, 1969). Home dialysis has been a partially satisfactory solution to some of these problems.

Lag Period

Though complete reversal of neuropsychiatric symptoms of uremia may occur following dialysis, it is important for the clinician to appreciate the lag period which exists between treatment and subsequent improvements or deteriorations. This is particularly crucial if decisions as to future management or placement are being made. This phenomenon is essentially a delay or lagging behind of the clinical picture and, particularly, of mental status changes when compared to alterations in blood chemistries. Thus, a patient may show unfavorable blood chemistry figures but feel well for a substantial period of time. The cycle has been described as: "chemical uremia → lag phase → clinical uremia → chemical reversal → lag phase → clinical reversal" (Schreiner, 1959). The length of the lag following treatment is extremely variable for different individuals or for the same individual at different phases of the illness. It may range from relatively immediate improvement after treatment to latent periods of up to six to eight days extending over several treatments. Finer measurements of nervous system functioning, such as conduction velocities, may demonstrate improvement only after many months following treatment (Reichenmiller et al., 1972).

No one knows why this lag occurs. It may represent a delay in cellular recovery, or in the distribution of toxic agents in the tissues (as opposed to in the blood). In some patients, the improvement seems to be directly related to the severity and duration of prior symptoms. In one report, the time required to awaken from the uremic coma following dialysis correlated with the duration of the oliguria prior to dialysis, rather than to the serum creatinine or urea nitrogen concentrations (Massey and Sellers, 1976).

Dialysis-Related Mental Status Changes

In addition to uremic encephalopathy, the clinician must keep in mind a variety of pathological conditions that may alter cerebral functioning. Schreiner (1959) has listed several: associated vascular disease, toxins of infection, water intoxication, hepatic coma, associated anemias, and nutritional deficiencies. Two cases of Wernicke's encephalopathy associated with the uremia have also been specifically described (Arieff and Massey, 1976; Faris, 1972). These, however, are part of the differential diagnosis of any prominent mental status change. Other possibilities that have been described are cerebral embolism secondary to shunt clotting, depletion syndrome, and copper intoxication (Arieff and Massey, 1976).

Following are several other conditions, found with relative frequency among dialysis patients, that deserve special mention.

Dialysis Disequilibrium Syndrome. Dialysis disequilibrium is a clinical pathological entity that may occur during or soon after dialysis. The syndrome is more severe when plasma urea is high before dialysis and may last for 24 hours after dialysis. Though reported in all age groups, it is more common among younger patients, the pediatric age group (Grushkin et al., 1972). Formerly called the reverse urea syndrome, it was thought to be due to the slower removal of urea from cerebrospinal fluid than from blood, which resulted in an abnormal urea gradient. This gradient caused the shift of fluid into the brain, and a rapid rise in intracranial pressure, with resulting clinical deterioration secondary to the brain edema. Subsequent studies, particularly in animals, demonstrated that it was unlikely to be so simple a mechanism. Some workers pointed to a paradoxical acidosis in the CSF secondary to differences in the rate of diffusion across the blood–brain barrier by carbon dioxide (CO_2) and bicarbonate (the former diffusing more rapidly than latter) (Couiee et al., 1962). Other studies implicated hypoglycemia and hyponatremia (Rigg and Berar, 1967; Wakins, 1969). A suggested summary hypothesis is that the cause of the dialysis disequilibrium syndrome is brain edema secondary to idiogenic osmoles (Arieff and Massey, 1976). The precise nature and mechanism are unclear at this time.

In its mildest form, the dialysis disequilibrium syndrome may be manifested only by restlessness, mild drowsiness, and headache. As severity increases, nausea, vomiting, blurred vision, and increased blood pressure may also occur. The mental status changes from lassitude and an apathetic appearance to disorientation and occasional agitation. Muscle irritability increases, and ultimately seizures, usually of the grand mal type, occur. In some patients, coma and death may follow if the syndrome is untreated. During the disequilibrium period, the EEG becomes abnormal in 75% of the patients, returning to predialysis levels in 8–48 hr (Tyler, 1968). This syndrome is now relatively well known by clinicians on dialysis units and can be avoided by slower dialysis over a longer period, by more frequent, shorter dialysis, or by dialysis against a high glucose concentration thereby not altering the osmolality as rapidly. Prophylactic administration of anticonvulsive agents such as barbiturates, diazepam, or diphenylhydantoin has been used to prevent seizures. The syndrome is characterized primarily by its tendency to be self-limiting and to be completely reversible in time if biochemical changes are not extreme.

Dialysis Dementia. In 1972, a clinical syndrome of a progressively fatal encephalopathy was reported in five patients on long-term dialysis (Alfrey et al., 1972). Later, seven more cases were added to that series, and, eventually, during the period between 1965 and 1975, 31% of the dialysis-related deaths at the dialysis unit in Denver demonstrated this constellation of symptoms (Burks et al., 1976). Subsequently, other centers have reported or confirmed similar phenomena (Mahurkar et al., 1973: Chokroverty et al., 1976; Scheiber and Ziesat, 1976).

Characterized by speech disorder, dementia, myoclonus and/or seizures, and behavioral changes, the time of onset is variable, ranging from 14 months to 4 years. The earliest and most characteristic clinical sign is the speech disturbance. Nursing personnel may initially note this change during dialysis treatment. Stuttering is usually the first sign, with dysarthria, dyspraxia, and dysphasia being recognized later. Mutism is also occasionally seen. Early in the illness, dialysis appears to markedly worsen the speech difficulty, with improvement following within 24 hr. Later, progression of the disturbance reaches a point of noncommunication, uninfluenced by the dialysis. Myoclonic jerks occur early in the course of the encephalopathy. Present bilaterally, they are often stimulus-sensitive. Asterixis and seizures may subsequently occur. Lederman and Henry (1978) recently summarized the neurologic features associated with this syndrome.

The dementia portion of the illness is of a global type, with confusion, disorientation, and impairment of memory. Behavioral disturbances include personality changes, paranoid ideation, hallucinations, and bizarre behavior. These changes do not appear to be specific. One group felt they could be differentiated from uremic encephalopathy by the subacute onset, the longer duration of illness, the lack of relationship to systemic biochemical changes, and the EEG (Chokroverty et al., 1976). They felt that the EEG was generally nonspecific but distinctive, with the bisynchronous rhythmic delta, frontocentral spike-and-slow waves, and photosensitivity characteristic of uremic encephalopathy. This group also believed that, following autopsy, pathologic changes could be determined that differentiate these syndromes. Others have noted no difference, their findings being more consistent with a diffuse toxic metabolic disorder (Burks et al., 1976).

The pathogenesis of dialytic encephalopathy is unknown. Several workers have argued for accumulation or depletion of trace metals such as aluminum, tin, and rubidium (Alfrey et al., 1972; Alfrey, LeGendre and Kaehuy, 1976; McDermott et al., 1978). An increasing amount of evidence seems to incriminate aluminum (Vaisrub, 1978). A viral disease, or dopamine or asparagine deficiencies have also been suggested (Burks et al., 1976; Wardle, 1977).

The illness progresses to coma and death, although a number of patients have died as a result of suicide, septicemia, or unexplained sudden deaths. All attempts at treatment thus far have failed including vigorous dialysis, and administration of phenobarbital, diphenylhydantoin, diazepam, L-dopa, or dexamethasone. Madel and Wilson (1976) reported some improvement in patients with classical features of dialysis dementia following the administration of parenteral diazepam. Subsequent authors have not found a similar response, although a transient reversal of certain components of this syndrome has occurred (Snider et al., 1979). Some suggest that early transplantation might be helpful, but, as yet, reports show that only two patients with this syndrome improved following transplantation (Burks et al., 1976; Sullivan et al., 1977).

Subdural Hematoma. Several reports have described the identification of subdural hematomas among patients on chronic dialysis (Leonard et al., 1969; Talalla et al., 1970). Two factors contribute to this possibility. First, many patients are given anticoagulant drugs to maintain the patency of their arteriovenous shunts against thrombosis. Secondarily, patients with advanced renal failure could have abnormal bleeding. Clinically, this is often seen as gastrointestinal hemorrhage, epistaxis, and ecchymosis. The cause has been attributed to circulating anticoagulants and to a qualitative deficit of the platelets (Talalla et al., 1970).

The symptoms of subdural hematoma may initially be similar to other dialysis syndromes: drowsiness, headaches, and nausea. Only later, focal signs such as neck stiffness (meningeal irritation), lateralizing signs, or progressive deterioration in mental functioning point to the correct diagnosis. Some differentiation can be made from the disequilibrium syndrome if the symptoms persist between dialyses or progressively worsen. Knowledge of, or an alertness to the possibility of an overdose of anticoagulants should also heighten clinical suspicion. The EEG is not very helpful (Leonard et al., 1969). More reliable are the brain scan or angiography. Early recognition of the condition can avert death or chronic invalidism.

Brain Injury and Renal Failure

There are a few reports that suggest that the relationship between renal failure and the central nervous system is not a one-way process. Several studies have noted an influence on renal function following intracerebral hemorrhage and injury (Fishberg, 1957; Steinmetz and Kiley, 1960). Several other reports have described renal failure subsequent to electroconvulsive therapy (ECT) (Goodman, 1950; McNichol, 1958; Selzer et al., 1963). These included several deaths and at least one case successfully treated with dialysis. Goodman noted that the relationship to ECT may be unsuspected because of the time interval between the treatment and onset of symptoms, 10 to 14 days (McNichol, 1958). Supportive evidence comes from laboratory work demonstrating renal vasoconstriction and alteration in electrolyte retention mechanisms with central electrical stimulation and experimentally produced lesions (Hoff et al., 1951).

Renal Failure and Associated Psychoses

There are several early clinicians who stoutly maintained that azotemia can be associated with different psychotic pictures but not be causal (Marchand and Courtois, 1935; Toulouse et al., 1930; Ey et al., 1960). "Azotemia acute psychotic encephalitis," acute delirium, and fatal catatonias have been described (Toulouse et al., 1930). The difficulties in interpreting these reports are considerable, for to some degree renal failure will be found in psychotic patients by chance. We also know that dehydration, catabolism of protein under stress, dieting, and a variety of other medical and surgical conditions causing varying degrees of renal failure can raise nonprotein nitrogen levels. The absence of validation of this work in the past 20 years suggests that azotemia occurring directly secondary to psychotic processes is unlikely.

Renal Disease and Sexual Dysfunction

Males

Disturbances in sexual function are common in patients with renal failure. Male patients experience decreased libido and varying degress of impotence, and there is a marked decline of intercourse frequency compared to pre-illness levels (Levy, 1973; Abram et al., 1975; Salvatierra et al., 1975). Chronic hemodialysis does not usually improve sexual functioning, even though the patient's subjective sense of better health and well-being is markedly improved. In fact, it is in this phase that sexual function often becomes problematic or further deteriorates (Kaplan De-Nour, 1969). Successful renal transplantation reverses this trend for some patients, but many remain partially or totally impotent (Abram et al., 1975; Levy, 1977). In addition, gynecomastia, decreases in testicular size, and alterations of testicular histology occur, with decreased or absent spermatogenesis (Schmidt et al., 1968; Nagel et al., 1973; Elstein et al., 1969; Freeman et al., 1968).

The causes of these phenomena are not clear and undoubtedly include both emotional and physical components. Some writers point to psychological factors such as conflict related to passivity and dependency, alterations in sexual identity, and other regressive aspects of chronic illness (Levy, 1973; Abram et al., 1975). Other observations suggest metabolic changes. One study found impotent male subjects to have prolonged nerve conduction velocities and absent bulbocavernosus reflexes (Sherman, 1975). Most studies demonstrate decreased plasma testosterone levels and increased levels of luteinizing hormone (LH) and follicle stimulating hormone (FSH) (Guevara et al., 1969; Chen et al., 1970).

It is believed that retention of uremic toxins is responsible for these changes. Recent reports suggest combined testicular dysfunction and inadequate hypothalamic response to end-organ insufficiency (Lim and Fang, 1975; Distiller, et al., 1975). Holdsworth et al. (1977) demonstrated that the primary deficit lies in testicular suppression.

Several directions for treatment are presently being explored. One group found uniformly improved libido, sexual potency, and general sense of well-being in five subjects treated with clomiphene citrate (Lim and Fang, 1976). This drug stimulates pituitary gonadotropin secretion and secondarily increases testosterone production. Other investigators, following reports of zinc deficiency in chronic renal patients and in those on hemodialysis, obtained similar results for four patients who were treated with zinc chloride added to the dialysis bath (Antoniou et al., 1977).

Females

Females, too, suffer sexual changes in renal failure. With progressive uremia, ovulation ceases, and absence of menstruation soon follows, along with the development of other uremic symptoms. Libido is decreased for most patients as measured by frequency of sex and quality (frequency of orgasm) (Levy, 1973). As in males, beginning and continuing hemodialysis is often associated with deterioration of sexual function (25% worsened compared with 6% reporting improvement) (Levy, 1977). Transplantation does not offer substantial improvement for most patients.

Following dialytic therapy, menses may return and ovulation has been demonstrated among these patients (Goodwin et al., 1968). There are also reports of successful pregnancies occurring both during end-stage renal failure and while on chronic dialysis (Ackrill et al., 1975; Nagle et al., 1975; Unzelman et al., 1973). Again, the exact mechanism of these changes is unclear, but contraceptive therapy may be needed. Hyperprolactinemia has been reported in females on dialysis, and lowering these levels with the dopamine agonist bromocriptine, has restored normal gonadal function (Thorner et al., 1975; Thorner et al., 1974).

PSYCHOTROPIC DRUGS AND RENAL DISORDERS

Adverse changes in mental status among renal patients may occur as a result of the effects of medication. An increasing degree of renal insufficiency increases both the frequency of occurrence and/or the severity of drug reactions. It is estimated that adverse drug reactions are two to three times more common for patients with mild elevations of blood urea nitrogen than for those with normal chemistries. Richet et al. (1970) found 178 episodes of neurologic derangement in 203 renal patients, with one third caused by drug intoxication.

The reasons for such responses to drugs are multiple. Because disorders of several systems are frequently encountered in patients with acute or chronic renal failure, they are likely to receive different kinds of drugs. A typical sequence involves prescribing a drug for mild symptoms, such as insomnia or nausea, which then creates new symptoms for which other drugs are subsequently added.

There are several other factors which may account for this increased incidence of drug reactions. Administration of drugs that are excreted in unchanged forms or as active metabolites will result in increased blood levels of active drug if renal function is significantly impaired. Reduced plasma protein binding, thus increasing the unbound or free fraction, will also increase blood concentrations, resulting in enhanced or prolonged drug effect. Such a reduction of binding may also occur in renal patients with low serum protein levels. Changes in volume of distribution or rate of metabolism will have the same effect. Increased sensitivity to drugs may occur either through changes in the blood–brain barrier, allowing increased uptake, or by alterations of central nervous system susceptibility when the patient is uremic (Bennet, 1975). Also, hemodialysis removes varying amounts of different drugs, further complicating management.

The exact effect of decreased renal function on all drugs given for neuropsychiatric symptoms is still unclear. Bennet et al. (1971), in their excellent series on drug therapy and renal failure, offer some guidelines. Fortunately, most psychotropic drugs have few relative contraindications and only rare absolute ones. For most, a standard loading dose equivalent to that given to patients without renal disease is prescribed initially, and future adjustments are made in dosage or interval to maintain proper blood levels. This is a clinical judgment, for blood level determinations are usually not feasible. Allowances must be made for factors which may alter drug absorption, such as nausea, vomiting, diarrhea, or gastrointestinal tract edema. Edematous patients tend to absorb drugs more slowly from intramuscular injection sites.

Barbiturates

Most barbiturate group drugs are metabolized by the hepatic route and may be used in normal dosages. Occasionally, increased sensitivity to sedative effects may be seen. When used chronically, the half-life of the barbiturates is reduced owing to hepatic microsomal-enzyme-induction. This may reduce effectiveness, but additional amounts of drugs seldom appear to be needed. This effect on microsomal enzyme systems may interfere with other drugs such as anticoagulants or anticonvulsants.

Long-acting barbiturates have relatively low protein binding and low lipid solubility, hence they are more dependent on renal function for excretion. Accumulation of these drugs may occur with glomerular filtration rates of less than 10 ml/min. To compensate for this phenomenon, the intervals of dosage must be lengthened. These particular barbiturates (long-acting type) are also partially removed by regular dialysis, requiring careful dosage adjustment in these patients.

Benzodiazepines

Though the major benzodiazepines appear to have some active metabolites excreted by the kidney, this does not usually require changes in either dosage or interval and they are considered safe within a wide therapeutic margin. Chlordiazepoxide, diazepam, and flurazepam all occasionally cause excessive sedation in renal patients. An exception to the relative comfort in using the benzodiazepines has been recently reported by Taclob and Needle (1976). They described five patients who had been on chronic maintenance hemodialysis who developed a syndrome involving altered consciousness, asterixis, and abnormal electroencephalograms after they had been given flurazepam and diazepam. There has not been further substantiation of this report. Chlordiazepoxide has been pointed out as a particular problem in this regard (Hansten, 1976). An increased central nervous system vulnerability may be responsible for this phenomenon.

Tricyclics

Amitriptyline, desmethylimipramine, and nortriptyline all have less than 5% drug excretion routes via the kidney; thus adjustments do not need to be made for renal failure. It should be noted, however, that all agents in this group are anticholinergic and may cause urinary retention. The development of urinary retention may further compromise impaired renal function. Orthostatic hypotension, occasionally a problem with these drugs, may be aggravated by the blood pressure fluctuations normally seen in patients on hemodialysis.

Because of drug–drug interactions, control of hypertension may be difficult to achieve with bethanidine and guanidinium drugs when they are used with tricyclic antidepressants (Bennet et al., 1971). Increased doses of these agents may suffice, or a change to a drug which exerts full hypotensive effects when used with tricyclics, such as methyldopa, may be needed. Reserpine's hypotensive effectiveness has also been reported as reduced, but it is less likely to be used because of its significant depressive side effects.

There is some suggestion that certain of the tricyclic antidepressants appear to impair the metabolism of the anticoagulants, thus increasing plasma levels (Koch, 1973). Thus, altered anticoagulant effects should be watched for when tricyclic antidepressants are started or stopped in patients receiving these drugs.

Antipsychotic Drugs

The major excretion route of the phenothiazines is hepatic, and these drugs are not effectively removed by dialysis; thus, no regular changes need to be made in dosage or interval. The same appears to be true of haloperidol and other antipsychotic drugs. All agents in this group have some anticholinergic properties and may cause urinary retention. Excessive sedation may also be a problem. Large parenteral doses should be avoided prior to hemodialysis because of the risk of hypotension. Extrapyramidal reactions, such as torticollis and Parkinsonian states, have been noted to be produced by relatively small doses of the phenothiazines (Tyler, 1968).

The phenothiazines may either augment or antagonize any of the antihypertensive drugs, depending on their mechanism of action. Careful blood pressure monitoring is indicated, and dosage adjustment may be needed.

Lithium Carbonate

Since lithium is excreted from the body almost entirely by the kidneys, its use in the presence of compromised renal function can be quite hazardous. In patients with advanced or unstable renal failure, consideration should be given to alternate treatments with medications whose excretion is not dependent upon renal function. However, with proper dose modification and careful medical followup, lithium has been used successfully even in patients with renal disease who are dependent on dialysis for survival.

A common side effect of lithium therapy is polyuria with secondary polydipsia caused by interference with antidiuretic hormone activity at the renal level. This side effect is generally mild and reversible, but occasionally a severe diabetes insipidus syndrome occurs, with urine volumes exceeding 6 liters per day. Recent work suggests that the impaired renal concentrating capacity caused by lithium may persist for long periods after drug discontinuation (Bucht and Wahlin, 1978).

Chronic renal structural damage attributable to lithium (especially with higher doses over longer periods of time) has been reported in a number of studies (Hestbech et al., 1977; Burrows et al., 1978; Ayd, 1979). These changes include interstitial fibrosis, tubular atrophy, and sclerotic glomeruli, and have been found in patients with and without histories of lithium toxicity. How prevalent these abnormalities are is not known, but preliminary studies suggest that 10–20% of patients on long-term lithium therapy may be affected. The likelihood of lithium causing renal failure (other than in situations of extreme toxicity) is quite low, and the morphological abnormalities are generally found in association with either normal renal function or mild reductions in creatinine clearance and increases in urine volume. Periodic assessment of renal function should, however, be an integral part of patient management.

A less common abnormality associated with the use of lithium has been a defect in urinary acidification, which, as yet, has not been found to be of clinical importance.

In addition to renal disease, a number of other factors alter renal lithium excretion (Jefferson and Greist, 1979). The most important of these are dietary sodium intake and the use of diuretic drugs. As was graphically illustrated in the late 1940's when lithium chloride was used as a salt substitute, marked dietary salt restriction will result in a decrease in lithium clearance and an increase in serum lithium levels (sometimes leading to toxicity). Thiazide diuretics have been clearly shown to have the same effect; namely, a reduced lithium clearance and increased serum lithium levels. The other classes of diuretics have been less thoroughly studied. There is some suggestion that potassium-sparing diuretics will increase serum lithium levels; loop diuretics cause no change, and osmotic diuretics cause a decrease. Nonetheless, caution should be exercised in any patient receiving lithium and drugs that will alter fluid–electrolyte balance.

REFERENCES

Abram HS: The psychiatrist, the treatment of chronic renal failure and the prolongation of life: I. Am J Psychiatry 124:1351–1358, 1968.

Abram HS: The psychiatrist, the treatment of chronic renal failure and the prolongation of life: II. Am J Psychiatry 126:157–167, 1969.

Abram HS, Hester LR, Sheridan WF, Epstein GM: Sexual functioning in patients with chronic renal failure. J Nerv Ment Dis 160:220–226, 1975.

Ackrill P, Goodwin FJ, Marsh FP, et al: Successful pregnancy in patients on regular dialysis. Br Med J 2:172–174, 1975.

Alfrey AC, LeGendre GR, Kaehny WD: The dialysis encephalopathy syndrome. N Eng J Med 1:184–188, 1976.

Alfrey AC, Mishell JM, Burks J, Continguglia RH, Lewin E, Holmes JH: Syndrome of dyspraxia and multifocal seizures associated with chronic hemodialysis. Trans Am Soc Artif Intern Organs 18:257–262, 1972.

Antoniou LD, Shalhaub RJ, Sudhakar T, Smith JC Jr: Reversal of uremic impotence by zinc. Lancet 2:895–898, 1977.

Arieff AI, Massey SG: Dialysis disequilibrium syndrome, in Massey SG, Sellers AL (eds): Clinical Aspects of Uremia. Springfield, Charles C Thomas, 1976.

Avram MM, Feinfeld DA, Huatuco H: Search for the uremic toxin: Decreased motor-nerve conduction velocity and elevated parathyroid hormone in uremia. New Eng J Med 298:1000–1002, 1978.

Ayd FJ: Lithium and the kidney. *Int Drug Ther Newsl* 14:25–28, 1979.

Balser AB, Knutson J: Psychiatric aspects of uremia. *Am J Psychiatry* 102:683–687, 1946.

Bennet WM: Principles of drug therapy in patients with renal disease (medical progress). *West J Med* 123:372–379, 1975.

Bennet WM, Singer I, Golper T, Feig P, Coggins CJ: Guidelines for drug therapy in renal failure. *Ann Intern Med* 86:754–783, 1971.

Bricker NS: On the pathogenesis of the uremic state: An exposition of the "trade-off hypothesis." *N Eng J Med* 286:1093–1095, 1972.

Bucht G, Wahlin A: Impairment of renal concentrating capacity by lithium. *Lancet* 1:778–779, 1978.

Burks JS, Alfrey AC, Huddlestone J, Narenberg MD, Lewin E: A fatal encephalopathy in chronic haemodialysis patients. *Lancet* **1**:764–768, 1976.

Burrows GD, Davies B, Kincaid-Smith P: Unique tubular lesion after lithium. *Lancet* 1:1310, 1978.

Callaghan N: Restless legs syndrome in uremic neuropathy. *Neurology* 16:359–363, 1966.

Chen JC, Vidt DG, Zorn EM, Hallberg MC, Wieland RG: Pituitary-Leydig cell function in uremic males. *J Clin Endocrinol* 31:14–17, 1970.

Chokroverty S, Bruetman ME, Berger V, Reyes MG: Progressive dialytic encephalopathy. *J Neurol Neurosurg Psychiatry* 39:411–419, 1976.

Couiee J, Lambie AT, Robson JS: The influence of extra-corporeal dialysis on the acid–base conjunction of blood and cerebrospinal fluid. *Clin Sci* 23:397–400, 1962.

Distiller La, Morley JE, Sagel J, Pokroy M, Rabkin R: Pituitary–gonadal function in chronic renal failure: The effect of luteinizing hormone–releasing hormone and the influence of dialysis. *Metab Clin Exp* 24:711–719, 1975.

Elstein M, Smith EKM, Curtis JR: Reproductive potential of patients evaluated by maintenance hemodialysis. *Br Med J* 2:734–736, 1969.

Ey H, Bernard P, Brisset CB: *Manuel de Psychiatrie*. Paris, Masson et Cie, 1960.

Faris AA: Wernichs' encephalopathy in uremia. *Neurology* 22:1293–1297, 1972.

Fishberg AM: Neurogenic nephropathy. *Arch Intern Med* 99:129–133, 1957.

Freeman RM, Lawton RL, Fearing MO: Gynecomastia: An endocrinologic complication of hemodialysis. *Ann Intern Med* 69:67–70, 1968.

Ginn HE, Teschan PE, Walker PJ, et al: Neurotoxicity in uremia. *Kidney Int* 7:357–360, 1975.

Goodman L: Lower nephron nephrosis following electroconvulsive treatment. *J Nerv Ment Dis* 112:130–131, 1950.

Goodwin NJ, Valenti C, Hall JE, et al: Effects of uremia and chronic hemodialysis on the reproductive cycle. *Am J Obstet Gynecol* 100:528–535, 1968.

Grushkin CM, Korsch B, Fine RN: Hemodialysis in small children. *JAMA* 221:869–871, 1972.

Guevara AD, Vidt DG, Hallberg MD, et al: Serum gonadotropin and testosterone levels in males undergoing intermittent hemodialysis. *Metabolism* 18:1062–1066. 1969.

HanstenPD (ed): *Drug Interactions*, ed 2. Philadelphia, Lea and Febriger, 1976.

Hestbech J, Hansen HE, Amdisen A, et al: Chronic renal lesions following long-term treatment with lithium. *Kidney International* 12:205–213, 1977.

Heyman A, Patterson JL Jr, Jones RW Jr: Cerebral circulation and metabolism in uremia. *Circulation* 3:558–563, 1951.

Hoff EC, Kell JF, Hastings N, et al: Vasomotor cellular and functional changes produced in kidney by brain stimulation. *J Neurophysiol* 14:317–322, 1951.

Holdsworth S, Atkins RC, de Kretzer DM: The pituitary-testicular axis in men with chronic renal failure. *N Eng J Med* 296:1245–1249, 1977.

Javid M, Settlage P: Effect of urea on cerebrospinal fluid pressure in human subjects. *JAMA* 160:943–949, 1956.

Jefferson JW, Greist JH: Lithium and the Kidney, in Davis JM, Greenblatt D (eds): *Psychopharmacology Update: New and Neglected Areas*. New York, Grune & Stratton, pp 81–104, 1979.

Kaplan De-Nour A: Some notes on the psychological significance of urination. *J Nerv Ment Dis* 148:615–618, 1969.

Kiley JE, Hines O: EEG evaluation of uremia, wave frequency evaluation on 40 uremic patients. *Arch Intern Med* 116:67–73, 1965.

Koch WJ: Hemorrhagic reactions and drug interactions in 500 warfarin-treated patients, abstracted. *Clin Pharmacol Ther* 14:139–141, 1973.

Lederman RJ, Henry CE: Progressive dialysis encephalopathy. *Ann Neurol* 4:199–204, 1978.

Leonard CD, Weil E, Schribner BH: Subdural hematomas in patients undergoing haemodialysis. *Lancet* 2:239–240, 1969.

Levy NB: Sexual adjustment to maintenance dialysis and renal transplantation: National survey. *Trans Am Soc Artif Intern Organs* 19:138–143, 1973.

Levy NB (ed): Living or Dying: Adaptation to Hemodialysis. Springfield, Thomas, 1974.

Levy NB: Letter to the editor. *N Eng J Med* 297:725–726, 1977.

Lim VS, Fang VS: Gonadal dysfunction in uremic men: A study of the hypothalamic-pituitary-testicular axis before and after renal transplantation. *Am J Med* 58:655–659, 1975.

Lim VS, Fang VS: Determination of plasma testosterone levels in uremic men with clomiphene citrate. *J Clin Endocrinol Metab* 43:1370–1377, 1976.

McDermott JR, Smith AI, Ward MK, et al: Brain-aluminum concentration in dialysis encephalopathy. *Lancet*, 901–903, 1978.

McNichol R: Delayed complications of ECT-crush syndrome. *Am J Psychiatry* 115:346–348, 1958.

Madel AM, Wilson WP: Dialysis encephalopathy: A possible seizure disorder. *Neurology* 26:1130–1134, 1976.

Mahurkar SD, Dhar SK, Salta R, et al: Dialysis dementia. *Lancet* 1:1412–1415, 1973.

Marchand L, Courtois A: *Les Encephalites Psychosiques*. Paris, Librairie E Le Francois, 1935.

Massey SG, Sellers AL (eds): *Clinical Aspects of Uremia and Dialysis*. Springfield, Charles C Thomas, 1976.

Merrill JP, Legrain M, Hoigne R: Observations on the role of urea in uremia. *Am J Med* 14:519–520, 1953.

Nagel TC, Freinkel N, Bell RH, et al: Gynecomastia, prolactin and other peptide hormones in patients undergoing chronic hemodialysis. *J Clin Endocrinol Metab* 36:428–432, 1973.

Nagle S, Winder E, Pinnock S: Successful pregnancy in home dialysis. *Proc Eur Dial Transplant Assoc* 3:89–92, 1975.

Reichenmiller HE, Dürr F, Bundschu HD: Neurologic disorders in uremia, in Kluthe R, Berlyne G, Burton B (eds): *Uremia*. Stuttgart, Gearg Thieme Verlag, 1972.

Richet G, Lopez de Novales E, Verroust P: Drug intoxication and neurological episodes in chronic renal failure. *Br Med J*, 394–395, 1970.

Rigg GA, Berar BR: Hypoglycemia: A complication of hemodialysis. *N Eng J Med* 277:1139–1141, 1967.

Salvatierra O, Fortmann JL, Belzar FO: Sexual function in males before and after renal transplantation. *Urology* 5:64–66, 1975.

Scheiber SC, Ziesat H: Dementia dialitica: A new psychotic brain syndrome. *Compr Psychiatry* 17:781–785, 1976.

Scheinberg P: Effects of uremia on cerebral blood flow and metabolism. *Neurology* 4:101–109, 1954.

Schmidt GW, Shehadeh I, Sawin CT: Transient gynecomastia in chronic renal failure during chronic intermittent hemodialysis. *Ann Intern Med* 69:73–79, 1968.

Schreiner GE: Mental and personality changes in the uremic syndrome. *Med Ann DC* 28:316–323, 1959.

Selzer ML, Reinhardt MJ, Deeney JM: Acute renal failure following EST. *Am J Psychiatry* 120:602–603, 1963.

Shea EJ, Bogdon DF, Freeman RB, et al: Hemodialysis for chronic renal failure. IV. Psychological consideration. *Ann Intern Med* 62:558–562, 1965.

Sherman FP: Impotence in patients with chronic renal failure on dialysis: Its frequency and etiology. *Fertil Steril* 26:221–223, 1975.

Snider WD, DeMaria AA, Mann JD: Dialysis and dialysis encephalopathy. *Neurology* 29:414–415, 1979.

Steinmetz PR, Kiley JE: Renal tubular necrosis following lesions of the brain. *Am J Med* 29:268–276, 1960.

Stenbäck A, Haapanen E: Azotemia and psychosis. *Acta Psychiatr Scand* 43(suppl):30–38, 1967.

Sullivan PA, Murnaghan DJ, Callaghan N: Dialysis dementia: Recovery after transplantation. *Br Med J* 17:740, 1977.

Taclob L, Needle M: Drug-induced encephalopathy in patients on maintenance hemodialysis. *Lancet* 1:704–705, 1976.

Talalla A, Halbrook H, Barbour BH, et al: Subdural hematoma associated with long-term hemodialysis for chronic renal disease. *JAMA* 212:1847–1849, 1970.

Thorner MO, McNeilly AS, Hagen C, et al: Long-term treatment of galactorrhoea and hypogonadism with bromocriptine. *Br Med J* 2:419–422, 1974.

Thorner MO, Besser GM, Jones A, et al: Bromocriptine treatment of female infertility: Report of 13 pregnancies. *Br Med J* 4:694–697, 1975.

Toulouse E, Marchand L, Courtois A: L'encephalite psychosique aigue azotemizue. *Presse Medicale*, April 12, 1930, pp 497–500.

Tyler HR: Neurologic disorders in renal failure. *Am J Med* 44:734–748, 1968.

Tyler R: Neurological complications of acute and chronic failure, in Merrill JP (ed): *The Treatment of Renal Failure*. London, Heinemann, 1965.

Unzelman RF, Alderfer GR, Chojnacki RE: Pregnancy and chronic hemodialysis. *Trans Am Soc Artif Intern Organs* 19:144–149, 1973.

Vaisrub S: Dangerous waters. *JAMA* 240:1630, 1978.

Wakins KG: Predominance of hyponatremia over hypo-osmolality in simulation of the dialysis disequilibrium syndrome. *Mayo Clin Proc* 44:433–437, 1969.

Wardle EN: Dialysis dementia, letter. *Lancet* 2:47, 1977.

Wise TN: The pitfalls of diagnosing depression in chronic renal disease. *Psychosomatics* 15:83–84, 1974.

Wright RG, Sand P, Livingston G: Psychological stress during hemodialysis for chronic failure. *Ann Intern Med* 64:611–618, 1966.

Gastrointestinal Disorders

ALIMENTARY TRACT DISORDERS

The organ system which has received the most attention from psychiatrists is the gastrointestinal (GI) tract, and the importance of emotional factors in the genesis or treatment of diseases in this organ system is well accepted by clinicians of most specialities. Despite repeated clinical observations and extensive research from a psychosomatic viewpoint, a definitive understanding of the exact circumstances and mechanisms of many of the GI illnesses has not been clarified.

At our present stage of knowledge, it does not appear that neuropsychiatric considerations in response to GI pathology are major. The GI system, while strongly affected by central nervous system processes, seems to have less capability of reciprocally and specifically influencing CNS functioning, i.e., it does not appear to produce products or metabolities which are known to have significant systemic or central nervous system effects.

Early writers have disagreed with this view, for Pinel wrote in 1899, "The primary seat of insanity generally is in the region of the stomach and intestines and it is from that center that the disorder of intelligence propagates itself" (Watson, 1923). The concept of autointoxication from the bowel, though attractive for many years, has, of course, not been substantiated. An exception occurs in liver failure, when absorption of amines or ammonia from the bowel contributes to encephalopathic states. Though psychiatrists have historically been involved most with the classic psychosomatic GI illnesses, there are other clinical situations in which psychiatric expertise may be sought.

Vomiting

Because vomiting is a symptom rather than a disease, occurs in such a large variety of disorders, and is often accompanied by few physical signs, its cause may be difficult to elucidate. The mechanisms resulting in the act of vomiting are complex and poorly understood. The psychological features of the patient may be causal and/or reactive, accounting for variable portions of the clinical picture. There are several major clinical situations in which psychiatric consultation may be sought for diagnostic or treatment purposes.

Psychogenic Vomiting

The psychophysiologic disorder of psychogenic vomiting appears to be quite common (Alvarez, 1951; Rivers and Ferreira, 1938; Leibovich, 1973). Except for scattered case reports in the literature, there has been remarkably little work done toward pinpointing the specific determinants of vomiting. Cleghorn and Brown ('1964) gave some attention to the psychogenesis, drawing on the sparse accounts and case histories that were available for a profile of these patients. They described them as dependent personalities with immature sexuality and impaired parental relationships. They felt that the episodes of vomiting were often related to fears of heterosexuality. How these common deficiencies of character formation can lead to vomiting, other than acting as general source of stress, is unknown. While personality characteristics may be highlighted, it is necessary to keep in mind that virtually any kind of personality and every psychiatric disorder may have psychogenic vomiting as a symptom.

A survey of the literature suggests that there are a number of features of vomiting that tend to lend support to the diagnosis of a psychogenic etiology. A series of 140 cases was reported by Wilbur and Washburn (1938) who felt that diagnosis of functional vomiting was not difficult. A typical picture was that of a relatively young woman with some signs of emotional instability who, without apparent reason or associated nausea or abdominal stress, had for long periods of time vomited within an hour after meals. Other features felt to be common were the characteristic ability of the patient to reach a receptacle before vomiting and the relative ease with which the vomiting occurs. Some authors describe regurgitation as occurring, rather than vomiting, meaning that there is an expulsion of food in the absence of nausea, and without the abdominal diaphragmatic muscular contraction that occurs normally with vomiting. A desire or ability to eat again immediately following vomiting is felt to be characteristic, a feature relatively rarely found when the vomiting is a result of organic disease. These patients are often able to postpone their vomiting if actively encouraged to do so, and there is seldom a significant weight loss or cachectic appearance.

A careful history will usually reveal that the vomiting takes place at certain times, and that there is a relationship to stressful events in the patient's life. Hill (1968) noted that a common feature of psychogenic vomiting was that the individual felt trapped in a hostile relationship and suggested that vomiting occurring chiefly at mealtime might be related to eating with someone who aroused strong feelings.

Hill also noted that his group of vomiters gave a history of being subject to recurrent spells of vomiting in childhood, suggesting a type of organ vulnerability. A similar finding has been noted among patients who experienced persistent nausea without organic cause (Swanson et al., 1976). Hill also found that there appeared to be an excessive amount of childhood parental loss among his group of patients.

A subgroup of vomiters are those patients who self-induce vomiting. This appears to be relatively rare except as a concomitant of anorexia nervosa, which must be suspected in this condition. Further examining this phenomenon, Beaumont et al. (1976), retrospectively studies "dieters" and "vomiters and purgers." They found that the "vomiters and purgers" were more outgoing and that most had previously been obese. As they had been unable to keep themselves thin by simply abstaining from food, they came to rely on vomiting as another means to control their weight. These patients seemed to have more histrionic personality traits and did less well in treatment.

Vomiting and Pregnancy

Approximately 50% of normal women living in industrialized societies experience nausea and vomiting during the first 10–12 weeks of pregnancy (Fairweather, 1968). A few women will develop a more severe type of vomiting early in pregnancy known as hyperemesis gravidarum. This condition can give rise to considerable morbidity and even mortality, but its relationship to the more commonly seen vomiting is unknown.

Several theories have been advanced to explain the presence or absence of first trimester vomiting. Though there appears to be a definite endocrinologic basis to this symptom, no physiologic theory alone can account for the phenomena. Kroger (1962) presents the widely held psychological theory that vomiting represents an unconsciousness attempt to reject the child. An opposing view has been suggested by Deutsch (1945) who felt that symptom-free pregnancy should be regarded with suspicion, being a demonstration that the reality of pregnancy was being denied. Tylden (1968) suggested a less specific explanation, saying that vomiting is a psychologically based response to high levels of stress caused by a wide range of physical and social difficulties. In general, however, studies using objective methods of assessment have failed to support the idea that there are pronounced psychological differences between women who experience mild vomiting during early pregnancy and those who do not (Palmer, 1973; Coppens, 1959; Uddenberg et al., 1971; Netter-Munkelt et al., 1972).

Vomiting and Cancer

In cancer patients, nausea and vomiting are common and are distressing complications of the disease or its treatments. The latter appears to be an increasing problem as therapeutic modalities become more aggressive. In advanced cancer, nausea and vomiting are undoubtedly multifactorial, with contributions from abnormalities of smell and taste, disorders of central hunger satiety mechanisms, and possible production of tumor metabolities that affect central and peripheral mediators of these symptoms. In addition, because radiation therapy and many of the agents used in chemotherapy induce nausea and vomiting, conditioned reflexes may develop and become ingrained as an inadvertent concomitant of the treatment. It is common for patients to become "sick to their stomachs" as they approach the hospital or cancer ward. Differentiation is often aided by the presence of nausea with the emesis, which suggests a larger biologic contribution to the symptom complex than that seen in the more "pure" psychogenic vomiter who seldom describes nausea.

Complications of Vomiting

Whether vomiting is of psychogenic origin or symptomatic of organic disease, repeated emesis may have serious deleterious effects. The process of vomiting may lead to traumatic rupture or tearing in the region of the cardioesophageal junction, resulting in massive bleeding: the Mallory–Weiss syndrome. There are also risks associated with weight loss and potassium depletion, which may lead to muscle paralysis (Hill, 1967; Mitchell and Feldman, 1968). Hill stresses the importance of bearing in mind the possibility of hypokalemia in patients suffering from psychogenic vomiting. There is a great tendency to ascribe all of their symptoms to "hysteria," especially when the symptoms are bizarre. Other authors have elaborated on the severe effects of hypokalemia occurring with surreptitious vomiting (Nicholls and Espiner, 1973; Wolff et al., 1968). Both functional and morphological changes may occur in the kidneys secondary to severe electrolyte disturbance (see section on Electrolytes) (Alvasaker et al., 1960).

Treatment

The complete treatment of vomiting is based on a definitive diagnosis of the underlying cause. Correctable organic lesions must be ruled out and a thorough investigation into possible psychological concomitants should be made when this is a possibility. In general, patients should be treated in a calm, reassuring environment, ideally alone and away from the sight or smell of food. Frequent small feedings are usually more desirable than large meals, and dietary supplements of various kinds may be useful. Psychotherapy of the patient and family, where warranted, is important, and behavioral kinds of approaches are frequently effective.

Proper use of anti-emetic drugs depends on an understanding of their dose response characteristics and pharmacokinetics. Harris (1978) recently reviewed these drugs from this viewpoint. Prominent anti-emetics include the phenothiazines which are good inhibitors of the apomorphine response (apomorphine is an emetic used to test the potency of anti-emetics.) Haldol has received a substantial amount of recent attention for the control of nausea and vomiting (Barton et al., 1975; Robbins and Nagle, 1975; Plotkin et al., 1973). These studies demonstrated that haloperidol, even in small dosages (2–4 mg), was effective in a significant number of patients. It is important to note that there have been several reports of vomiting occurring 24–48 hr after the abrupt withdrawal of several different neuroleptics. The frequency of these reports suggests that this may be a common phenomenon (Lacoursiere et al., 1976; Brooks, 1959; Gallant et al., 1964). A variety of other drugs have received both anecdotal and experimental support to suggest some effectiveness as anti-emetics. An isolated case reported by Reid and Leonard (1977) describes the treatment with lithium of cyclical vomiting in a mentally defective patient. The authors suggest that it may be worthwhile to use lithium to treat resistant cases of cyclical vomiting in children.

Dysphagia

Dysphagia, or difficulty in swallowing, is a common symptom. One of the original formulations of an "esophageal neurosis" resulting in dysphagia was "an unconscious rejection of incorporation resulting from aggressive impulses, often sexual in nature, such as castration wishes" (Kronfeld, 1934). Ambivalence between the desire and the attempt to swallow appeared to lead to dysphagia or regurgitation. Cardiospasm was also regarded as an "organ neurosis—deeply rooted in the unconscious life of the individual" (Weiss and English, 1957). Sexual, hostile, and self-punitive acts were felt to be operative in achalasia (failure to relex the smooth muscle fibers of the gastrointestinal tract at points of juncture). The belief in the predominantly emotional genesis in these disorders has been held even though symptom relief may be obtained by bouginage (dilatation with a bougie).

Perhaps because of an original report by Vinson (1922), which attributed cervical dysphagia in 59 female patients to conversion hysteria because radiologic and endoscopic abnormalities were not seen, a priori assumptions of this kind persist. The Plummer–Vinson (Kelly–Patterson) syndrome, or sideropenic dysphagia, was later elucidated more fully and found to be associated with anemia, mucosal changes, and esophageal webs.

Many esophageal diseases are now recognized as causing dysphagia. They include motility disturbances attributed to causes such as achalasia, diffuse spasm, scleroderma, neuropathy secondary to diabetes or alcoholism, myotonia dystrophica, polymyositis, and myasthenia gravis. Drug-induced loss of peristalsis with phenothiazine treatment has also been described (Cohen, 1973). Mechanical narrowing of the esophageal lumen due to pharyngeal diverticula, esophageal webs, esophageal compression secondary to benign tumors of carcinoma, Schatzki rings, or strictures secondary to chronic reflux will also produce symptoms. A more complete listing of differential etiologies can be found in Cohen's excellent review (Cohen, 1973).

Globus Hystericus

Globus is another major esophageal symptom with multiple causes. The term globus hystericus is used to define the subjective sensation of discomfort, a choking feeling or "lump in the throat," for which no causal organic factors can be found. *Hystericus* infers a neurotic basis, and psychoanalytic accounts of cases usually describe unconscious fantasies of hysterical women in which forbidden impulses are associated with the mouth. Most often, however, patients presenting with these symptoms lack a hysterical personality (Cohen, 1973). Globus is a rather common symptom in the general population; Elwood et al. (1964) found a prevalence of 1.5% in males and 5% in females in a study of 4805 subjects aged 40 to 75. In spite of this, controlled studies of the emotional basis for globus using objective psychiatric and esophageal testing methods are lacking.

It appears that any organic or motor disorder of the esophagus that causes either esophageal distention or late emptying can cause these symptoms. Many of the above mentioned conditions resulting in dysphagia will also cause complaints of globus. Gastroesophageal reflex appears likely to be responsible for a large number of globus complaints. In two recent studies, gastroesophageal reflux was identified radiologically in 11 of 12 and 22 of 25 patients complaining of globus (Delahunty and Ardran, 1970; Cherry, 1970). Perfusion of the distal esophagus with hydrocholoric acid (0.1 N) reproduced the globus sensation in 10 of the 12 patients. Moreover, intensive treatment of the reflux esophagitis completely relieved the globus sensations in all patients in both studies.

The exact impact of emotions on sphincter function in the globus syndrome has not been clarified. There is some suggestion that affect may directly alter esophageal motility (Ruben et al., 1962). As in general contemporary psychosomatic medicine, studies focusing on how emotional stress alters the physiology of organ systems are more likely to be fruitful than those that attempt to link emotional stress to the genesis of specific symptoms. However, most gastrointestinal specialists continue to feel that there are a significant number of patients whose esophageal symptoms have a primary psychogenic basis. When such emotional causes are actually present, they most often take the form of conversion symptoms, somatic delusions, and hypochondriasis (Cohen, 1973).

Detailed questioning aimed at eliciting specifics, such as the type of food that brings on the symptom, the amount of liquid needed to wash the food down, frequency of occurrence, when and where the sensation is felt, what the nature of the sensation is, and the length of time it persists, is most helpful. Neurotic symptoms are often vague. Even infrequent and intermittent symptoms may have an organic basis. For example, patients with minimal esophageal narrowing may sense dysphagia only when a large bolus of food is swallowed. Complete and occasionally repeated diagnostic workups may be needed. Psychogenesis should not be assumed.

Gastric and Intestinal Disorders

The psychosomatic literature abounds with studies of dynamics and personality characteristics of patients with varying kinds of GI disorders. In addition to the classic studies of peptic ulcer and ulcerative colitis, other intestinal disorders such as regional enteritis (Crohn disease), nontropical sprue (celiac disease), idiopathic steatorrhea, and irritable bowel have been examined. Most of these studies appear to be conflicting and inconclusive, though it appears to be widely accepted that there are changes in mood and personality among patients with gastrointestinal disorders. Paulley (1959) observed: "Even colleagues not interested in psychosomatic disorders have commented on their mental peculiarities," referring to patients with idiopathic steatorrhea. However, Goldberg (1970), found mental and psychological abnormalities associated with diseases of the small intestine to be many and varied, but not significantly different from those in the general population.

There are a number of reports of neurologic and psychiatric changes found in association with disordered function of the stomach and/or small intestine which might properly be called somatopsychic in that the physical disorder appears to be causal of neuropsychiatric changes. In most of the reported cases, the changes appear to have been caused by malabsorption of required nutrient substances leading to metabolic defects. In many, however, the exact mechanism is not understood.

Postgastrectomy States

There are several reports of serious neurologic disease as a late complication of gastric surgery and a suggestion that these complications are more common than might be expected (Banjeri and Hurwitz, 1971; Olivarious and Roos, 1968). In 1969, Williams et al. described 14 patients with neurologic disease occurring after partial gastrectomy. In this study, the psychiatric manifestations were not reported in detail, but the authors commented that psychopathic disturbances were a notable feature, and that many patients were difficult to treat due to their resistance to supervision. They reported 10 of 14 patients as having either depression or psychosis. Predominant neurologic symptoms consisted of difficulty walking, unsteadiness, muscular weakness, and paresthesias. Attacks of loss of consciousness were reported by five patients, while other common findings included muscle weakness and wasting, loss of vibration sense, and deficits in proprioception.

A particularly significant finding in this series and in other reports is that the average time of onset of the neurologic findings occurred ten or more years beyond the original surgery, highlighting the importance of obtaining an adequate history of surgical procedures. In the series of Williams et al., there was a preponderance of patients whose original operation had been for gastric ulcer as compared to those with duodenal ulcer (9:5). One patient had had a gastrojejunostomy and the others had Billroth II procedures (bypassing the duodenum).

There was evidence of vitamin B_{12} malabsorption with serum levels below normal in "most patients" (three of the patients had normal B_{12} levels). Response to vitamin B_{12} was variable, with three of the patients showing a good response. These appeared to be the patients with more florid neurologic disease typical of "subacute combined degeneration." The other patients had a rather poor overall response, although some appeared to improve temporarily with vitamin B_{12} or additional multivitamin preparations.

There are several reports in the literature of neurologic changes believed to be secondary to hypoglycemia following a gastrectomy (Hafken et al., 1975; Bacon and Myles, 1971; Belding and Freedman, 1960). Hypoglycemic convulsions, coma, and dementia have been described. The chronic organic brain changes have an insidious onset, with progression continuing many years after the surgery. (See Hypoglycemia section.)

Malabsorption Disorders

The principal intestinal disorders that have been associated with malabsorption syndromes include small intestinal diverticulosis, tropical sprue, regional enteritis, celiac disease, and Whipple disease. When neuropsychiatric symptoms are found in conjunction with these disorders, the usual symptoms of alimentary disturbances are likely to be present, including anorexia, abdominal pain of varying severity and location, vomiting, constipation and/or diarrhea, and abdominal distension. Bloating, weight loss, and arthralgia are also common findings in some of these illnesses.

None of these symptoms are specific for a particular intestinal disorder, and since the mechanism for production of neuropsychiatric symptoms is not completely known, they may be discussed as a group. The principal effects of the malabsorption syndrome are seen in peripheral nerve and spinal cord changes. The neuropathy affects the limbs primarily, the legs in particular, with numbness, tingling, pain, weakness, and unsteadiness of gait being the major complaints. Ataxia is often a primary problem. Evidence of posterior column involvement in the legs is marked with ankle jerk reflex being lost early, and sensory impairment of the glove and stocking type frequently found. The arms are less commonly affected, but common motor skills become difficult when there is impairment. Attacks of unconsciousness occur in many patients.

The course of these symptoms appears to be slowly progressive, and in a few patients Cooke (1978) noted that the course suggests an ascending polyneuritis of infectious origin leading to death from respiratory failure.

The mental status changes which have been described as associated with these diseases of the small intestine are quite variable. There are no studies which have specifically assessed psychiatric functioning other than Goldberg's (1970) study which examined idiopathic steatorrhea, Crohn disease and alactasia. In the study done by Cooke and Smith (1966) on neurologic disorders associated with adult celiac disease, two patients complained of memory loss and one other demonstrated confusion, with agitation and hallucinations. In all of these patients, the mental status changes were of late onset following considerable deterioration in the patient's general physical condition. Morris et al. (1970), investigating the incidence of neurologic disorder in 30 patients with adult celiac disease, found that three of the patients had severe depression and one suffered from transient attacks of loss of consciousness. It is not known where in the course of the illness these findings occurred. Cooke (1978) stated that it is "widely accepted that there are changes in mood and personality in the untreated celiac patients, particularly in children, mainly of a depressive nature." He also observed that this was profoundly influenced by the dietary gluten load, and he described striking improvement in "mental capacity" in one such patient following a gluten-free diet. Cooke further noted that in those celiac patients who had been followed to postmortem, there were some with progressive mental deterioration, some who had been diagnosed as suffering from an organic dementia, and some with evidence of cerebral atrophy. In 1976, he described two similar patients under treatment with a gluten-free diet in whom the progressive mental deterioration appeared to have been halted for four years (Cooke, 1976).

Similar findings have been noted among patients with Whipple disease, which is a rare adult-onset multisystem disorder, typically manifested by diarrhea, malabsorption, and other abdominal complaints, as well as arthritis, anemia, malaise, and fever, Present evidence points to an infectious cause. The most common neurologic signs noted have been myoclonus, supranuclear ophthalmoplegia, and ataxia. Hearing loss, dizziness, ocular inflammation, and papilledema have also occurred. The neuropsychiatric symptoms described by most investigators are those of organic cerebral impairment with memory loss, irritability, withdrawal and loss of interest, confusional states, and impaired memory being prominent. Progression of the illness seems to be that of dementia, although treatment interventions in several cases have reversed the cerebral manifestations (Feurle et al., 1979; Finelli, 1977; Knox et al., 1976). Significantly, Knox reported neurologic signs and symptoms occurring in patients more than one year after they had been treated with antibiotics for their proven Whipple disease.

The Carcinoid Syndrome

Carcinoid tumors are slowly-growing neoplasms of enterochromaffin cells. Occurring as small primary tumors of the ileum and appendix, the metastatic tumors associated with the carcinoid syndrome are the most common tumors found in this area. They may also be found in other tissue such as stomach, pancreas, thyroid, and lung. Unlike most metastatic cancers, carcinoid tumors have a very slow rate of growth, with most patients surviving five to ten years after the disease is recognized. Most morbidity results from the endocrine function of the tumor, though death may occur from complications secondary to tumor growth.

As with other types of tumors, the overall incidence of carcinoid tumor is highest in middle and old age, though appendiceal carcinoids occur most often in the 25- to 35-year-old age group. There is no apparent difference in sex distribution.

The carcinoid syndrome is mediated by release of biologically active agents by the tumor. Serotonin was the first such agent to be discovered, and overproduction of this amine is the most consistent biochemical indicator of the carcinoid syndrome. A variety of other indoles and chemically unrelated agents may also be synthesized and be partial mediators of the clinical syndrome. These agents include bradykinin, histamine, and adrenal corticotropic hormone (ACTH). Because of the great diversity in the production of biologically active substances, there is a varied spectrum of clinical manifestations.

Clinical Features.   The most common early symptom of the carcinoid syndrome is cutaneous flushing. This flushing may appear spontaneously or be precipitated by excitement, exertion, eating, alcohol, or epinephrine administration. It may also be produced by direct pressure upon the tumor. The typical flush is erythematous and involves the head and neck, and occasionally the entire upper half of the body. These episodic flushes may be accompanied by attacks of abdominal cramping pain, with either intermittent or chronic diarrhea. Symptoms vary according to the site of the primary tumor and the biochemical agent which is produced. Cardiopulmonary symptoms may be seen, consisting of bronchospasm with wheezing and dyspnea, as well as tachycardia or other signs of high cardiac output. These symptoms are usually most pronounced during the flushing attack. In addition to the endocrine effects, tumors may cause intestinal obstruction and secondary bleeding owing to their mass.

Laboratory Findings.   The diagnostic hallmark of carcinoid syndrome is an overproduction of 5-hydroxyindoles with increased urinary excretion of 5-hydroxyindoleacetic acid (5-HIAA). Thus, a quantative determination of 24-hour urinary excretion of 5-HIAA is usually diagnostic, although certain foods may contain enough serotonin to produce abnormally elevated urinary levels. Normal excretion of 5-HIAA does not exceed 9 mg daily.

Neuropsychiatric Features. Although the carcinoid syndrome has been long ascribed to excesses of serotonin, there has been little in the literature describing psychiatric symptoms. Often, when noted, symptoms have been attributed to the psychologic stress of chronic illness or explained on the basis of other somatic problems (Thorson, 1958; Wooley, 1962). In 1966, Sokoloff indicated that the incidence of mental abnormalities in patients with carcinoid tumors is far greater than generally assumed, and that the mental aberrations were a reflection of disturbed brain metabolism of 5-hydroxytryptamine. Lehmann (1966) reported an instance of carcinoid tumor in a women who had had a number of episodes of mental disturbance including severe depression, hypomania, and periodic confusion. Feedings of tryptophan appeared to reduce the symptoms. Major et al. (1973) reviewed the charts of 20 patients with the documented diagnosis of carcinoid tumor. Most of these patients had not received thorough evaluations of their mental status. Despite this handicap, the investigators concluded that 50% of the patients had evidence of depression, 35% evinced anxiety, and 35% had episodes of confusion or defects in sensorium. The three groups of symptoms were not mutually exclusive. Nevertheless, they felt that 15 of the 20 patients demonstrated disturbances in at least one of these three areas. In addition, a high percent of patients were receiving sleeping and tranquilizing medications.

The authors went on to try to explain these findings by noting evidence that serotonin is decreased in the brain in the presence of carcinoid tumors, and this may cause both depression and confusion. There appears to be two possible explanations for low levels of serotonin in the brain. First, brain serotonin may be decreased because the carcinoid tumor uses large quantities of tryptophan, which is then unavailable to cross the blood–brain barrier. Secondly, adrenal hormones may lower brain serotonin by inducing tryptophan pyrrolase in the liver, thus shunting the metabolism of tryptophan into kynurenine production. The authors felt that depression of brain 5-hydroxytryptamine levels may result in weakening of the inhibition process on the amygdaloid complex, the activation of which in man produces increases in the plasma 17-hydroxycorticosteroids.

Major et al. concluded their paper by quoting Bean and Funks' (1968) rhyme and by adding a second verse of their own:

> The man was addicted to moaning,
> Confusion, edema and groaning,
> Intestinal rushes,
> Great tricolored blushes
> And died from too much serotonin.
>
> Much peripheral serotonin production,
> Can lead to a striking induction
> Of depressive affects,
> Sleeping defects
> And abnormal mental perceptions.

Irritable Bowel Syndrome

Irritable bowel syndrome accounts for half the gastrointestinal complaints brought to the attention of the physician, and ranks second among the causes of industrial absenteeism due to illness (Almy, 1957; Ruoff, 1973). Despite numerous clinical investigations, no organic etiology for this syndrome has been discovered. Conversely, most physicians working in this area stress the eminence of psychological factors in the genesis of the condition.

The most pragmatic information gained from previous observations and studies suggest that the irritable bowel syndrome is often associated with a psychiatric disorder. Haffernon and Lippincott (1966) reported that psychotic depression may be masked by the irritable colon syndrome. Dorfman (1967) and Diamond (1964) suggested that spastic colon may be a symptom of depression. Young et al. (1976) found a 72% incidence of psychiatric illness among subjects with irritable bowel syndrome as compared to a control group (18%). Hysteria and depression were the most prevalent syndromes. The most methodologically sound study of the irritable bowel syndrome was done by Hislop (1971). Examining 67 patients with this syndrome, Hislop concluded that the syndrome complex is considered to be a concomitant of an affective disorder. Fifty-six percent of the patients received treatment with antidepressants, and 80% of these reported significant improvements. However, similar kinds of findings have been suggested by others (Feldman, 1965; Kasich, 1965). The average time of followup in this series was only three months.

Psychotropic Drugs and Alimentary Tract Disorders

Because psychiatric conditions, particularly affective disorders, are found in patients with gastrointestinal disease, these patients are very likely to be treated with psychotropic drugs. All psychotropic drugs appear to act on the gastrointestinal tract, causing combinations of central and peripheral effects. Depending on the illness, these effects may have beneficial results or may complicate or interfere with other therapeutic regimens. Knowledge in this area is still fragmentary, but some potential problems can be anticipated.

Tricyclic Antidepressants

The major effects of tricyclics that are pertinent to gastrointestinal illness are caused by their anticholinergic properties. Peripheral toxicity is marked by tachycardia, mydriasis, flushing of the skin, decreased sweating, increased temperature, decreased bronchial, pharyngeal, nasal, and salivary secretions, urinary retention, and decreased motility of the bowel. Certain of these effects, such as decreased bowel motility, may be desirable. The marked improvement reported in a study of patients with irritable colon syndrome may be partially attributable to this "side effect" (Hislop, 1971). Anticholinergic influences resulting in the inhibition of gastric acid secretion may be helpful in peptic ulcer disease or may inhibit nausea and vomiting in other conditions (Bonfils et al., 1962; Avery, 1976).

The significant possibility of adverse consequences in gastrointestinal disease is also related to anticholinergic phenomena. Because other drugs, particularly the antispasmodics, such as methantheline (Banthine) and propantheline (Probanthine), also have anticholinergic properties, additive effects are possible when they are used with tricyclics. This is especially likely if an additional psychotropic medication, such as an antipsychotic drug, is being used. Neuropsychiatric disturbances may occur centrally with an anticholinergic syndrome. Central toxic effects include anxious agitation, restless hyperactivity, delirium, disorientation with hallucinations, defects of recent memory, dysarthria, and seizures. The elderly are particularly susceptible. Management of this syndrome is now feasible with physostigmine (Granacher and Baldessarini, 1976).

Peripheral effects occur at various levels of the gastrointestinal tract. Drugs that produce anticholinergic effects are contraindicated in the presence of esophageal reflux or pyloric stenosis because they inhibit the "clearing" of acid contents of the esophagus (Avery, 1976). Heartburn may also be aggravated if the patient has a hiatal hernia. Similar effects on the large bowel must also be considered. Constipation is a common complaint among patients receiving tricyclics, although it is often difficult to determine whether it is secondary to the drug or to the underlying depression (Ayd, 1960). Decreased intestinal motility and chronic constipation may lead to ileus, particularly in the elderly. Amitriptyline (Elavil) and nortriptyline (Aventyl) have been reported to be associated with paralytic ileus in several cases (Gander and Devlin, 1963; Burkitt and Sutcliff, 1961; Milner and Hills, 1966).

Awareness of the anticholinergic potential of drug combinations as well as the strength of individual drugs will allow drug selection to minimize these effects. Animal experiments suggest that the order of anticholinergic potency of the tricyclics is (in descending order): amitriptyline (Elavil), doxepin (Sinequan), nortriptyline (Aventyl), imipramine (Tofranil), and desipramine (Norpramin) (Granacher and Baldessarini, 1976). Amitriptyline has approximately eight times the antimuscarinic potency of imipramine, and 17 times that of desipramine. The monoamine-oxidase inhibitor group of antidepressants appears to have no clinically significant anticholinergic effects.

Antipsychotics

The effects of antipsychotic drugs on patients with gastrointestinal illness are also largely related to their anticholinergic properties. The antipsychotics have substantially less anticholinergic effect than the tricyclics; however, since they are often combined with antiparkinsonian drugs, which have high antimuscarinic potency, this potential cannot be ignored. Both central and peripheral effects may occur. Decreased gastrointestinal tract motility at all levels is also present. Megacolon, intestinal dilatation, and abdominal distention have also been described with long-term chlorpromazine (Thorazine) therapy (Greiner and Nicholson, 1964; Ritama et al., 1969). Evans et al. (1979) reviewed the literature in this area and added a case report of a fatality secondary to intestinal dilatation. Thioridazine (Mellaril) and chlorprothixene (Taractan) have also been implicated. Based on animal studies, thioridazine clearly has the strongest anticholinergic effect, approximately seven times that of chlorpromazine. These two drugs are followed in magnitude of anticholinergic effect by perphenazine (Trilafon), fluphenazine (Prolixin), and trifluoperazine (Stelazine). Haloperidol (Haldol) has the least effect, approximately one three-hundredth that of thioridazine (Granacher and Baldessarini, 1976).

Some studies have suggested that liquid chlorpromazine should not be given with antacids because of absorption by the antacid (aluminum-magnesium hydroxide gel and magnesium trisilicate-aluminum hydroxide gel) (Fann, 1973; Forrest et al., 1970). The exact significance of these reports for long-term administration is not clear, and no reports on absorption when chlorpromazine is given in the tablet form have appeared.

Antianxiety Drugs

Antianxiety agents are commonly used for gastrointestinal disturbances. Since the anticholinergic effects of these drugs are minimal, they do not constitute contraindications to their use. It appears that beneficial responses to treatment with antianxiety agents result from reduction of anxiety rather than from peripheral autonomic effects. The rate of absorption of chlordiazepoxide (Librium) has been reported as being slowed by concomitant administration of the antacid magnesium-aluminum hydroxide gel. However, the total amount absorbed and the rate of elimination remained the same. This interaction is probably significant only in treatment of acute anxiety states, when the desired rapid absorption of a single dose of chlordiazepoxide might be prevented by the presence of an antacid. The steady state level of the drug in longer term administration appears to remain unchanged. Similar findings have been reported for clorazepate (Tranxene).

Neuropsychiatric Effects of Alimentary Tract Drugs

Cimetidine

The competitive histamine H_2 receptor antagonist, cimetidine, is widely used to decrease gastric acid secretion in the treatment of duodenal ulcer and pathological hypersecretory syndromes. Experimental uses include the treatment of benign gastric ulcer, gastroesophogeal reflex, acute gastric hemorrhage, and pancreatic insufficiency.

Although the drug is generally well tolerated, there is a low but real incidence of neuropsychiatric toxicity. The most common manifestation is that of a classic organic brain syndrome with findings such as lethargy, coma, restlessness, disorientation, confusion, agitation, delirium, unsteadiness, slurred speech, visual impairment, visual hallucinations, and incontinence (McMillen et al., 1978; Schentag et al., 1979; Barnhart and Bowden, 1979). One case of cimetidine-induced depression has been reported, suggesting that under proper conditions the organic mental disorder can have an affectiform presentation (Jefferson, 1979).

Although cimetidine-induced central nervous system toxicity can occur in the absence of predisposing factors, the presence of one or more of the following is likely to render a patient more susceptible to toxicity:

1. Advanced age
2. Renal dysfunction
3. Hepatic dysfunction
4. Associated serious medical problems
5. Higher than recommended dosage
6. Associated use of psychotropic medication
7. Preexisting organic brain syndrome
8. Co-existing psychiatric illness

If promptly recognized, this drug-induced organic mental disorder is readily reversible. Misdiagnosis, on the other hand, will result in increased risk of morbidity, needless suffering, unnecessary diagnostic procedures, and inappropriate and potentially dangerous treatment.

The use of cimetidine has also been associated with male sexual dysfunction. Decreased libido and erectile dysfunction were reported in four patients, two of whom improved when the drug was discontinued (Wolfe, 1979; Peden et al., 1979). The available data are insufficient to establish a firm cause and effect relationship. There is also some evidence that cimetidine can effect male fertility, as evidenced by one study which found a 30% reduction in sperm count after treatment, which was felt to reflect dysfunction of the hypothalamic–pituitary–gonadal axis (Van Thiel et al., 1979).

PANCREATIC DISORDERS

Carcinoma

Pancreatic carcinoma, which represents about 4% of all malignancies in the general population (12% in diabetics), occurs approximately twice as often among males, with the highest incidence in the sixth and seventh decades of life (Gullick, 1959). The disease is seldom seen before age 40, with a history of chronic alcohol intake frequently being found (Ansari, 1970). A high index of clinical suspicion in addition to techniques such as pancreatic angiography and radioisotope photoscanning are helpful in diagnosis.

When only "medical" symptoms are considered, pancreatic cancer has a very rapid progression. Most patients have had these symptoms for less than four months before hospitalization; some patients (41% in one series) first have symptoms only in the previous month (Lowe and Palmer, 1967; Thamsen et al., 1950). Following the first hospital admission, a large majority of patients with pancreatic carcinoma die within 10 months, and many die earlier (Lowe and Palmer, 1967). Although considered by some to be an "incurable disease," prolonged survivals of pancreatic carcinoma lasting five or more years are now being reported. Palliative surgery may further lengthen this interval. Success depends upon early diagnosis.

It has long been known that psychiatric symptoms occur in association with carcinoma of the pancreas, but this knowledge has had little practical impact. Neuropsychiatric manifestations early in the course of the illness have usually been viewed either as an error in diagnosis or as an example of the misleading early presentation of this disease. The possible positive diagnostic value of initial psychiatric signs and symptoms in an illness in which early diagnosis is imperative has thus been largely ignored.

Clinical Features

The most common clinical features of carcinoma of the pancreas are pain, weight loss, and jaundice. The most frequent presenting complaint is pain (though this may not be the initial symptom). It is also the most common symptom, eventually occurring in 77% to 87% of patients (Ansari, 1970). Occasionally, pain may be the only symptom, particularly when the tumor originates in the body or tail of the pancreas. Typically the pain is described as epigastric or central abdominal, boring in quality, and radiating to the back. Some patients complain only of back pain. The reported pain lacks absolute characteristics. It may range from vague to intense, may be episodic or constant, and may vary in location, occasionally being experienced in the chest. It is often relieved by sitting up and bending forward and increases in intensity at night. These phenomena appear related to pressure exerted on associated structures, particularly the celiac plexus, when the patient is in a lying position. The pain usually bears no relationship to meals.

Weight loss is a frequent symptom and is usually rapid and severe. Twenty to forty pounds' loss in a two- to six-month period is common. Anorexia may be present but is not invariable and doesn't appear to account for all of the weight loss. In the early stages, patients may describe only vague dyspeptic symptoms, although nausea and vomiting can occur later, depending on the growth of the tumor. Weakness and fatigue usually accompany the weight loss.

Jaundice is the next most frequent presenting sign, occurring much less often than commonly believed (in 16–28% of patients) (Rash, 1969). Painless, progressive jaundice is rare, occurring most often with carcinoma of the head of the pancreas. It is generally a late sign.

Other symptoms include changes in bowel habits, most often constipation (which is difficult to separate from that found in depression), but occasionally diarrhea. Thrombophlebitis migrans, a condition in which multiple lesions affect short portions of veins scattered throughout the body, is also seen. These lesions, which are reddened, inflamed, and tender, disappear in a week or two, only to reappear elsewhere. This syndrome has also been described in association with carcinoma of various other organs. Other symptoms depend on the extent and direction of invasion by the advancing tumor.

A careful abdominal examination commonly reveals tenderness, enlargement of the liver, and/or a palpable mass. In one series, approximately one half of the patients presented with a mass, although this is generally a late finding (Lowe and Palmer, 1967). Other late manifestations are a palpable gall bladder or ascites.

Laboratory Findings

Laboratory findings vary considerably, depending on the site and extent of tumor encroachment. None is a reliable diagnostic guide. Anemia is common; one study reported that 33% of patients had a hemoglobin concentration of less than 12 g% (Ansari, 1970). A hematocrit of less than 35% in 30% of patients with carcinoma of the head of the pancreas has also been reported (Gullick, 1959).

Serum amylase and lipase levels may be elevated, normal, or decreased. Changes in serum lipase levels appear to be more consistently correlated with abnormalities secondary to pancreatic cancer. Liver function studies may also be abnormal in a direction indicating an extrahepatic biliary obstruction. Lowered serum protein is also common.

Pancreatic cancer has a dual relationship with diabetes, in that it occurs most often in diabetic patients and also occasionally produces diabetes. However, neither fasting blood sugars nor glucose tolerance tests are clinically very useful in diagnosing pancreatic cancer. Stool guaiac tests are positive when bleeding into the gut occurs.

Neuropsychiatric Features

In 1931 Yaskin wrote a paper titled, "Nervous Symptoms as Earliest Manifestations of Carcinoma of the Pancreas," in which he described depression with crying spells, insomnia unresponsive to sleeping medications, and anxiety with premonitions of serious illness among patients who were later diagnosed as having pancreatic carcinoma. Since then others have described similar findings (Perlas and Faillace, 1964; Savage and Noble, 1954; Latter and Wilbur, 1937; Kohn, 1952; Rickles, 1945). Perhaps because of the anecdotal nature, these reports appear to have had little impact on either psychiatrists or nonpsychiatric physicians.

In 1967, Fras et al., in a study of 46 consecutively admitted patients with carcinoma of the pancreas, provided remarkable support for earlier writings. Fras and Litin (1967) searched diligently for earliest symptoms, being careful not to exclude psychological experiences; they then compared those symptoms to those found in patients with other intra-abdominal neoplasms. Forty-six percent of patients with pancreatic cancer first experienced only mental symptoms, which preceded physical symptoms by an average of six months, with a range of 1 to 43 months. Symptoms of depression were most frequent. The incidence of these symptoms was substantially higher than in a control group consisting of patients with carcinoma of the colon and a "mixed" group. The overall incidence of psychiatric symptoms in the course of illness prior to surgery was 76% in the pancreatic carcinoma group, compared to 17% and 20% in the others. Data from the Minnesota Multiphasic Personality Inventory supported the clinical findings of increased depression in the pancreatic group.

Although the described depression was not specifically characteristic of pancreatic carcinoma, there were common features worth reviewing. In general, the depression was mild or moderate. They noted "loss of ambition" (often the patient's exact words) as the most frequently reported first symptom. Patients also used terms such as "lack of go," "loss of initiative," and "loss of push" to describe this feeling. They spoke of the feeling as unusual in their lives and clearly differentiated it from fatigue or physical illness. Later this feeling was accompanied by depressive-like sadness ("feeling lowdown," "being in the dumps," etc.). The ability to concentrate was only minimally impaired for these patients, and there appeared to be no change in perception, memory, or judgment. Self-accusatory ideation, paranoid features, delusions, and feelings of guilt or worthlessness were not present. Hopelessness, when present, was not complete, and help was sought and accepted. Suicidal ideation was infrequent and not acted upon.

A very specific type of anxiety has often been noted by internists and even labeled "pancreatic anxiety" (Savage and Noble, 1954). Frequent clinical reports describe patients who sit upright, holding their knees and rocking to and fro in an extreme state of anxiety or panic. Sometimes this anxiety coincides with the onset of pain, but more often it seems related to the conviction of some "imminent physical danger which no amount of suggestion or persuasion could allay" (Yaskin, 1931). These patients are convinced there is something seriously wrong with their health and often specifically believe it is cancer.

The usual vegetative signs of depression are difficult to separate from those associated with the pancreatic lesion itself. Early reports described a characteristic insomnia not relieved by usual methods, which is likely to be related to pain and the additional distress of lying down. Symptoms such as anorexia, weight loss, fatigue, and constipation may be directly related to the cancer, especially late in the course of illness.

Most patients have no history of depression, no family history of psychiatric illness, and no obvious precipitating events. Although relatives and physicians often ascribe the illness to various external events or psychogenic causes, the patient is not inclined to do so. In some cases the depressive symptoms have responded to treatment (Savage and Noble, 1954).

The reasons for the increased incidence of psychiatric symptoms in patients with carcinoma of the pancreas are unknown. Since they occur well before physical symptoms or a definitive diagnosis, they do not appear to be a reaction to the symptoms or to knowledge of the malignancy. Various hypotheses have been suggested. Yaskin quotes William James, who maintained that emotions are the sensation of body changes registered in the cortex; emotions are "sensory qualities arising from visceral or body changes duplicated in imagery." (Yaskin, 1931). Might the retroperitoneal location somehow affect the autonomic system? One study comparing symptoms of retroperitoneal lymphomas, lymphoma in other locations, and pancreatic carcinomas was performed at least in part to answer this question. The finding of a higher incidence of psychiatric symptoms in pancreatic carcinoma patients than in those with retroperitoneal lymphomas suggests that other factors still need to be considered. Does the neoplastic process affect an unknown function of the pancreas? Could the loss of ambition be correlated with the giving-up stance often seen following object loss and thus be facilitating the neoplastic process?

In summary, psychiatric symptoms appear to precede somatic ones by a substantial period of time. The diagnosis of pancreatic carcinoma might be made earlier if physicians had a high index of suspicion of patients who are 50–70 years old, usually male, lack psychiatric history or definitive external causal factors, and present with an uncharacteristic depressive complex. They often describe a feeling that there is something wrong (described as a loss of ambition or premonition of impending doom), have pain of the abdomen or back, and have weight loss that is often extreme, with or without anorexia. In the early period the depression lacks vegetative signs. At this point, proceeding with a more thorough physical examination of the abdomen, basic laboratory tests, and consultation will improve diagnostic yield. Recognizing pancreatic carcinoma by means of the psychiatric picture may provide the margin necessary to substantially prolong life in this deadly illness.

Pancreatitis

A well-known clinical entity, pancreatitis is the inflammation and destruction of pancreatic tissue. It usually results from anatomic or physiologic destruction of the ampulla of Vater, causing reflux of pancreatic secretions. Acute attacks tend to become recurrent and may progress to a chronic form with irreversible tissue damage. Although in a significant portion of cases causes are unknown, pancreatitis often occurs in association with chronic alcoholism and other diseases of the biliary system.

An association between mental functioning and both the acute and chronic forms of pancreatitis has been repeatedly observed. In 1941, eight cases of a specific syndrome of acute pancreatitis and encephalopathy were reported by Rothermich and von Hamm, who first coined the term pancreatic encephalopathy. The clinical picture was described as resembling an acute toxic psychosis with rather abrupt onset, disorientation, marked agitation, incoherency, and vivid auditory and visual hallucinations. However intervals of marked lucidity were common. Other authors have noted similar findings in less detailed reports (Schuster and Iber, 1965; Rickles, 1945; Savage et al., 1972). These authors suggest that high circulating levels of pancreatic enzyme are at fault, either by virtue of their inherent toxicity or their effect on cerebral fat or carbohydrate metabolism. There have been no later reports dealing specifically with psychoses and pancreatitis, although many general studies mention psychiatric symptoms.

One interesting case report suggests that pancreatitis represents a psychophysiologic response to a specific psychiatric conflict and its affects (Tripp and Agle, 1968). It attempts to document the effect of mental functioning on pancreatic disease rather than the converse. Seven episodes of pancreatitis occurring as a response to a specific conflict in specific situations were documented in a patient seen in ongoing psychotherapy. Lawton and Phillips (1955) also attempted to demonstrate more objectively the existence of psychopathology in a group of patients with chronic relapsing pancreatitis and further explored possible patterns of psychodynamics.

HEPATIC DISORDERS

Hepatic Encephalopathy

If the liver is unable to carry out its appropriate functions (because of advanced hepatocellular disease and/or extensive portal–systemic collateral shunting), profound neuropsychiatric complications can occur. Among the terms used to refer to this condition are "hepatic encephalopathy," "hepatic coma," and "portal–systemic encephalopathy." The earlier phase of the syndrome is called "impending hepatic coma" or "hepatic precoma."

Clinical Features

The clinical course of hepatic encephalopathy can be acute or chronic, mild or severe, intermittent or progressive, or self-limiting. Because the course will have a modifying effect on the manifestations, the overview that follows should be considered a generalization requiring adaptation to specific situations.

Stages of Hepatic Coma. As an aid in assessing clinical course and prognosis, the progression of hepatic encephalopathy has been divided into stages (Table 5-1).

Prodrome. The prodromal phase of hepatic coma may be so subtle that it is apparent only to those who know the patient well or is recognized in retrospect only after more serious manifestations occur. There is no characteristic presentation, and mental status alterations may be nonspecific and misleading. Patients have been described as apathetic, depressed, or euphoric. Hallucinations have been reported preceding the onset of coma. Excessive daytime drowsiness may be an early manifestation, followed later by reversal of the sleep cycle, with nocturnal wandering and confusion. Although the patient may appear normal to the casual observer, formal mental status testing will usually reveal organic deficits. Establishing the presence of organic deficits at this stage is quite important, since otherwise the mood changes may suggest a functional affective disorder.

The onset of the prodromal stage may be so gradual as to defy recognition until it is well established and it may wax and wane in severity for days or weeks. The addition or removal of precipitating factors is probably responsible for much of the variability. If the clinical course of liver failure is fulminant, the prodromal phase may be compressed into a very brief period.

Precoma. The classic findings in the precoma stage are:

1. Mental confusion
2. Asterixis (flapping tremor)
3. EEG abnormalities

While none of these is diagnostic of hepatic coma, and while all three need not be present in this stage, their combined presence in someone with severe liver disease is virtually diagnostic of impending hepatic coma.

The **mental status alterations** are those of a progressive organic brain syndrome, with paranoid features often present. Constructional apraxia is a characteristic finding, as exemplified by the patient's inability to construct a star from five matches, copy diagrams, or reproduce a design.

Asterixis, sometimes known as "liver flap," is a characteristic tremor which is usually, but not always, present in this stage. The tremor is caused by an inability to maintain posture and is best demonstrated by having the patient hold his arms outstretched, fingers extended and wrists dorsiflexed. The movements are arrhythmic and rapid, with lateral finger deviations and flexion–extension at the wrist and metacarpophalangeal joints. The presence of asterixis is *not* diagnostic of liver disease, and can occur in renal failure, respiratory failure, heart failure, and with other metabolic imbalances. If deep coma ensues, the patient will no longer be able to maintain the posture necessary to produce the flapping tremor and it will disappear. If the patient

TABLE 5-1. Stages in Onset and Development of Hepatic Coma[a]

	Mental state	Tremor	EEG changes
Prodrome (often only in retrospect)	Euphoria, occasionally depression Confusion, absent or difficult to detect Slight slowing on mentation Untidiness	Often present but slight	Usually absent
Impending coma	Confusion Usually euphoria Drowsiness Inappropriate behavior	Usually present and easily elicitable	Almost always present
Stupor	Sleeps most of time but arousable Confusion, marked	Usually present if patient can cooperate	Almost always present
Semicoma or coma	Unconsciousness May respond to noxious stimuli or, when deep, may not respond	Usually absent (no muscle tone)	Often present

[a] From Davidson and Gabuzda (1975) with permission of authors and publisher.

recovers, the tremor eventually disappears, although it may persist for days or weeks.

Adams and Foley (1953) described the characteristic **EEG alteration** in hepatic coma as a "paroxysmal bilaterally synchronous slow wave abnormality superimposed on a background of relatively normal features." These findings are *not* specific for impending hepatic coma, since they are found in a wide variety of toxic–metabolic conditions. They are also not inevitably present in this stage of hepatic coma. Adams and Foley (1953), for example, found typical slow waves in only 22 of 25 patients.

The EEG is a valuable tool in both the diagnosis and monitoring of hepatic encephalopathy. In the early phases of the illness, a fasting EEG may be normal, where a recording after protein or ammonium chloride loading or sedative administration is likely to reveal characteristic changes. Serial EEGs are also useful in evaluating response to various treatment interventions.

The course of the precoma stage can be quite variable, ranging from hours to weeks, with wide fluctuations in severity. Diagnosis of precoma is quite important because treatment at this stage can prevent progression to coma with its attendant high mortality.

Stupor and Coma. With progression of the illness, the patient becomes more obtunded, more difficult to arouse, and less responsive to noxious stimuli. Although the patient may appear to be sleeping peacefully, severe metabolic derangements are present. Abnormal reflexes, limb rigidity, and convulsions are common, yet deep coma may be accompanied by areflexia, loss of rigidity, and unresponsiveness to any stimuli. Death may occur from secondary complications such as bleeding or overwhelming sepsis, or a more chronic course may ensue.

Other Forms of Hepatic Coma. While the four stages of hepatic coma provide a general background, there are many variations on this theme. Chen and Chen (1977) described several patterns which are determined, in part, by the underlying hepatic disease. The **acute pattern** usually occurs in association with fulminant liver failure due to virus, drugs, or other toxins although it may also be seen with alcoholic hepatitis and chronic active hepatitis. The mortality rate approaches 75%. Onset may be "dramatic with delirium, violent behavior, convulsions, and a clouding of consciousness, which rapidly passes into coma in hours or days."

A second pattern consists of apathy, drowsiness, intellectual impairment, and progressive stupor, which has a slow, subtle onset, is often associated with precipitating causes, and is usually reversible.

The authors also refer to a less common third pattern known as "**acquired (nonWilsonian) chronic hepatocerebral degeneration**," which is characterized by relatively irreversible neurological disturbances such as dementia, dysarthria, ataxia, intention tremor, and choreoathetosis.

Portal–Systemic Encephalopathy. If blood is shunted, either surgically or by disease processes, so that the liver is bypassed, marked central nervous system abnormalities can occur, even in the presence of a relatively normal liver. This can be demonstrated in animals by ligating the portal vein and shunting blood directly into the inferior vena cava (an Eck fistula). A meat diet (protein load) in this setting can cause ataxia, convulsions, and impaired consciousness.

When portal hypertension in man is treated surgically by portal–systemic shunting, the incidence of hepatic encephalopathy is quite high. Sherlock et al. (1970) found that over a five-year period, 80–90% of shunted patients developed encephalopathy.

The symptoms of portal–systemic encephalopathy are variations of those described under the stages of hepatic coma. However, since the clinical course may be quite protracted and varied, and since severe intrinsic liver disease is not necessarily present, accurate early diagnosis may be a problem. Sherlock et al. (1954) and Summerskill et al. (1956) mention the following misdiagnoses:

1. Anxiety state
2. Psychotic depression
3. Hysterical ataxia
4. Psychomotor epilepsy
5. Frontal lobe tumor
6. Narcolepsy
7. Multiple sclerosis
8. Cerebral arteriosclerosis
9. Wilson disease
10. Parkinson disease

Patients, unfortunately, have been admitted to psychiatric hospitals by physicians unaware of the true diagnosis (Havens and Child, 1955; Summerskill et al., 1956). Leevy (1974) described such a case—a 56-year-old woman with no history of liver disease, jaundice, alcoholism, or toxin exposure who developed depressions which were aggravated by eating (worsening after a protein load should have suggested the correct diagnosis). Symptoms of both mania and depression, coupled with hallucinations and poor grooming led to psychiatric hospitalization. Examination at that time revealed asterixis, constructional apraxia, and EEG slowing, and the correct diagnosis of hepatic encephalopathy was finally made.

The neuropsychiatric changes following portal–systemic surgical shunts may be quite atypical. Read et al. (1967) reported 21 cases of encephalopathy, 5 of whom were diagnosed as schizophrenia and 1 as hypomania and dementia. Those patients were considered unusual, in that their psychiatric manifestations did not change with dietary protein manipulations that characteristically improve or worsen hepatic encephalopathy. Since they also showed more conventional findings of encephalopathy that could be distinguished from the psychosis, the role of the shunt in causing the schizophrenic or hypomanic symptoms can be questioned.

Of interest is the theory of Kroll and Fog (1968) that certain mental disorders are actually caused by "autointoxication" secondary to portal–systemic shunts. The theory was developed from evidence obtained by postmortem portography studies in psychiatric and senile patients and has not been further substantiated.

It should be emphasized that **personality changes** may be the first manifestations of hepatic coma (Kornfeld, 1973). Proper diagnosis at this time depends on a high index of suspicion, coupled with a thorough mental status examination, physical evaluation for stigmata of liver disease and portal hypertension, and appropriate laboratory testing (the EEG is especially helpful).

Acquired, Chronic Hepatocerebral Degeneration. A less common manifestation of portal-systemic shunting is a relatively *irreversible* neurological syndrome which was first described by Victor et al. (1965). Findings included dementia, dysarthria, ataxia, intention tremor, grimacing, and choreoathetosis. Additional manifestations include pyramidal and extrapyramidal signs, muscular rigidity, grasp reflexes, nystagmus, paraplegia, and permanent myelopathy. Mental status findings are those of an organic brain syndrome, which may vary from quite severe to intermittent and barely detectable. In some patients, delusions and hallucinations are also present. Read et al. (1967) described five patients with paraplegia and upper motor neuron signs and five with basal ganglia and cerebellar disturbances, none of whom responded favorably to standard hepatic coma treatment.

Victor et al. (1965) distinguished this syndrome from hepatic coma because of its irreversibility, and also because it became well established in some patients before the first episode of hepatic coma occurred. Most workers, however, consider these syndromes to be different stages of the same process, all of which have in common deranged hepatic function and/or portal–systemic shunting. It would be wise to consider any neuropsychiatric syndrome developing in the presence of those conditions to be etiologically related until clearly proven otherwise.

Laboratory Findings

The usual laboratory tests of hepatic function (serum bilirubin, enzymes, prothrombin activity, etc.) tend to be abnormal and to reflect activity of the liver disease, but do not correlate well with the diagnosis or prognosis of hepatic coma. The absence of jaundice or the presence of a normal serum bilirubin does not exclude the possibility of hepatic coma.

Arterial blood ammonia levels have been a more useful laboratory guide to hepatic coma, with the ammonia level correlating well with the severity of coma. Also, interventions which increase or decrease blood ammonia tend to cause corresponding changes in the level of coma. The correlation is not perfect, however, and 10% of patients with hepatic coma do not have elevated blood ammonia levels (Chen and Chen, 1977). In addition, technical difficulties with the determination can produce misleading and unreliable results.

Precipitating Factors

A precipitating factor can be identified in over half of the patients who develop hepatic coma, and, once identified, appropriate treatment may readily reverse the coma. Chen and Chen (1977) list the following factors:

1.   Protein excess (dietary, gastrointestinal hemorrhage)
2.   Ammonia overload (diuretics, hypokalemic alkalosis, uremia, frequent paracenteses)
3.   Cerebral depressants (sedatives, narcotics, anesthetics)
4.   Increased tissue catabolism (infections, acute pancreatitis, hepatoma)

Pathogenesis

A number of theories have evolved to explain the pathogenesis of hepatic encephalopathy but none, as yet, has been universally proven. The most important studies and speculations have concerned:

1.   Ammonia
2.   Amino acid inbalance
3.   Short chain fatty acids
4.   Mercaptans
5.   Biogenic amines

For a more detailed discussion of these theories, the reader is referred to Schenker et al. (1974), Davidson and Gabuzda (1975), Chen and Chen (1977), and Baldessarini and Fischer (1977).

Differential Diagnosis

Hepatic precoma and coma must be distinguished from the other complications of alcoholism. Since delirium tremens is treated with sedatives, and since sedatives can aggravate hepatic coma, this distinction is especially important. Findings suggestive of delirium tremens include appearance following alcohol withdrawal, agitation, vivid visual hallucinations, and a coarse rhythmic nonflapping tremor. Other alcohol-associated disorders include Wernicke encephalopathy, Korsakoff psychosis, alcoholic hallucinosis, and alcohol-induced hypoglycemia.

The cerebral consequences of head trauma can also be confused with hepatic coma. Subdural hematoma is a common complication of alcoholism, and since a clear history of trauma is not always available, it is wise to proceed to more definitive testing (computerized axial tomography) in case of doubt.

The hepatic and neurological findings in Wilson disease may be suggestive of hepatic encephalopathy. The tremor in Wilson disease tends to be choreoathetoic rather than flapping, and, *if sought*, the diagnostic Kayser–Fleischer corneal ring will be found.

The "functional" psychiatric disorders are less likely to be confused with hepatic coma, yet, given the varied neuropsychiatric presentations of the latter (see above), misdiagnosis remains a possibility.

Treatment

Treatment of hepatic coma is directed toward (1) preventing further damage to the liver, (2) controlling precipitating factors, and (3) reducing nitrogenous substances in the blood (Chen and Chen, 1977). A detailed discussion of these measures and elaboration upon more speculative and heroic approaches is beyond the scope of this book. Of both pathogenic and therapeutic interest is the finding that L-dopa (Parkes et al., 1970; Loiudice et al., 1979) and the dopamine receptor agonist, bromocriptine, (Morgan et al., 1977) may produce striking, although sometimes temporary, improvement in hepatic encephalopathy.

Posthepatitis Syndrome

A particularly troublesome condition occupying the borderland between "functional" and "organic" is the posthepatitis (or prolonged convalescence) syndrome (Kornfeld, 1973). Some patients who appear to have recovered from an episode of viral hepatitis (with normalization of biochemical and morphological tests) continue to have persistent complaints. Symptoms include:

1. Depression
2. Listlessness
3. Easy fatigability
4. Weakness
5. Anorexia
6. Lack of libido
7. Abdominal pains
8. Backache
9. Fatty food intolerance
10. Anxiety

When compared to asymptomatic posthepatitis patients, this group shows no difference in isolated abnormalities of liver function or morphological changes on liver biopsy.

The syndrome was first reported in soldiers during World War II, and was felt, in general, to represent a maladaptive emotional response to illness. Benjamin and Hoyt (1945) reported on 200 soldiers who, despite resolution of acute illness, were unable to return to duty five to nine months later. Of the 135 who had psychiatric evaluations, 115 were diagnosed as having a psychoneurosis. Others, however, appeared more physically ill and had a higher number of abnormal physical and laboratory findings. It is unfortunate that this large study took place at a time when more sophisticated biochemical and morphological studies were not available.

Whether this syndrome of prolonged convalescence is an intrinsic feature of viral hepatitis (there are similarities to the postinfluenza syndrome) or whether it represents an emotional response to a physical illness in a properly predisposed patient is unresolved (Mosley and Galambos, 1969). Because the syndrome gradually resolves in most patients, reassurance coupled with measures to discourage reinforcement of illness behaviors are important aspects of treatment.

Psychotropic Drugs and the Liver

Psychotropic Drug Disposition and Elimination

General Considerations. The disposition and elimination of drugs that are metabolized in the liver can be expected to be altered in the presence of liver disease. Detecting and quantitating the contribution of altered liver function may be difficult, however, due to the presence of nonhepatic factors such as age, sex, nutritional status, renal function, urinary pH, and the presence of other drugs which can also alter drug metabolism (Schenker et al., 1975; Hoyumpa et al., 1978). Other problems include lack of adequately matched control groups and difficulty determining the extent of liver damage. Finally, the elimination half-life of a drug depends not only on clearance of the drug by the eliminating organs but also on the volume of distribution of the drug in the body (Schenker et al., 1975). Hepatic clearance of a drug, in turn, is a reflection of hepatic blood flow, amount of free drug available, the extent of portal–systemic shunting, and hepatic metabolizing enzyme activity. With these considerations in mind, the effect of liver disease on disposition and elimination of the different classes of psychiatric drugs will be discussed.

Barbiturates. Schenker et al. (1975) state:

> In summary then, the present information on the fate of barbiturates in patients with liver disease is limited and at times conflicting. It would appear, however, that the elimination of these drugs in general is impaired in patients with chronic liver disease, particularly if it is of a severe nature, but that the extent of the abnormality (at least for pentobarbital and phenobarbital) is only modest.

Although 30% of a dose of phenobarbital is excreted unchanged by the kidneys, the elimination half-life of the drug in cirrhotic patients was 130 hr compared to 86 hr in controls (Alvin et al., 1975). The same study found no significant prolongation of half-life in patients with acute viral hepatitis.

Benzodiazepines. Liver-disease related alterations in benzodiazepine metabolism have been summarized by Hoyumpa et al. (1978). The elimination half-life of **diazepam** is prolonged in the presence of alcoholic cirrhosis, acute viral hepatitis, and hepatic malignancy, but not with extrahepatic obstruction. The difference in diazepam half-life in alcoholic cirrhosis and viral hepatitis as compared to age-matched controls is shown in Figure 5-1 (Klotz et al., 1975). Both the appearance and elimination of desmethyldiazepam, the major metabolite of diazepam, is delayed in patients with cirrhosis. In the presence of liver disease, the elimination half-life of diazepam may be increased two- to fivefold.

These changes in elimination half-life do not correlate well with conventional tests of liver function, and such tests cannot be used as a guide to estimate the proper diazepam dose. In addition, while recovery from acute viral hepatitis results in the normalization of elimination half-life, this occurs *more slowly* than normalization of tests such as SGOT and serum bilirubin.

Although **chlordiazepoxide** has not been as extensively studied as di-

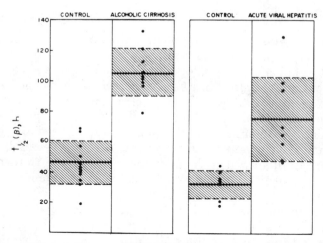

Figure 5-1. Comparison of diazepam half-life ($t_{1/2}(\beta)$) in patients with alcoholic cirrhosis and acute viral hepatitis, and their age-matched controls. Each point represents an individual subject, and the hatched area indicates the mean $\pm$ SD. The $t_{1/2}(\beta)$ values in both the cirrhotic and acute viral hepatitis groups were significantly longer ($P < 0.001$) than in the corresponding age-matched control groups. [From Klotz et al. (1975) with permission of author and publisher.]

azepam, marked prolongation of elimination half-life has been found in the presence of cirrhosis and hepatitis (Roberts et al., 1977).

Lorazepam, unlike diazepam and chlordiazepoxide, has no active metabolites, being converted in the liver to a glucuronide which is then excreted by the kidney. The elimination half-life of intravenous lorazepam was doubled in patients with alcoholic cirrhosis, probably as a result of reduced protein binding leading to an increased volume of distribution. Lorazepam kinetics were not significantly changed in the presence of viral hepatitis. In general, metabolism of lorazepam is less impaired by liver disease than is that of diazepam or chlordiazepoxide (Kraus et al., 1978).

Oxazepam is the benzodiazepine of choice for oral use in patients with parenchymal liver disease. It has a relatively short half-life (6–8 hr), no active metabolites, and its elimination half-life, clearance, protein binding, and urinary excretion remain unchanged in the presence of acute viral hepatitis or cirrhosis (Schull et al., 1976). It is unfortunate that a parenteral form of oxazepam is not available, but should this route of administration be necessary, lorazepam offers a reasonable alternative.

Antipsychotics. Antipsychotic drug disposition in the presence of liver disease has not been adequately studied. In compensated cirrhotic patients, plasma disappearance of a 25 mg intravenous dose of **chlorpromazine** did not differ from matched controls (Maxwell et al., 1972). Metabolic products and protein binding were not studied.

Antidepressants—No studies.

Lithium—No studies.

Cerebral Sensitivity

Liver disease may be associated with a greater cerebral sensitivity to the effects of psychotropic drugs. This appears to be especially true in patients predisposed to hepatic encephalopathy, in whom electroencephalographic and/or clinical deterioration has been observed with morphine, chlorpromazine, diazepam, and tranylcypromine (Hoyumpa et al., 1978). Extensive testing has not been done with these or other drugs but, pending evidence to the contrary, one should assume that all drugs with sedative or analgesic properties have the potential for adversely affecting cerebral function in patients who are disposed to hepatic encephalopathy. Morgan and Read (1972) showed that patients with cirrhosis had a heightened sensitivity to the CNS effects of tranylcypromine, especially if there was a prior history of hepatic encephalopathy. Although amitriptyline appeared to be better tolerated in a similar group of patients, experimental limitations prohibit generalizations from these findings.

Conclusion

Creatinine clearance provides a reasonable measure of the ability of the kidney to excrete drugs and, hence, appropriate dosage adjustments can be made in the presence of renal disease. Unfortunately, such a correlation does not exist between conventional liver function tests and the ability of the liver to metabolize drugs. Hence, clinical judgment and, when appropriate, drug blood levels must guide the physician until better predictive tests become available.

Much remains to be learned about the fate of psychotropic drugs in patients with liver disease and about the sensitivity of these patients to the drugs. Even with those few drugs that have been formally studied, there is a need for more extensive testing with larger populations, a wider range of doses and durations of treatment, and greater attention to neurophysiologic effects. For example, oxazepam, whose elimination half-life is unchanged in the presence of liver disease, has not been studied with regard to its effect on cerebral sensitivity.

Psychotropic Drug-Induced Liver Disease

There is no firm evidence that patients with preexisting liver disease are more susceptible to hepatotoxicity from psychotropic drugs (Dujovne, 1977). The biochemical and morphological changes caused by the preexisting disease may, however, interfere with the diagnosis and evaluation of superimposed drug-induced hepatotoxicity.

The true incidence of psychotropic drug-induced hepatotoxicity is difficult to determine, both in terms of subclinical alterations of liver function tests and clinical manifestations. Considering the widespread use of these drugs and the paucity of reports of hepatotoxicity, the likelihood of a serious adverse reaction to any of the drugs in current use is quite low. The review by Ebert and Shader (1970) provides a comprehensive survey of the area and, except for certain updatings, serves as the base for this summary.

Antipsychotic Drugs. Reports of antipsychotic drug-induced hepatotoxicity have focused primarily on **chlorpromazine**. The incidence of chlorpromazine-associated jaundice ranges from 0.1% to 2%, with a trend in recent years toward the lower value. Clinical manifestations include a prodromal phase of about five days, consisting of fever, chills, nausea, malaise, and upper abdominal pain, followed by jaundice, which appears in most cases during the first month of treatment. The severity of the clinical illness varies greatly from patient to patient, but the duration tends to be relatively short (60% recovered within four to eight weeks) and resolution complete. Fatalities are rare, and it is unlikely that chlorpromazine hepatotoxicity can lead to biliary cirrhosis.

Laboratory findings in chlorpromazine-induced hepatotoxicity are those found with cholestatic jaundice and are not specific for chlorpromazine. Baseline evaluation of liver function is important, since a high incidence of preexisting abnormalities may be present and thereby complicate evaluation of drug effects (Dickes et al., 1957). Of interest is the observation that abnormal liver function tests occurring during the course of chlorpromazine therapy may return to normal despite continuation of the drug. This approach is not advised, however, in view of the availability of structurally unrelated and equally effective substitutes.

The histological findings on liver biopsy during the acute phase of chlorpromazine-induced jaundice are a mixture of both "cholestatic changes and evidence of inflammation and parenchymal cell destruction" (Ebert and Shader, 1970).

Hepatotoxicity from chlorpromazine does not appear to be related to dose, age, sex, or preexisting liver disease. Although rare, jaundice has been reported following a single dose of the drug. While the etiology is not fully understood, chlorpromazine-induced hepatitis appears to be due to a hypersensitivity reaction.

Reports of hepatotoxicity from other phenothiazines or from nonphenothiazine antipsychotic drugs are uncommon or nonexistent. For example, Ebert and Shader (1970) found no cases of cholestatic hepatitis in 638 patients taking trifluoperazine alone, or in 197 patients on thioridazine alone.

Because of the extremely low incidence of clinical jaundice in antipsychotic drug treated populations, it is difficult to tell if the incidence really differs from that found in the untreated general population. To ascribe causality to the drug would require drug withdrawal followed by rechallenge once the dysfunction had resolved. Given the availability of effective alternative drugs, such a procedure would be difficult to justify.

Antidepressants. The incidence of jaundice in patients treated with **tricyclic antidepressants** is very low and, hence, establishing a causal relationship between drug and liver dysfunction is difficult. Yon and Anuras (1975) rechallenged a patient with amitriptyline and were able to confirm its role in causing liver function test abnormalities. When jaundice does occur in association with use of tricyclic antidepressants, it tends to be mild and clears rapidly following drug discontinuation. Lethal hepatic necrosis did occur in an 80-year-old woman after treatment with imipramine and desipramine, and the authors speculated that this was a hypersensitivity reaction to the drugs (Powell et al., 1968).

Unlike the cholestatic hepatitis associated with antipsychotic drugs and tricyclic antidepressants, the **monoamine oxidase inhibitors** (MAOI) can cause severe hepatocellular damage that is morphologically similar to that of viral hepatitis. Most reports of MAOI-induced hepatitis involve iproniazid (Marsilid), a hydrazine derivative that has been withdrawn from the market. Approximately 1.4% of patients receiving this drug developed hepatitis, with an associated mortality rate of 15–20% (Ebert and Shader, 1970). Iproniazid-induced hepatitis is independent of dose and duration of therapy, tends to develop after the fourth week of therapy, and, in nonfatal cases, resolves slowly over several months. It is felt to be a hypersensitivity reaction.

The currently available hydrazine derivatives, isocarboxazid and phenelzine, can cause iproniazid-like hepatitis, although the incidence is considerably lower than with the latter drug. The nonhydrazine MAOI, tranylcypromine, has rarely been associated with the development of hepatitis.

Antianxiety Drugs. There have been isolated reports of cholestatic jaundice associated with the use of benzodizepines (Ebert and Shader, 1970; Fang et al., 1978). A causal relationship was not firmly established.

Lithium. There have been no reports of hepatic dysfunction associated with the therapeutic use of lithium.

Hepatic Drug Metabolizing Enzymes

The hepatic microsomal enzymes that metabolize drugs can be induced or inhibited by other drugs. For example, methylphenidate inhibits the metabolism of phenothiazines and tricyclic antidepressants, leading to increased blood levels of these drugs; phenobarbital, through enzyme stimulation, can lower the blood level and reduce the clinical effectiveness of a phenothiazine; the neuroleptics inhibit the metabolism of the tricyclic antidepressants; while benzodiazepines and lithium do not appear to cause any clinically important alterations in hepatic drug metabolism. While it is clear that the liver plays a major role in psychotropic drug metabolism, the clinical implications of these interactions are not fully understood and much work remains to be done.

REFERENCES

Adams RD, Foley JM: The neurological disorder associated with liver disease, in Merritt HH, Hare CC (eds): *Metabolic and Toxic Diseases of the Nervous System.* Baltimore, Williams & Wilkins, 1953, vol 32, 198–237.

Almy TP: What is the irritable colon? *Am J Dig Dis* 2:93–97, 1957.

Alvarez WC: *On Neuroses.* Philadelphia, Saunders, 1951.

Alvasaker JO, Brodwall E, Haarstad J: Nervous vomiting as the cause of electrolyte disturbances, kidney damage—and general tissue damage? *Acta Med Scand* 166:331–336, 1960.

Alvin J, McHorse T, Hoyumpa A, et al: The effect of liver disease in man on the disposition of phenobarbital. *J Pharmacol Exp Ther* 192:224–235, 1975.

Ansari A: Carcinoma of the pancreas. *Geriatrics* 25:91–99, 1970.

Avery GS (ed): *Drug Treatment: Principles and Practice of Clinical Pharmacology and Therapeutics.* Sydney, Adis Press, 1976.

Ayd FJ: Amitriptyline (Elavil) therapy for depressive reactions. *Psychosomatics* 1:320–325, 1960.

Bacon PA, Myles AB: Hypoglycaemic coma after partial gastrectomy. *Postgrad Med J* 47:134–136, 1971.

Baldessarini RJ, Fischer JE: Substitute and alternative neurotransmitters in neuropsychiatric illness. *Arch Gen Psychiatry* 34:958–964, 1977.

Banjeri NK, Hurwitz LJ: Nervous system manifestations after gastric surgery. *Acta Neurol Scand* 47:485–513, 1971.

Barnhart CC, Bowden CL: Toxic psychosis with cimetidine. *Am J Psychiatry* 136:725–726, 1979.

Barton MD, Libonati M, Cohen PJ: The use of haloperidol for treatment of post-operative nausea and vomiting—A double blind placebo-controlled trial. *Anesthesiology* 42:508–512, 1975.

Bean WB, Funk D: *Serotonin.* Chicago, Yearbook Medical Publishers, 1968.

Beaumont PJ, George JC, Smart DE: "Dieters" and "vomiters and purgers" in anorexia nervosa. *Psychol Med* 6:617–622, 1976.

Belding WL, Freedman DA: Postprandial hypoglycemia presenting as a neurologic problem. *Neurology* 10:613–618, 1960.

Benjamin JE, Hoyt RC: Disability following postvaccinal (yellow fever) hepatitis. *JAMA* 128:319–324, 1945.

Bonfils S, Dubrasquet M, Lambling A: Comparisons of two iminodibenzil derivatives on restraint-induced ulcers and gastric secretion. *J Appl Physiol* 17:299–300, 1962.

Brooks GM: Withdrawal from neuroleptic drugs. *Am J Psychiatry* 115:931–932, 1959.

Burkitt E, Sutcliff EC: Paralytic ileus after amitriptyline. *Br Med J* 2:1648–1651, 1961.

Chen TS, Chen PS: *Essential Hepatology.* Massachusetts, Butterworth, 1977, pp 137–154.

Cherry J: Pharyngeal location of symptoms of gastroesophageal reflux. *Ann Otol Rhinol Laryngol* 79:912–915, 1970.

Cleghorn RA, Brown WT: Psychogenesis of emesis. *Can Psychiatr Assoc J* 9:299–310, 1964.

Cohen CR: *Emotional Factors in Gastrointestinal Illness.* Lindner AE (ed). A Roche Medical Monograph Series. New York, American Elsevier Co, 1973, p 42.

Cooke WT: Neurological manifestations of malabsorption, in Vinken J, Bruyn GW (eds): *Clinical Handbook of Neurology* 28:225–227, Amsterdam, North–Holland Publishing Co., 1976.

Cooke WT: The neurologic manifestations of malabsorption. *Postgrad Med J* 54:760–762, 1978.

Cooke WT, Smith WT: Neurologic disorders associated with adult coeliac disease. *Brain* 89:683–722, 1966.

Coppens AJ: Vomiting in early pregnancy. *Lancet* 1:172–173, 1959.

Davidson CS, Gabuzda GJ: Hepatic coma, in Schiff L (ed): *Diseases of the Liver.* Philadelphia, Lippincott, 1975, pp 466–499.

Delahunty JE, Ardran GM: Globus hystericus—a manifestation of reflux of oesophagitis. *J Laryng* 84:1049–1064, 1970.

Deutsch H: *The Psychology of Woman.* New York, Grune & Stratton, 1945.

Diamond S: Amitriptyline in the treatment of gastrointestinal disorders. *Psychosomatics* 5:221–224, 1964.

Dickes R, Schinker V, Deutsch L: Serial liver-function and blood studies in patients receiving chlorpromazine. *N Eng J Med* 256:1–7, 1957.

Dorfman W: Somatic components of depression. *Psychosomatics* 8:4–5, 1967.

Dujovne CA: A clinical pharmacologist's view of drug hepatotoxicity. *Pharmacol Res Commun* 9:1–15, 1977.

Ebert MH, Shader RI: Hepatic effects, in Shader RI, DiMascio A (eds): *Psychotropic Drug Side Effects: Clinical and Theoretical Perspectives*. Baltimore, Williams & Wilkins, 1970, pp 175–196.

Elwood PC, Jacobs A, Pittman RG, et al: Epidemiology of Patterson-Kelly Syndrome. *Lancet* 2:716–720, 1964.

Evans DL, Rogers JF, Peiper SC: Intestinal dilatation associated with phenothiazine therapy: A case report and literature review. *Am J Psychiatry* 136:970–972, 1979.

Fairweather DV: Nausea and vomiting in pregnancy. *Am J Obstet Gynecol* 102:135–138, 1968.

Fang MH, Ginsberg AL, Dobbins WO: Cholestatic jaundice associated with flurazepam hydrochloride. *Ann Int Med* 89:363–364, 1978.

Fann WE: Chlorpromazine: Effects of antacids on its gastrointestinal absorption. *J Clin Pharmacol* 13:388–391, 1973.

Feldman PE: The mask of depression. *J Kans Med Soc* 66:6–10, 1965.

Feurle GE, Bolk B, Waldherr R: Cerebral Whipple's disease with negative jejunal histology. *N Eng J Med* 300:907–908, 1979.

Finelli PF, McEntree WJ, Lussell S, et al: Whipple's disease with predominantly neuroophthalmic manifestations. *Ann Neurology* 1:247–252, 1977.

Forrest FM, Forrest IS, Serra MT: Modification of chlorpromazine metabolism by some other drugs frequently administered to psychiatric patients. *Biol Psychiatry* 2:53–59, 1970.

Fras I, Litin EM: Comparison of psychiatric manifestations in carcinoma of the pancreas, retroperitoneal malignant lymphoma and lymphoma in other locations. *Psychosomatics* 8:275–277, 1967.

Fras I, Litin EM, Pearson JS: Comparison of psychiatric symptoms of carcinoma of the pancreas with those in some other intraabdominal neoplasms. *Am J Psychiatry* 123:1553–1562, 1967.

Gallant DM, Edwards CG, Bishop MP et al: Withdrawal symptoms after abrupt cessation of antipsychotic compounds: Clinical confirmation in chronic schizophrenics. *Am J Psychiatry* 121:491–493, 1964.

Gander DR, Devlin H: Ileus after amitriptyline. *Br Med J* 1:1160–1161, 1963.

Goldberg D: A psychiatric study of patients with diseases of the small intestine. *Gut* 11:459–465, 1970.

Granacher RP, Baldessarini RJ: The usefulness of physostigmine in neurology and psychiatry, in Klawans HL (ed): *Clinical Neuropharmacology*. New York, Raven Press, 1976, vol 1, pp 63–79.

Greiner AC, Nicholson GA: Pigment deposition in viscera associated with prolonged chlorpromazine therapy. *Can Med Assoc J* 91:627–635, 1964.

Gullick HD: Carcinoma of the pancreas: A review and critical study of 100 cases. *Medicine* 38:47–84, 1959.

Hafken L, Leichter S, Reich T: Organic brain dysfunction as a possible consequence of postgastrectomy hypoglycemia. *Am J Psychiatry* 132:1321–1324, 1975.

Harris JG: Nausea, vomiting and cancer treatment. *CA-A Cancer J Clinicians* 28:195–201, 1978.

Havens LL, Child CG: Recurrent psychosis associated with liver disease and elevated blood ammonia. *N Engl J Med* 252:756–759, 1955.

Heffernon EW, Lippincott RC: Gastrointestinal response to stress (irritable colon). *Med Clin North Am* 50:591–595, 1966.

Hill OW: Psychogenic vomiting and hypokalaemia. *Gut* 8:98–101, 1967.

Hill OW: Psychogenic vomiting. *Gut* 9:348–352, 1968.

Hislop IG: Psychological significance of the irritable colon syndrome. *Gut* 12:452–457, 1971.

Hoyumpa AM, Branch RA, Schenker S: The disposition and effects of sedatives and analgesics in liver disease. *Ann Rev Med* 29:205–218, 1978.

Jefferson JW: Central nervous system toxicity of cimetidine: A case of depression. *Am J Psychiatry* 136:346, 1979.

Kasich AM: Management of emotional disorders and depression in patients with gastrointestinal disease. *J Ther Res* 7:542–547, 1965.

Klotz U, Avant GR, Hoyumpa A, et al: The effects of age and liver disease on the disposition and elimination of diazepam in adult man. *J Clin Invest* 55:347–359, 1975.

Knox DL, Bayless TM, Pittman FE: Neurologic disease in patients with treated Whipple disease. *Medicine* (Baltimore) 55:467–476, 1976.

Kohn LA: The behavior of patients with cancer of the pancreas. *Cancer* 5:328–330, 1952.

Kornfeld DS: Psychiatric aspects of liver disease, in Lindner AE (ed): *Emotional Factors in Gastrointestinal Illness.* Amsterdam, Excerpta Medica, 1973, pp 166–181.

Kraus JM, Desmond PV, Marshall JP, et al: Effects of aging and liver disease on disposition of lorazepam. *Clin Pharmacol Ther* 24:411–419, 1978.

Kroger WS: Psychosomatic Obstetrics, Gynecology and Endocrinology. Springfield, Charles C Thomas, 1962.

Kroll J, Fog R: Portal-systemic shunts and mental disorders. *Acta Psychiatr Scand* 44:255–260, 1968.

Kronfeld A: Oesophagus-neurosen-psychotherapeut. *Praxis* 1:21–27, 1934.

Lacoursiere RB, Spohn HE, Thompson K: Medical effects of abrupt neuroleptic withdrawal. *Compr Psychiatry* 17:285–294, 1976.

Latter KA, Wilbur DL: Psychic and neurologic manifestations of carcinoma of the pancreas. *Staff Meetings Mayo Clin* 12:457–462, 1937.

Lawton MP, Phillips RM: Psychopathological accompaniments of chronic relapsing pancreatitis. *J Nerv Ment Dis* 122:248–253, 1955.

Leevy CM: Exploring the brain–liver relationship. *Mod Med* 42:17–22, 1974.

Lehmann J: Mental disturbances followed by stupor in a patient with carcinoidosis. *Acta Psychiatr Scand* 42:153–161, 1966.

Leibovich MA: Psychogenic vomiting. *Psychother and Psychosom* 22:263–268, 1973.

Loiudice TA, Tulman A, Buhac I: L-Dopa and hepatic encephalopathy. *NY State J Med* 79:364–366, 1979.

Lowe WC, Palmer ED: Carcinoma of the pancreas. *Am J Gastroenterol* 47:412–420, 1967.

McMillen MA, Ambis D, Siegel JH: Cimetidine and mental confusion. *N Eng J Med* 298:284–285, 1978.

Major LE, Brown GL, Wilson WP: Carcinoid and psychiatric symptoms. *South Med J* 66:787–790, 1973.

Maxwell JD, Carrella M, Parkes JD, et al: Plasma disappearance and cerebral effects of chlorpromazine in cirrhosis. *Clin Sci* 43:143–151, 1972.

Milner G, Hills NF: Adynamic ileus and nortriptyline. *Br Med J* 1:841–842, 1966.

Mitchell W, Feldman F: Neuropsychiatric aspects of hypokalaemia. *Can Med Assoc J* 98:49–51, 1968.

Morgan MH, Read AE: Antidepressants and liver disease. *Gut* 13:697–701, 1972.

Morgan MY, Jakobovits A, Elithorn A, et al: Successful use of bromocriptine in the treatment of a patient with chronic portalsystemic encephalopathy. *N Engl J Med* 296:793–794, 1977.

Morris JS, Ajdukiewicz AB, Reed AE: Neurologic disorders and adult coeliac disease. *Gut* 11:549–554, 1970.

Mosley JW, Galambos JT: Viral hepatitis, in Schiff L (ed): *Disease of the Liver,* ed 3. Philadelphia, Lippincott, 1969, pp 410–497.

Netter-Munkelt P, Mau G, Konig B: The dementia of neuroticism as a modifying factor in the association between biologic conditions and nausea in pregnancy. *J Psychosom Res* 16:395–399, 1972.

Nicholls MG, Espiner EA: Surreptitious vomiting causing severe kypokalaemia: Case report. *N Z Med J* 77:248–250, 1973.

Olivarius B, Roos D: Myelopathy following partial gastrectomy. *Acta Neurol Scand* 44:1347–1362, 1968.

Palmer RL: The psychosomatic study of vomiting of early pregnancies. *J Psychosom Res* 17:303–308, 1973.

Parkes JD, Sharpstone P, Williams R: Levodopa in hepatic coma. *Lancet* 2:1341–1343, 1970.

Paulley JW: Emotion and personality and etiology of steatorrhea. *Am J Dig Dis* 4:352–360, 1959.

Peden NR, Cargill JM, Browning MCK, et al: Male sexual dysfunction during treatment with cimetidine. *Br Med J* 1:659, 1979.

Perlas AP, Faillace LA: Psychiatric manifestations of carcinoma of the pancreas. *Am J Psychiatry* 121:182, 1964.

Plotkin DA, Plotkin D, Okun R: Haloperidol in the treatment of nausea and vomiting due to cytotoxic drug administration. *Curr Ther Res Clin Exp* 15:599–601, 1973.

Powell WJ, Koch-Weser J, Williams RA: Lethal hepatic necrosis after therapy with imipramine and desipramine. *JAMA* 206:642–644, 1968.

Rash RM: Observations and the clinical features of carcinoma of the pancreas. *Am J Gastroenterol* 51:235–245, 1969.

Read AE, Sherlock S, Laidlaw J, et al: The neuro-psychiatric syndrome associated with chronic liver disease and an extensive portal-systemic collateral circulation. *Quart J Med* 36:135–150, 1967.

Reid AH, Leonard A: Lithium treatment of cyclical vomiting in a mentally defective patient. *Br J Psychiatry* 130:316, 1977.

Rickles NK: Functional symptoms as first evidence of pancreatic disease. *J Nerv Ment Dis* 101:566–571, 1945.

Ritama V, Vapaatalohi, Neuvongn PJ, et al: Phenothiazines and intestinal dilatation. *Lancet* 1:470–472, 1969.

Rivers A, Ferreira AE: Incidence and causes of chronic dyspepsia at various ages; an analysis of 4223 cases. *JAMA* 110:2132–2136, 1938.

Robbins EL, Nagle JD: Haloperidol parenterally for treatment of vomiting and nausea from gastro-intestinal disorders in a group of geriatric patients: Double-blind placebo-controlled study. *J Am Geriatr Soc* 23:38–41, 1975.

Roberts R, Wilkinson GR, Branch RA, et al: Effect of age and cirrhosis on the disposition and elimination of chlordiazepoxide (Librium). *Gastroenterol* 73:1245/1243, 1977.

Rothermich NO, von Hamm E: Pancreatic encephalopathy. *J Clin Endocrinol* 1:872–881, 1941.

Ruben J, Nagler R, Spiro HM, et al: Measuring the effects of emotions on esophageal motility. *Psychosom Med* 24:170–175, 1962.

Ruoff M: The irritable colon syndrome, in Lindner AE (ed): *Emotional Factors in Gastrointestinal Illness.* Amsterdam, Excerpta Medica, 1973, pp 156–164.

Savage C, Butcher W, Noble D: Psychological manifestations in pancreatic disease. *J Clin Exp Psychopathol* 13:9–12, 1972.

Savage C, Noble D: Cancer of the pancreas: Two cases simulating psychogenic illness. *J Nerv Ment Dis* 120:62–65, 1954.

Schenker S, Breen KJ, Hoyumpa AM: Hepatic encephalopathy: Current status. *Gastroenterol* 66:121–151, 1974.

Schenker S, Hoyumpa AM, Wilkinson GR: The effect of parenchymal liver disease on the disposition and elimination of sedatives and analgesics. *Med Clin North Am* 59:887–896, 1975.

Schentag JJ, Cerra FB, Calleri G, et al: Pharmacokinetic and clinical studies in patients with cimetidine-associated mental confusion. *Lancet* 1:177–181, 1979.

Schuster MM, Iber FL: Psychosis with pancreatitis. *Arch Intern Med* 116:118–233, 1965.

Sherlock S, Howligan K, George P: Medical complications of shunt surgery for portal hypertension. *Ann NY Acad Sci* 170:392–405, 1970.

Sherlock S, Summerskill WHJ, White LP, et al: Portal-systemic encephalopathy, neurological complications of liver disease. *Lancet* 2:453–457, 1954.

Shull HJ, Wilkinson GR, Johnson R, et al: Normal disposition of oxazepam in acute viral hepatitis and cirrhosis. *Ann Intern Med* 84:420–425, 1976.

Sokoloff B: *Recent Results in Cancer Research: Carcinoid and Serotonin.* New York, Springer–Verlag, 1966, vol 15.

Summerskill WHJ, Davidson EA, Sherlock S, et al: The neuropsychiatric syndrome associated with hepatic cirrhosis and an extensive portal collateral circulation. *Quart J Med* 25:245–266, 1956.

Swanson DW, Swenson WN, Huizenga KA, et al: Persistent nausea without organic cause. *Mayo Clinic Proc* 51:257–262, 1976.

Thamsen L, Hjorth N, Christianson AR, et al: Cancer of the pancreas: A clinical and pathologic study. *Acta Med Scand* 139:28–41, 1950.

Thorson A: Studies on carcinoid disease. *Acta Med Scand* 161 (suppl 334):1–146, 1958.

Tripp LE, Agle DP: Acute pancreatitis as a psychophysiologic response: A case study. *Am J Psychiatry* 124:1253–1257, 1968.

Tylden E: Hyperemesis and physiologic vomiting. *J Psychosom Res* 12:85–89, 1968.

Uddenberg N, Nilsson A, Almgren PE: Nausea and pregnancy: Psychological and psychosomatic aspects. *J Psychosom Res* 15:269–271, 1971.

Van Thiel DH, Gavaler JS, Smith WI, et al: Hypothalamic–pituitary–gonadal dysfunction in men using cimetidine. *N Eng J Med* 300:1012–1015, 1979.

Victor M, Adams RD, Cole M: The acquired (nonWilsonian) type of chronic hepatocellular degeneration. *Medicine* 44:345–396, 1965.

Vinson PO: Hysterical dysphagia. *Minn Med* 5:107–112, 1922.

Watson E: The role of auto-intoxication or auto-infection in mental disorders. *J Ment Sci* 69:52–57, 1923.

Weiss E, English OS: Cardiospasm, in *Psychosomatic Medicine.* Philadelphia, WB Saunders Co, 1957, pp 285–289.

Wilbur DL, Washburn RN: Clinical features and treatment of functional or nervous vomiting. *JAMA* 110:477–480, 1938.

Williams J, Hall GS, Thompson AG, et al: Neurologic disease after partial gastrectomy. *Br Med J* 3:210–212, 1969.

Wolfe MM: Impotence on cimetidine treatment. *N Eng J Med* 300:94, 1979.

Wolff HP, Kruck F, Vecsei P, et al: Psychiatric disturbance leading to potassium depletion, sodium depletion, raised plasma-renin concentration, and secondary hyperaldosteronism. *Lancet* 10:257–261, 1968.

Wooley OW: *The Biochemical Basis of Psychosis.* New York, John Wiley and Sons, 1962.

Yaskin JC: Nervous symptoms as earliest manifestations of carcinoma of the pancreas. *JAMA* 96:1664–1668, 1931.

Yon T, Anuras S: Hepatitis caused by amitriptyline therapy. *JAMA* 232:833–834, 1975.

Young SJ, Elpers DH, Norland CC, et al: Psychiatric illness and the irritable bowel syndrome. *Gastroenterol* 70:162–166, 1976.

6

Endocrine Disorders

ADRENAL DISORDERS

Hyperadrenalism

Several distinct clinical syndromes may be produced by the secretion of excess adrenal cortical hormones. Excessive production of the principal mineralocorticoid, aldosterone, results in clinical and chemical signs of aldosteronism, and adrenal virilism may result from excessive production of adrenal androgens. Neuropsychiatric changes are most prominently associated with an excess of the principal glucocorticoid, cortisol.

In 1932, Harvey Cushing first described a disease occurring in association with a basophilic adenoma of the pituitary gland, subsequently named Cushing disease. Since it was later recognized that the characteristic picture was associated with a wide variety of endocrinopathies, it became customary to speak of Cushing syndrome. In approximately 70% of cases, adrenal hyperplasia occurs secondary to hypersecretion of adrenocorticotrophic hormone (ACTH) from the anterior pituitary, because of either a tumor or a hypothalamic neuroendocrine disturbance (Sacher, 1975). In these situations, both ACTH and cortisol are present in excessive amounts. Adrenal hyperplasia is three times more frequent in females, with the most common age of onset the third or fourth decade (Williams et al., 1977).

The remainder of cases producing Cushing syndrome are caused by tumors of the adrenal gland, such as adrenal adenomas or carcinomas (causing excessive cortisol production and consequent suppression of ACTH), or by nonadrenal tumors that secrete substances biologically indistinguishable from ACTH. "Oat cell" carcinomas of the lung are the most common example of this latter group.

Clinical Features

Signs and symptoms of Cushing syndrome usually present in an insidious manner, making the exact date of onset unclear. The syndrome is often found while patients are being evaluated for such diverse entities as diabetes mellitus, hypertension, obesity, and osteoporosis. Occasionally, when a tumor is present, the onset may be more rapid. Early changes include weight gain, usually in the trunk, alteration or cessation of menses, muscle weakness, and rounding of the face (the classic "moon" facies). In fact, many clinicians feel that the diagnosis can be made solely by the changes in the face. Fat may accumulate over the upper dorsal vertebrae, resulting in a "buffalo hump." Skin changes include acne, hirsutism, ecchymoses, easy bruising, and striae over the hips and abdomen. Bone collapse secondary to osteoporosis, hypertension leading to edema and congestive heart failure, and carbohydrate intolerance occur in later stages.

Laboratory Findings

The diagnosis of Cushing syndrome depends on the direct or indirect determination of increased cortisol production in the absence of stress. Once increased production is determined, further tests are employed to establish whether ACTH control of the adrenal glands is physiologically normal. In these suppression tests, specific amounts of potent glucocorticoids are given, and subsequent reduction of ACTH secretion is measured by analysis of urinary steroid values. Exogenous administration of ACTH also aids in identifying the specific location of the lesion contributing to the excessive cortisol production. Final confirmation of the syndrome rests on key laboratory determinations, including ACTH and cortisol plasma levels, and urinary levels of 17-hydroxycorticoids, 17-ketosteroids, and 17-ketogenic steroids. Free cortisol measurement can be done, but it requires radioimmunoassay techniques.

Neuropsychiatric Features

Since Cushing's first paper (1932), significant mental disturbances associated with Cushing syndrome have been noted. The incidence of these changes is difficult to determine, for one must rely on small numbers of case reports or on summaries by authors who use varying criteria for reporting psychiatric symptomatology. The incidence is high, however, and mental changes may be seen early in the illness.

It appears that approximately 5–24% of patients experience major mental changes, 22–54% experience significant (moderate) changes, and 32–40% demonstrate minor changes (Borman and Schmallenberg, 1951; Goolker and Schein, 1953; Hurxthal and O'Sullivan, 1959; Spillane, 1951; Starr, 1952; Trethowan and Cobb, 1952; Smith et al., 1972). Depending largely upon whether these changes are specifically sought, the overall percentage of patients with mental disturbance ranges from 44% to 88% (Mills, 1964; Spillane, 1951).

There is no specificity to mental changes secondary to hyperadrenalism and, as in all endocrinopathies, premorbid or underlying personality is important in determining the features and course of the clinical presentation.

In the past, emotional changes were thought to be secondary to the social disruption and maladjustment caused by the repulsive appearance of these patients. This is clearly an insufficient explanation, since neuropsychiatric manifestations often precede overt body changes, especially the more striking ones.

Depression. The most frequently encountered state is depression, the severity of which ranges from a moderately depressed mood with some overreaction to life stresses, to a severe depressive illness with associated delusions (Starr, 1952). Fawcett and Bunney (1967), in a review of 94 patients with psychiatric complications, showed that in over half of them severe depression was a prominent feature. Trethowan and Cobb (1952) felt that behavioral retardation is prominent in these depressive disorders. When it is absent, it often appears to be replaced by irritability, in the form of agitation, crying spells, or noncooperative behavior. Both irritability and retardation may occur in the same patient. A patient's emotional state may fluctuate rapidly and show similarities to manic-depressive disease. However, the euphoria reported with exogenous administration of ACTH or steroids appears rare. Spillane (1951) noted that the depression can often reach serious proportions. He reported four suicides and two serious attempts in 50 cases of psychiatric complications associated with Cushing syndrome. Starr (1952) noted suicide attempts in 10% of his cases. In several of these patients there was no indication of prior psychiatric difficulty, and they appeared to be improving medically when they rather suddenly became agitated and depressed and committed suicide.

Psychoses. Psychosis is the next most commonly associated psychiatric picture, although less severe disturbances of perceptual and cognitive abilities seem common to most patients. Paranoid states, hallucinations, associated memory deficits, and confusion suggest that these states are acute organic brain syndromes, although they often have affective components. These reactions occur more frequently when medical complications of the syndrome are present, such as severe hypertension with encephalopathy, uncontrolled diabetes, congestive heart failure, or electrolyte disturbances.

Exogenous Steroids

In the early 1950s, the introduction of cortisone and ACTH as therapeutic agents stimulated investigation of the effects of exogenous steroids. Since then, steroid analogues have been developed that share the same basic properties but differ in such qualities as biologic half-life, cost, dosage, and mineralocorticoid effect. There have been no reliably demonstrated differences in effect on mental processes among these agents and other exogenous steroids.

In addition to substitution therapy in adrenal insufficiency. ACTH and corticosteroids are used in the symptomatic treatment of a wide variety of disorders, including the following: arthritis; rheumatic heart disease; renal disease; systemic lupus erythematosus; bronchial asthma; ulcerative colitis; inflammatory diseases of the eyes, skin, and other organ; cerebral edema; and increased intracranial pressure. A variety of allergic reactions and general inflammatory conditions are also treated with corticosteroids. In general, mental disturbances are very similar to those associated with Cushing syndrome, although there are some differences, and the clinical picture may be influenced by the underlying disease.

A substantial number of patients receiving ACTH or steroids demonstrate mental status alterations. Again, the incidence depends on the strictness of the criteria used and the diligence with which these changes are sought. Early reports tended to describe a higher incidence of changes, particularly severe ones; this may be due to increased use of synthetic high-potency steroids instead of cortisone and hydrocortisone in recent years, even though a clear difference between these agents has not been demonstrated. The Boston Collaborative Drug Surveillance Program (1972) noted that acute psychiatric reactions occurred in 21 patients of the 676 prednisone recipients (3.1%). Michael and Gibbons (1963) suggest that serious psychological disturbances occur at a rate of about 25% of that seen in spontaneous hypercortisolism. Whether this higher incidence is due to differences in plasma levels of biologically active steroids, or to the long, continued chronic elevation of steroids in Cushing syndrome, is not known. Glaser (1953) estimated that psychotic reactions occur in about 5% of patients.

Minor initial changes seem quite common. Clark et al. (1952) reported increased joviality and optimism in "nearly all cases." Goldman (1950) reported "an improvement in morale and sense of well being" in all of his series of nine patients. Sixty percent of the patients of Hoefer and Glaser (1950) experienced increased feelings of well-being and alertness together with some tension and irritability. Seventy-five percent of these patients were mildly elated or euphoric. The patients of Rome and Braceland (1952) made statements such as "I'm on the top of the world," "I never felt better in my life," and "I feel more vigorous than I really am." They felt less fatigue and claimed to think faster and concentrate better. It is not clear whether this "typical euphoria" is an effect of the drug or a psychological response to improvement in the underlying physical condition.

The more prominent changes fall into two general groups of symptom patterns, although overlap may be present. In one, affective symptoms predominate. A progression of the early "normal" and "positive feelings" may occur, with restlessness, insomnia, increased motor activity, flight of ideas, and talkativeness (Goolker and Schein, 1953; Clark et al. 1952; Rome and Braceland, 1952; Glaser, 1953). During this hypomanic period judgment may be impaired. Patients may minimize their illnesses and become management problems. Although euphoria is present, it is neither consistent nor pleasant, for patients are often anxious, emotionally labile, irritable, and restless. Depression may also be present, and alternate with periods of elation. A consistently depressed affect is more common in the endogenous forms of hyperadrenalism (Fawcett and Bunney, 1967). With more severe reactions, affective changes are of psychotic proportions. Full-blown manic storms, with assaultiveness, suicidal tendencies, and physical exhaustion may occur (Glaser, 1953). Some psychotic depressions have been reported.

A second pattern of responses with less of an affective flavor includes symptoms such as paresthesias (often of the forehead), "hazy feelings," depersonalization, anxiety with obsessional or ruminative features, and phobic behaviors. These may shade into responses having organic components such as bewilderment, flatness of affect, memory disturbance, and disorientation (Glaser, 1953). Several studies have found EEG changes suggestive of generalized metabolic alterations (Hoefer and Glaser, 1950; Freyberg et al., 1951). There is disagreement in this area about the presence or absence of organic features among these patients. While changes in the EEG are present, the correlation with psychic changes is not consistent, and patients have been noted to have EEG changes without significant mental disturbances. Some workers felt that most cases did not exhibit the type of confusion, disorientation, recent memory impairment, or sensorial disturbance characteristic of delirium, but rather thought that the patient seemed overwhelmingly involved with illusory or hallucinatory experiences (Clark et al., 1952; Clark et al., 1953). In one study, the patients indicated no decrement in intellectual functioning when tested with a Kohs Block Test (Lidz et al., 1952). As the severity of the reaction increases more complex pictures are seen, with organic components and associated paranoid–hallucinatory features. Clinical states resembling paranoid schizophrenia may occur (Sacher, 1975; Glaser, 1953).

The unpredictability of response to steroid therapy severely hinders a priori clinical decision making. Clinical predictions about patients' psychiatric responses are difficult, for correlations between the daily dose and acute reactions are not well documented. An exception to this is the Boston Collaborative Drug Surveillance Program (1972) which did find a significant correlation for prednisone. Psychiatric reactions were recorded in 1.3% of 463 patients receiving 40 mg per day or less, 4.6% of 175 patients receiving 41–80 mg per day, and 18.4% of 38 patients who received more than 80 mg per day. At this time there are insufficient data to suggest that personality factors predispose patients to mental disturbances from ACTH or corticosteroids, although some earlier workers did suggest a causative association. There is also no known relationship of personality features to the duration or severity of disorders (Clark et al., 1952). Although there are reports of patients with prior histories of psychosis, statistical comparison do not permit the inference of increased susceptibility to psychosis (Goolker and Schein, 1953). Conversely, the absence of a history of psychosis or emotional maladjustment during prior courses of steroid treatment is no guarantee against subsequent neuropsychiatric disorders (Clark et al., 1952). Goolker and Schein (1953) felt that a primary mental change occurred, with ACTH or cortisone producing a state of cerebral excitability characterized as a "ready state." They felt this state may occur within the first four to six hours and, following a mean period of 3.6 days after the beginning of treatment, may merge with a more formed psychic reaction.

Mental changes may begin within several days of starting treatment or may occur only after a prolonged course of several months or even years. These mental changes may be difficult to anticipate, but Freyberg et al., (1951) regarded the onset of insomnia as a particularly important indication for reducing the dosage. Abrupt withdrawal or decreases in dosage also seem to be associated with psychiatric complications. Freyberg et al., (1951) described a "withdrawal syndrome" associated with abrupt discontinuation of treatment, consisting of relapse of the underlying disease manifested by fatigue, weakness, discouragement, and depression. Gupta and Ehrlich (1976) also noted organic brain syndromes associated with steroid withdrawal in their patients with rheumatoid arthritis, but suggested that this response may be related to a flare-up of an underlying central nervous system vasculitis.

Treatment

Recovery from severe psychiatric reactions appears to occur in almost all cases with reduction of dosage or cessation of the administration of steroids (Clark et al., 1953). An exception to this (Glaser, 1953) may be that some manic storms do not abate with the discontinuation of the corticosteroids. A frequent pattern of recovery in psychotic patients is the occurrence of progressively longer and more frequent lucid intervals punctuated by psychotic relapses. Because of this tendency to relapse, patients should remain under careful observation for a reasonable period after apparent recovery.

Not all mental disturbances that arise during the course of steroid treatment are drug induced. Should neuropsychiatric abnormalities appear, a patient should be evaluated carefully for alternative etiologies, such as metabolic conditions, electrolyte imbalance, intracranial disorders, or other circumstances that may disturb cerebral function. This is particularly important since cessation of therapy may seriously jeopardize the welfare of the patient.

The treatment of choice for psychiatric disturbances associated with Cushing disease is, of course, correction of the underlying disorder. For neuropsychiatric manifestations secondary to the administration of exogenous steroids, reducing or discontinuing the drug is most likely to produce remission of the symptoms, but often this is not possible for pressing medical reasons. In many of these situations, however, certain behavioral symptoms must be controlled. Systematic studies of the effectiveness of psychotropic drugs in these conditions are not available. The literature generally suggests that psychotropic drugs and occasionally electroconvulsive therapy are helpful in bringing about the remission of this psychiatric condition, even in the continued presence of hyperadrenal corticism. An exception to this generalization may be contained in the recent report by Hall et al. (1978) of four patients with a steroid psychosis demonstrating a predominantly affective mood change who were treated with tricyclic antidepressants. In each case, the patient's mental state deteriorated rapidly, following the initiation of tricyclics in mid-range doses. The patients experienced visual hallucinations, threatening and accusatory auditory hallucinations, and general exacerbation of psychotic features. Phenothiazines reversed these symptoms. In another recent communication, it was suggested that treatment with lithium may control steroid-induced hypomania that would otherwise prevent the use of medically effective doses of the steroid (Siegal, 1978).

Falk et al. (1979) treated 27 multiple sclerosis and retrobulbar neuritis patients empirically with lithium carbonate in addition to the corticotropin. None of these patients developed psychotic symptoms, while in a comparable group of 44 patients treated identically with corticotropin but without lithium, six (14%) became psychotic.

Hypoadrenalism

Hypofunction of the adrenal cortex may be associated with a primary inability of the adrenal gland to produce sufficient quantities of adrenocortical hormone or may be secondary to deficient pituitary production of ACTH. A primary deficiency, Addison disease, is produced by slow, progressive destruction of the adrenal cortex, called idiopathic atrophy. Historically, this was caused predominantly by infections of varying kinds; at present it is more likely to be due to an autoimmune mechanism. Ninety percent of the gland's capacity must be destroyed before clinical signs of insufficiency appear. In primary adrenocortical failure, there is secondary hypersecretion of ACTH due to the absence of cortisol feedback inhibition. Acute adrenocortical insufficiency, which may be a medical emergency, may result from several different processes, such as hemorrhage into the gland or sudden withdrawal of administered steroids.

Secondary adrenocortical insufficiency can occur in association with pituitary trophic hormone deficiencies (hypopituitarism) or may be caused by prolonged or excessive administration of glucocorticosteroids, resulting in ACTH suppression. The frequency of this phenomenon has increased with the growing use of exogenous steroids. Secondary adrenocortical insufficiency due to pituitary deficits is associated with signs and symptoms suggestive of other hormone deficiencies, and near-normal levels of aldosterone secretion because of the presence of the intact adrenocortical gland. Adrenal atrophy may occur with a long-term use of steroid therapy even in the presence of physical findings indicating Cushing syndrome because of the loss of endogenous ACTH stimulation. The deficit will then be exposed when the exogenous steroid is withdrawn. Thus most of these patients will have two deficits, a loss of adrenal responsiveness to ACTH and a failure of pituitary ACTH release.

Clinical Features

The syndrome of hypoadrenalism is most frequently characterized by slowly progressive fatigability and weakness. In the early stages, the asthenia may be periodic and evident only with stress, but as the disease progresses, fatigue becomes more constant, may severely limit activities, and may require bed rest. Dizzy spells and posturally related fainting secondary to arterial hypotension may compound the clinical picture. These episodes have been mistaken for hypoglycemia. Symptoms related to gastrointestinal function may include anorexia (insidious at first, later severe), nausea, vomiting after meals, intermittent abdominal pain, and weight loss. Diarrhea or constipation have also been reported.

Hyperpigmentation usually appears early and is the most striking physical evidence of the disease. It may present as a diffuse tanning with increased pigmentation over pressure points such as knees, elbows, and knuckles. There may be a bluish-black pigmentation of the mucous membranes and multiple dark freckles. Patients occasionally notice unusually persistent tanning following exposure to the sun. Hyperpigmentation characteristically does not occur in patients with secondary adrenocortical hypofunction.

Laboratory Findings

The diagnosis of adrenal insufficiency requires the direct or indirect demonstration of decreased cortisol production in the basal or ACTH stimulated state. Final confirmation of the syndrome rests upon key laboratory determinations including plasma ACTH and cortisol levels, and urinary levels of 17-hydroxycorticoids, 17-ketosteroids, 17-ketogenic steroids, and free cortisol.

A definitive diagnosis can be made only with ACTH stimulation, which tests the adrenal capacity for steroid production. ACTH testing also helps establish whether adrenal insufficiency is primary or secondary.

Neuropsychiatric Features

Perhaps because of the rareness of Addison disease, little systematic study has been done of neuropsychiatric manifestations, although this association with hypoadrenalism has long been noted. Addison's original paper (1855) described mental status alterations. In most reports, mental status findings are presented as incidental observations, while the authors focus on the medical aspects of the illness.

The literature does not suggest that patients with the syndrome of hypoadrenalism are likely to present initially complaining of psychiatric symptoms, even though early symptoms have a similarity to neurasthenia or depression. The most common early symptoms are loss of initiative, fatigue, and weakness (Cleghorn, 1951; Ebaugh and Drake, 1957). Patients complain of being too tired to participate in their usual activities, "too tired to read," or even too tired to talk. The voice is usually weak and may be whiney. Addison (1855) called it an "indescribable" whine. Apathy, negativism, and seclusiveness may be present but difficult to differentiate from the fatigue state. Michael and Gibbons (1963) note that memory impairment forms a major feature in up to three quarters of cases. The mental anergia, poverty of thought, and general air of indifference may simulate early dementia. Anorexia may also point to a diagnosis of depression, although nausea and vomiting are common.

Engle and Margolin (1941) and Cleghorn (1951), in their separate reviews of two groups of 25 patients with Addison disease, suggest that psychiatric disturbances relatively unrelated to medical complications can be recognized. Most commonly these symptoms include anxiety, depression, and suspiciousness. A characteristic feature of these disturbances is their fluctuating and episodic nature, with relatively symptom-free intervals in between.

More severe disturbances have often been described in association with adrenocortical insufficiency, although there is no proof of a causal relationship with the psychoses. Various psychotic symptoms have been reported, including those associated with organic brain syndrome, i.e., dulling of the intellect, impaired judgment, disorientation, and visual hallucinations (Sorkin, 1949). Engle and Margolin (1941) found EEGs to be abnormal in five of eight patients and proposed that the disturbance was secondary to hypoglycemia. Hoffman et al. (1942), observed that 18 of 25 patients with Addison disease exhibited definite abnormalities in their resting EEGs.

Other psychotic symptoms have been reported. They include a variety of delusions, paranoia, bizarre posturings, and occasional catatonic states (Cleghorn, 1951; Sorkin, 1949). These findings appear to be rare, have no specific response pattern, and are most often secondary to changes in underlying metabolic processes, such as hypoglycemia or electrolyte disturbances. It should be noted, however, that correction of these disturbances inconsistently or only partially alleviates the psychic manifestations (Woodbury, 1958; Cleghorn, 1951). With appropriate corticosteroid therapy (which also suppresses excessive ACTH secretion), the physical and mental disturbances associated with hypoadrenalism are nearly always reversed.

Mechanisms of Neuropsychiatric Symptom Production

There is little doubt that much of the psychopathology seen with both excess endogenous and exogenous ACTH and corticosteroids is due to their effects on the brain. Beyond this little is known. Quarton et al. (1955), in an exhaustive review of the many hypotheses purporting to explain mental disturbances associated with ACTH or cortisone, concluded that there are no completely satisfactory hypotheses. That was in 1955; since then relatively little has been added, but tools such as sleep encephalography are providing additional information (Kales et al., 1968; Krieger and Gewirtz, 1974). It has also become apparent that certain " naturally" occurring states, such as psychoses and severe depression illness, are associated with excessive secretion of cortisol. The exact meaning of this information is unclear, but it remains possible that the increased ACTH and cortisol secretions may be having a secondary effect on CNS function, perhaps aggravating the existing psychopathology.

A similar lack of knowledge exists regarding the changes found with hypoadrenalism. Sacher (1975), in noting the paradox that depression is a common feature of both Cushing and Addison diseases, wonders whether the fact that ACTH is hypersecreted in both is significant. Other theories of mechanisms of action revolve around electrolyte metabolism, carbohydrate, protein, and fat metabolism, and the effects of cerebral blood flow and oxygen consumption. The observation that the patient suffering from a severe defect in steroid secretion experiences a more marked stimulus from hormonal treatment than those with normal or slightly reduced levels suggests that sudden changes in hormone level may be an etiologic factor.

THYROID DISORDERS

The normal function of the thyroid gland is to secrete the active thyroid hormones L-thyroxine (T_4) and 3,5,3-triiodo-L-thyronine (T_3), which influence a diversity of metabolic processes. Diseases of the thyroid gland are manifested by qualitative and quantitative alterations in hormonal secretion, enlargement of the thyroid (goiter), or both. Insufficient secretion results in the syndrome of hypothyroidism, in which decreased oxygen consumption (hypometabolism) is a classic manifestation. Conversely, excessive secretion of active hormone results in hyperthyroidism with hypermetabolism.

Regulation of thyroid function is affected by two general mechanisms, one suprathyroid and one intrathyroid. The mediator of suprathyroid regulation is thyrotropin, or thyroid-stimulating hormone (TSH), which is secreted by the anterior pituitary gland. TSH stimulates, accelerates, and enhances most aspects of glandular activity.

Regulation of TSH secretion is affected by two opposing influences. Thyrotropin-releasing hormone (TRH) is secreted by the hypothalamus, and, upon reaching the pituitary, stimulates synthesis and secretion of TSH. The effects of TRH are in turn inhibited (negative feedback) by thyroid hormone action on the pituitary. There is also an intrathyroid autoregulatory function that is important but poorly understood.

Laboratory Findings

There is now a variety of laboratory tests permitting evaluation of many aspects of thyroid functioning. The following are the most common (Ingbar and Waeber, 1977). The thyroid radioactive iodide uptake (RAIU) is most often used as a direct test of thyroid gland function. The RAIU is usually measured 24 hr after ^{131}I administration; test results vary inversely with the amount of endogenous stable iodide. Due to the widespread use of iodine-enriched foods, the RAIU is no longer of value in discriminating hypothyroidism, but it remains useful in indicating thyroid hyperfunction. Normal values vary in differing geographical areas (average range is 5% to 45%).

Among tests related to hormone concentration and binding in blood are measurements of triiodothyronine (T_3) (normal range of 80–160 µg/100 ml) and thyroxine (T_4) measured by its ability to displace stable T_4 and called T_4(D) (normal range of 4–11 µg/100 ml). Measurement of serum protein-bound iodine (PBI) concentration (normal level 4–8 µg/100 ml) has generally been superceded by the T_4(D), which has more specificity.

Several tests of more general metabolic functioning have been traditionally used, but these are of comparatively less value than recent, more specific tests. They include the basal metabolic rate (BMR), serum cholestrol level, and measurements of the Achilles reflex time.

Among tests of homeostatic control, measurement of TSH has become important in the diagnosis of hypothyroidism and diminished thyroid reserve. The normal range is less than 5 microunits/ml. This test is of value in distinguishing between untreated hypothyroidism of thyroidal origin, in which the values are increased, and of pituitary or hypothalamic origin, in which the values are within the normal range. Use of the TSH stimulation test and the TRH stimulation test permits further discrimination of the type of thyroid dysfunction. The thyroid suppression test is also used to measure homeostatic control mechanisms. Further information about these tests may best be obtained from standard medical textbooks.

Hyperthyroidism

Hyperthyroidism may be defined as the constellation of signs and symptoms that occur when there is an excessive supply of thyroid hormone to the tissues. Although hyperthyroidism is most commonly associated with Graves disease (toxic goiter), it may also be caused by excessive administration of thyroid hormone or by autonomous nodules of toxic nodule goiter. All forms of hyperthyroidism are marked by an increased rate of tissue metabolism and by certain disturbances of the neuromuscular system. Graves disease has certain additional distinguishing characteristics.

Graves disease is relatively common; its etiology is unknown. It is especially frequent in the third and fourth decades of life and is more frequent in women. Although it has long been considered a classic psychosomatic disease, recent investigations (Hermann and Quarton, 1965; Robbins and Vinson, 1960) have cast doubt on proposed psychological explanations, especially those that postulate specific predisposing personality features. Recent evidence suggests the presence of an immunologic blood factor (LATS) of extrapituitary origin. Variations in the presentation and course of the disease suggest the possibility of multiple etiological factors.

Clinical Features

Hyperthyroidism (thyrotoxicosis) may be seen in all grades of severity and may begin suddenly or slowly. The disease is classically characterized by "nervousness," sensitivity to heat, sweating (though palms may remain dry), restless overactivity, a fine tremor, and weight loss (usually associated with increased appetite). Hyperdefecation and occasional nausea and vomiting may occur. Fatigue and weakness are often present, and are occasionally manifested by an inability to climb stairs. Severe muscle wasting may be seen. Tachycardia and arrhythmias causing dyspnea and palpitations are common. In general, symptoms referable to the nervous system are more likely to dominate the clinical picture in younger individuals, whereas cardiovascular and muscular symptoms predominate in older subjects.

Other findings may include velvety textured skin with palmar erythema. The hair tends to be fine and silky; hair loss is a common complaint. The thyroid is diffusely enlarged, and often a thrill or bruit may be heard.

Clinical signs particularly associated with Graves disease are ophthalmopathy and dermopathy. The eye signs, such as exophthalmos, may be a striking feature in Graves disease, but usually definitive findings are subtle. Associated signs of lid lag, globe lag, diminished blinking, and retraction of the upper or lower eyelid are noted, with weakness or paresis of the extraocular muscles. In more advanced cases of ophthamopathic types of Graves disease, peribulbar edema, conjunctivitis, and diminution in visual acuity occur.

Another specific sign of Graves disease is a localized myxedema or pretibial myxedema occuring over the dorsum of the legs or feet. Affected areas are demarcated from the normal skin by being raised, thickened, and pigmented. These signs may rarely be seen over the fingers and hands.

Patients with severe, prolonged thyrotoxicosis may enter a phase of the disease called thyroid crisis or storm. Often precipitated by surgery to the neck region, it may also occur with other kinds of trauma, such as infection. Classically, it occurs suddenly, resulting in great restlessness, high fever, sweating, shock, vomiting and dehydration, and associated delirium. In recent years, with adequate treatment, this particular kind of picture has become rare.

Neuropsychiatric Features

The literature dealing with mental disturbances and hyperthyroidism is less extensive than that dealing with hypothyroidism and most of it is oriented toward exploring psychogenic etiologies of the syndrome. The relative paucity of literature in this area, as well as several comparative studies suggest that mental changes are less common and extreme in hyperthyroidism than in hypothyroidism. The possibility of pre-existing or concurrent psychiatric illness also makes the statistical estimation of psychiatric changes in hyperthyroidism difficult.

When physical symptoms of hyperthyroidism are present, some mental symptoms are almost always found. Patients presenting with only mental changes have not been reported, though signs of thyroid dysfunction are occasionally overlooked. The patient is typically hyperactive and complains of nervousness or anxiety. This general self-assessment appears to be prompted by a generalized fine tremor, described as jitteriness or shakiness, and by a subjectively perceived irritability and emotional lability. Other autonomic symptoms may contribute to this conclusion. This "nervousness" is unlike that of the chronically anxious patient: it is characterized by restlessness, shortness of attention span, and a need to move about. Some authors (Kleinschmidt et al., 1956) have used the terms *destructive aggressiveness* and *impulsivity* to describe these patients, but these characteristics do not appear to be common.

Uitert and Russakoff (1979) described a case of a 26-year-old woman who presented herself as constantly nervous and restless with a tendency toward marked agitation and tremulousness. After hospitalization, her condition progressed to quick, jerky purposeless movements of the distal extremities, neck, and facial muscles, and, under stress, she developed choreiform movements. Examination revealed diffuse hyperreflexia and a rapid low-amplitude tremor of the extremities and tongue. Because of the concurrent psychodynamic issues in her life, this relatively rare manifestation of thyrotoxicosis, hyperthyroid chorea, led several physicians to consider her illness to be entirely psychiatric. An exaggerated startle reaction may also be seen or reported by the patient. Even when encouraged by physicians or relatives, most patients are usually unable to attach specific ideational content to their anxiety, referring to it more as a sensation. Another important clinical note in differentiating hyperthyroidism from anxiety neurosis, is that in the hyperthyroid state, appetite is characteristically increased, whereas in anxiety states it tends to be reduced.

The emotional lability results in episodes of unexpected tearfulness and crying. Patients often state that they have nothing to cry about and seem bewildered by their personality changes. They may attribute these changes to frustration from their lessened ability to carry out tasks requiring long attention spans, due to heightened distractibility and fatigue. MacCrimmon et al. (1979) have demonstrated evidence that in addition to the marked emotional disturbance, there is a subtle disturbance of cognitive function substantially related to the actual levels of excessive thyroid hormone. These changes are not present upon euthyroid followup. Wilson et al. (1964) demonstrated similar changes by giving 11 normal subjects exogenous T_3 for three days and noted that they showed marked changes in feeling tone and significant changes in the direction of increased depression, increased jitteriness, and decreased friendliness.

Depression is mentioned in the literature, but seems to have a less pervasive and severe quality than that found in hypothyroid patients. Whybrow's group (1969) were not found to be particularly depressed by either clinical observation or self-rating scales. Kleinschmidt et al. (1956) described a type of depression that preceded the fully developed toxic state. Hyperactivity may produce a clinical picture similar to agitated depression, but a consistent depressed mood is usually lacking.

Despite complaints of fatigue, insomnia is also common. Careful inquiry shows that patients are describing a shortened sleep period and alteration in sleep pattern, with easier arousability. It does not sound like typical neurotic insomnia with its inability to screen out upsetting thoughts. Other somatic complaints apparently unrelated to the basic hyperthyroid condition are common. Whybrow (1969) described deviated MMPI profiles, suggesting a hysterical elaboration of somatic complaints, but MacCrimmon et al. (1979), while finding similar scale elevations, noted the return to normal after treatment. Their findings thus suggest that manifestations of neurotic or even psychotic features in the presence of thyrotoxicity may well be related to biochemical abnormalities in cerebrospinal fluid and brain tissue and should not be used to infer previous personality patterns.

There is an exception to the usual hyperkinesis of the hyperthyroid patient. Almost 50 years ago, a form of thyrotoxicosis was identified in which "nonactivation" was a dominant clinical feature. It was designated "apathetic hyperthyroidism" (Lackey, 1931); it is also called "masked" thyrotoxicosis because it lacks the usual clinical characteristics of excessive activation, enlarged gland, and typical ocular manifestations. This type is most often found in the elderly. Instead of the usual findings, substantial fatigue and weakness, excessive weight loss, and cardiovascular complications are most prominent.

Mental status findings reveal an apathy or placidity often mistaken for depression. The patient may appear disinterested and detached, almost resigned to death (Thomas et al., 1970). (This type of picture may also be seen in hypothyroidism.) Patients with apathetic thyrotoxicosis may quietly lapse into coma and die, thus early differentiation from severe depression may be critical. Suspicion of thyroid dysfunction should lead to appropriate thyroid function studies to confirm the diagnosis.

Psychosis. Patients who simultaneously exhibit symptoms of hyperthyroidism and overt psychosis have been noted often enough to prompt studies of the relationship between the two sets of symptoms. Estimates of the incidence of this association depend heavily on the definition of psychosis and how the study was done, i.e., whether the studied patients are on medical units or are from a psychiatric population. Lidz (1949) described 20% of hyperthyroid patients in a medical outpatient setting as having psychotic symptomatology; however, the criteria in this study were soft, since none of these patients was felt to be sufficiently decompensated as to require hospitalization. Kleinschmidt (1956) also found that 9% of 84 thyrotoxic patients had been diagnosed as schizophrenic and 11% as "borderline." Most workers, however, maintain that it is rare to find psychosis among medical hyperthyroid populations (Michael and Gibbins, 1963; Bursten, 1961; Smith et al., 1972; Burch and Messervy, 1978).

When psychiatric populations are examined, the coincidence of symptoms seems quite low. Bluestone (1957) found one patient out of 1000 in a large public mental hospital to have hyperthyroidism. Bursten (1961) noted ten cases of thyrotoxicosis among 8000 overtly psychotic patients. The studies of Clower et al. (1969) also confirmed the rarity of this finding. However, a recent report found three patients with elevated serum thyroid hormone levels among 50 patients screened from a general psychiatric service (Weinberg and Katzell, 1977).

No single psychotic picture is typical, and diagnoses include schizophrenia, toxic psychoses, and manic-depressive disease. Bursten (1961) pointed to the hyperactivity of the hyperthyroid patient as providing a "manic veneer" to psychotic pictures. Suspiciousness and paranoid symptoms are prominently mentioned in the literature. Both the paranoia and schizophrenia scales of the MMPI have been reported as raised (Whybrow et al., 1969). Recent work (Robbins and Vinson, 1960; Kleinschmidt et al., 1956; Whybrow et al., 1969) stressing cognitive changes and the fact that these changes resolve with treatment, suggests that the psychosis is basically a toxic phenomenon. Whether the psychosis results from a direct toxic effect of thyroid hormone or by interference with metabolic processes, or whether hyperthyroidism is a nonspecific psychological stress that precipitates a "latent psychosis" is not known. In all likelihood either phenomenon might occur in different patients.

Treatment

The treatment of hyperthyroidism takes two major approaches. In the first, antithyroid agents are used to block hormone synthesis. In the second, the ablation of thyroid tissue by means of surgery or radioactive iodine achieves limitation of hormone production. Each mode of therapy has advantages and disadvantages, as well as varying indications.

There are no specific studies other than that by Whybrow et al. (1969) that report on mental status following treatment of patients with hyperthyroidism. Most studies imply that neuropsychiatric symptoms resolve to the extent that they are related to organic changes, with personality traits and constellations remaining relatively unaffected. In the study by Whybrow et al. (1969), a general reduction of psychiatric symptomatology could be seen on total scores of the Brief Psychiatric Rating Scale, Implied Mood Scale, and MMPI main profiles. The Trailmaking and Porteus Maze tests also showed significant improvement. There is no suggestion in the literature that irreversible changes occur, although this conclusion would be difficult to document in the case of psychoses that are likely to be of uncertain etiology. There are several reports of either an organic psychosis or a schizophrenic-like psychosis making an appearance during treatment with antithyroid drugs. It is not known whether this occurs in response to the toxic effect of the drug or to a period of drug-induced hypothyroidism (Herridge and Abey-Wickrama, 1969; Brewer, 1969; Bessher, 1971).

Hypothyroidism

Hypothyroidism is a clinical state resulting from a variety of structural or functional abnormalities that lead to insufficient synthesis of thyroid hormone. Abnormalities may occur at the pituitary or hypothalamic levels or in the thyroid gland itself. The most common cause is surgical or radioiodide ablation in the treatment of Graves disease. When hypothyroidism dates from birth and results in developmental abnormalities, it is termed cretinism. The term myxedema refers to a severe form of hypothyroidism with changes in the skin and other tissues.

Clinical Features

In the adult, early general symptoms are insidious and nonspecific. They include fatigue, cold intolerance, constipation, and menorrhagia. In succeeding months, slowing of intellectual and motor activity begin to appear. Appetite lessens, even though weight gain may occur. Other complaints include dry skin, hair loss or dryness, muscle aching, and fatigue. The voice may become hoarse and deeper. Finally, the clinical picture of myxedema appears, with a dull expressionless face, periorbital puffiness, dry sparse hair, large tongue, and pale, rough, and doughy skin. This slowed metabolic picture may, if untreated, pass into a stuporous state that can be fatal.

Neuropsychiatric Features

Almost every type of psychiatric reaction has been described as associated with hypothyroidism. Because most reports are case descriptions, it is difficult to determine accurately either the incidence or prevalence of various neuropsychiatric manifestations. Nearly all patients with clinical hypothyroidism have some minor cognitive changes. Conversely, many reports describe patients presenting initially or solely with psychiatric symptoms. Clower et al. (1969) did PBI determinations of 3011 patients hospitalized in a state mental hospital. Forty-seven patients (1.5%) had PBIs of less than 3.5 μg/100 ml (normal values range from 4 to 8 μg/100 ml).

There is a clear spectrum of symptoms ranging from mild, barely noticeable changes, to psychosis or delirium. Disturbances are described in cognitive, affective, and behavioral spheres. Early in the illness, a progressive slowing of all mental processes predominates. Sir William Gull (1873), in reporting the first cases of hypothyroidism, said of a patient, "The mind which previously had been active and inquisitive assumed a gentle, placid indifference." In another report (Schon et al., 1961), a patient stated, "I used to think clear, now I let someone else do the thinking for me. Before my thinking was vivid, now it is dull and veiled."

Memory for recent events is impaired, and patients complain of losing things and of making stupid mistakes while doing everyday chores. The ability to concentrate is also diminished, and simple mathematics becomes difficult. Tests using serial threes or sevens are particularly helpful in assessing this deficit. Whybrow et al. (1969), confirmed profound difficulty with psychological tests that demand attention, abstraction, and memory. Although reports of patients' responses to their deficit vary, it appears that they are initially very frustrated by their helplessness, but with time and the increasing severity of the dysfunction they come to appear indifferent.

Significant depressive affect is mentioned in nearly all clinical reports and is highlighted in studies using psychological tests or rating scales (Clower et al., 1969; Whybrow et al., 1969; Pitts and Guze, 1961; Jain, 1972; Bernstein, 1965; Tonks, 1964; Logothetis, 1963; Gibson, 1962). In cases presenting initially as psychiatric illness, the diagnosis of severe or psychotic depression is often made. In several reports (Pitts and Guze, 1961; Bernstein, 1965) antidepressant medication or electroconvulsive therapy was administered prior to the diagnosis of hypothyroidism (with occasional positive results).

It is interesting to note that, although many medical descriptions of hypothyroid patients use terms such as flat, somnolent, stuporous, or pathetic, psychiatric descriptions highlight a different aspect of patient behavior. They are frequently seen as anxious, markedly irritable with labile affect, and suffering from insomnia. One group of patients was described (Schon et al., 1961) as having "oppositional tendencies." A patient noted, "I did not want anyone to do anything for me, but I was annoyed if they did not do it. I wanted people to come and see me but when they came I could not wait for them to leave." Frequently, they were argumentative and emotionally explosive, with outbursts of screaming and yelling at family members. These behaviors were ego-dystonic and the patients were surprised, and puzzled, and deeply regretted their actions.

Psychosis. More severe manifestations have long been considered characteristic of hypothyroidism. Perhaps it was A. J. Cronin's (1937) vivid description of "myxedema madness" in *The Citadel* that prompted much of subsequent medical attention. Since that time, many cases of psychoses associated with hypothyrodism have been reported. Two early authors (Beck, 1926; Von Jauregg, 1912) indicated that psychotic symptoms are present in 15–26% of myxedematous patients. Eight of the 47 patients reported on by Clower et al. (1969) were felt to be psychotic. The difficulty of determining whether these symptoms were independent of the myxedema, the use of variable criteria for psychosis, and a relative paucity of appropriate laboratory methods leading to the diagnosis of hypothyroidism suggest that these frequency figures may not be accurate. In most reports, the psychosis is associated with severe hypothyroidism, but this is not always the case, since the severity of mental symptoms and physical symptoms is not closely correlated (the relationship of mental symptoms to laboratory values has not been reported) (Jain, 1972). For most patients, several months to a few years elapse between the appearance of clinical myxedema and psychiatric symptoms. However, in a substantial number of reported cases, mental symptoms were the initial indication and no clinical signs of myxedema were present.

No uniform type of psychosis appears to be specific to hypothyroidism. Most recent observers feel that the psychosis of myxedema resembles that seen in many different disturbances of cerebral metabolism caused by a multiplicity of agents or diseases. It is felt to be fundamentally an organic psychosis with basic sensorial disturbances, with mood, thought content, and behavioral changes superimposed, and representing a "release" phenomenon (Browing et al., 1954). General clouding of sensorium, disorientation, recent memory deficits, and visual hallucinations are prominent. As with all organic psychoses, the specific presentation is affected by situational variables, emotional conflict, and personality structure.

Initial misdiagnosis is common. The syndrome has similarities to depressive psychoses, and panpsychotic symptomatology may easily be mistaken for schizophrenia. It may include difficulty with abstractions, auditory hallucinations, persecutory delusions, and behavioral regression. Paranoid features have been frequently emphasized. Several reports (Clower et al., 1969; Pitts and Guze, 1961, Logothetis, 1963; Asher, 1949) describe hyperactive behavior, "restless violence," and occasional hypomania, again contradicting the common picture of a withdrawn, somnolent, myxedematous patient.

Dementia may develop as an extension of the acute organic brain syndrome. It may progress insidiously in a manner indistinguishable from primary presenile dementia, and, if not proceeded by an acute phase, may reach an advanced degree by the time the diagnosis is made. Olivarus and Roder (1970) consider myxedema to be the most important and most frequently overlooked of the metabolic causes of reversible organic intellectual impairment.

Neurologic Symptoms

Specific attention to neurosensory related complaints and to the neurologic history may be particularly useful. Both increased and decreased auditory acuity have been reported (Schon et al., 1961; DeVos, 1963; Post, 1964). Complaints referrable to the eyes, such as feeling "cross-eyed," haziness, double vision, and difficulty reading, are common, as are alterations in sense of smell and taste (Schon et al., 1961; McConnell et al., 1975). Acroparesthesias, in addition to neurologic signs such as pseudomyotonic reflexes and mild incoordination, are common in myxedematous patients (Logothetis, 1963). All of these symptoms have a hypochondriacal flavor, calling for alertness in interpretation.

Treatment

The response of neuropsychiatric symptoms to administration of thyroid replacement therapy is variable. Most patients report subjective improvement, which is verified by psychometric testing and clinical observation (Schon et al., 1961; Whybrow et al., 1969; Jain, 1972; Browning, 1954). Improvement appears to occur most often among patients with mental changes of a cognitive, nonpsychotic quality (Tonks, 1964). There have been no reports of recovery in patients with mental changes lasting more than two years. This is consistent with the view that basic mental changes are due to an organic brain syndrome secondary to altered cerebral metabolism. In several studies (Logothetis, 1963; Browning, 1954), EEG changes were closely correlated with improvement in the clinical picture.

In psychotic patients, improvement following return to a euthyroid state is less certain. Marked improvement in 75% has been estimated as an average (Logothetis, 1963). There are several explanations for this lower improvement rate. Irreversible changes may have occurred. Despite early beliefs that the adult central nervous system is refractory to thyroid hormone deficiency (Whybrow et al., 1969; Tonks, 1964), it appears that a chronic deficiency does leave a residual deficit. It is also possible that a relatively independent psychiatric disorder was coincidentally present along with the hypothyroidism; this possibility is a continuing problem in interpreting any of the studies in this area. As might be expected, patients who do not improve substantially show various clinical pictures. It has been suggested that paranoid symptoms are particularly refractive to replacement therapy (Tonks, 1964), and affective disorders may also be resistant. Electroconvulsive therapy has been effectively used in several patients with affective disorders (Pitts and Guze, 1961).

There are some reports suggesting that replacement therapy sometimes causes a worsening of the emotional state of myxedematous patients. In one study (Easson, 1966) 11 of 19 patients had a temporary deterioration of emotional adjustment soon after institution of replacement therapy. In several cases, psychosis developed after the start of the thyroid medication (Malden, 1955). Josefson and Mackeanzie (1979) described a patient with a history of affective disorder who developed a manic psychosis in the early stages of treatment with thyroxine. These changes appear temporary, and it is generally recommended that thyroid replacement be continued despite heightened disturbance. These sorts of problems and exceptions to smooth recovery emphasize the need for psychiatric and medical collaboration in the treatment of the hypothyroid patient.

Mechanisms of Neuropsychiatric Symptom Production

The mechanism of production of mental symptoms associated with either an excess or a deficit of thyroid hormone is not clear. Although it is well known that thyroid hormones are necessary for the normal development of the CNS, it was initially thought that the mature brain was refractory to direct influence by thyroid hormones and that changes were secondary to effects on other organ systems. This belief was based largely on studies (Scheinberg et al., 1950; Sasenbach et al., 1954) that demonstrated an alteration in cerebral blood flow without apparent alteration of oxygen consumption.

However, an increasing number of clinical reports (Tonks, 1964; Whybrow et al., 1969) demonstrate that irreversible damage to the CNS can occur, that chronic deficiency does leave a residual deficit, and that the CNS may be extremely sensitive to the effects of thyroid hormone. The evidence (Treadway et al., 1967; Williams, 1968) includes observations that in some patients the CNS is the first organ system to respond to thyroid hormone replacement therapy and that some "typical" symptoms can be reproduced when thyroid hormone is given to normal subjects.

Other research evidence (Voth et al., 1970; Axelrod, 1973) allows further speculation. Thyroid hormone increases the sensitivity of neuroreceptors to catecholamines, decreases monoamine oxidase activity, and decreases the turnover rate of norepinephrine. A resulting deficiency of catecholamine at central adrenergic receptor sites may account for the common association of depression with hypothyroidism and for the relative absence of profound depression in hyperthyroid states. Recent interest in the treatment of some depressive disorders with thyroid hormone stems from these observations.

Psychotropic Drugs and the Thyroid

Antianxiety Drugs

There are no known contraindications to the use of antianxiety drugs in thyroid illness. Early reports (Baron, 1967; Mazzaferri and Skillman, 1964) suggested that both diazepam and chlorodiazepoxide affected the handling of thyroid hormones. Subsequent studies (Clark and Ormston, 1971; Schussler, 1971; Barnes et al., 1972) have failed to confirm interference at a level that would significantly alter thyroid function studies.

Tricyclic Antidepressants

The interaction of thyroid hormone and tricyclic antidepressants appears to be beneficial. It was believed (Prange et al., 1970; Wilson et al., 1970) that the administration of thyroid hormone (or thyroid thyrotropin-releasing hormone) enhanced the response from this group of antidepressants. These hormones both seemed to accelerate the response, particularly in females; this was thought to be of aid in treating resistant depressions (Wheatley, 1972; Earle, 1970). The mechanism is felt to be secondary to the increase in receptor sensitivity to catacholamines and the enhancement of catecholamine metabolism. Hollister (1978) notes, however, that the initial reports of dramatic efficacy have not been confirmed by a great number of controlled studies. Conversely, there is some (unconfirmed) suggestion (Prange et al., 1976) that hyperthyroid patients are somewhat refractory to antidepressants.

Phenothiazines

Harmful drug–drug interactions have not been reported. In a preliminary study, Park (1974) suggested that T_4 may enhance the antipsychotic effects of chlopromazine. There is evidence (Davis, 1966) to indicate that phenothiazines may have an antithyroid effect, with decreases in PBI following large doses. Chlorpromazine also has been shown to increase thyroid uptake of ^{131}I (Blumberg and Klein, 1969).

Haloperidol

In 1973, Lake and Fann reported on a patient with hyperthyroidism who developed severe life-threatening neurotoxic symptoms (parkinsonlike rigidity) and symptoms of thyroid storm following treatment with haloperidol. Other similar cases (Hamadah and Teggin, 1974; Yosselson and Kaplan, 1975; Hoffman et al., 1978) have subsequently been reported. Since there have been reports demonstrating that thyroxine treatment sensitizes the CNS of rats to the toxic effects of haloperidol (Selye and Szabo, 1972), it is felt that a synergistic effect results in an extremely toxic picture and/or clinical thyroid storm. Weiner (1979) reported a patient with psychotic behavior who was treated with haloperidol and later discovered to have hyperthyroidism. The patient subsequently developed a bulbar-palsy-like syndrome with difficulty in swallowing and died.

In all of the reported cases (with the exception of Weiner's, in which the doses ranged from 5 to 25 mg/day), the doses of haloperidol were relatively small (4–8 mg/day); symptoms appeared to occur up to three weeks after administration of the drug, and discontinuation of the drug and administration of antiparkinsonian agents seems to be helpful. These cases suggest that haloperidol should not be used in patients who are known to be hyperthyroid and that a diagnosis of thyrotoxicosis should be considered when patients develop suggestive symptoms during haloperidol administration.

Lithium

Although lithium affects thyroid function at a number of sites, its predominant effect at therapeutic levels is to inhibit iodine release (including T_3 and T_4) from the gland (Jefferson and Greist, 1977). Thyroid-related complications of lithium therapy include euthyroid goiter, hypothyroidism with or without goiter, or merely abnormalities of laboratory tests in the absence of clinical manifestations.

The incidence of goiter consequent to lithium therapy is about 4%, and rarely does the thyroid enlarge to the extent that it becomes a cosmetic problem. The goiter is usually adequate to compensate for the lithium-induced depression of thyroid function but occasionally a patient becomes clinically hypothyroid.

Hypothyroidism due to lithium may develop in the presence or absence of goiter. The onset can occur at any time during the course of treatment and symptoms may vary from minimal to those of severe myxedema. The syndrome is reversible if lithium is discontinued, but should it be necessary to continue the drug, the appropriate amount of exogenous thyroid hormone will restore euthyroidism.

There have been a number of case reports of hyperthyroidism developing during the course of lithium therapy. (Lindstedt et al., 1977; Brownlie et al., 1976; Rosser, 1976; and Reus et al., 1979). This apparently paradoxical response may be coincidental, although it is possible that it represents a "break-through" of lithium-caused hormonal buildup in the gland. On the other hand, lithium has been used successfully in the treatment of thyrotoxicosis either alone or in combination with thiocarbamide drugs.

Serum TSH (thyroid stimulating hormone) levels are often elevated in patients taking lithium. The higher elevations tend to occur in association with a low serum T_4 level and clinical hypothyroidism, while lesser elevations may be found with normal serum T_4 levels in asymptomatic patients. Even if serum TSH levels are normal, patients on lithium are likely to show an exaggerated TSH response to intravenous TRH suggesting that thyroid function alterations (usually subclinical) occur in almost all patients.

PARATHYROID DISORDERS

Hyperparathyroidism

Parathyroid hormone promotes the absorption of calcium from the gastrointestinal tract, the absorption of calcium ion from bone, and the excretion of phosphate from the kidney, all of which increase the concentration of circulating calcium ions. In primary hyperparathyroidism, an increased amount of hormone is secreted directly from the gland. The cause is usually a benign adenoma occurring in one gland (81%), but may be carcinoma (4%), or a generalized hyperplasia of all of the glands (15%) (Ingbar and Waeber, 1977).

There is also evidence that a clinical syndrome resembling primary hyperparathyroidism may result from production of parathyroid-hormone-like peptides by some nonparathyroid tumors. This syndrome is called pseudoparathyroidism. Many types of tumors have been associated with this syndrome, lung and renal tumors being most common.

Most of the signs and syptoms of hyperparathyroidism reflect the consequences of hypercalcemia. The following discussion of hyperparathyroidism describes the effects of elevated serum calcium levels *regardless* of the underlying cause. There are many other conditions that may produce hypercalcemia, such as pheochromocytoma, hyperthyroidism, renal failure, sarcoidosis, excessive ingestion of vitamin D, adrenal insufficiency, bone disease, and lengthy immobilization from prolonged bed rest or containment in a body cast.

It has been estimated that up to 20% of all patients with carcinoma will have hypercalcemia at some point during their illness, usually in the terminal stages. The most common tumors which produce hypercalcemia are those of the lung, breast, and kidney. Among hematologic malignancies, multiple myeloma is a frequent cause (Singer et al., 1977). Transient increases in serum total calcium and inorganic phosphorus levels have also been observed during periodic recurrent exacerbations of psychotic agitation and mania (Carmen and Wyatt, 1979).

Primary hyperparathyroidism occurs most commonly in adults, with the peak incidence between the third and fifth decade, although it has been detected in young children and in the elderly as well. It is generally a chronic disease with insidious onset, but it may appear abruptly. An estimate of the incidence in the general population is one case per 1000 per year (Ingbar and Waeber, 1977).

Clinical Features

Although many organ systems may be involved, renal and skeletal systems are most prominent in the production of signs and symptoms. Kidney involvement due to deposition of calcium in the renal parenchyma or to production of renal stones is found in 60–70% of patients. Bone changes are usually in the form of osteitis fibrosa cystica, in which there is an altered pattern of bone formation. These changes are not likely to give specific symptoms, but the characteristic patterns in the bone of the hand, skull, or margins of the teeth may be demonstrated by x-ray. Other general features of the disease include neuromuscular involvement, with specific muscle weakness, occasional atrophy, and general easy fatigability. Anorexia, nausea, vomiting, constipation, and symptoms related to duodenal ulcer are common gastrointestinal complaints.

Laboratory Findings

The most important screening test for hyperparathyroidism is the serum calcium, which is now part of the routine admission screening battery in many hospitals (normal level is 9–11 mg/100 ml). The serum phosphorus is also important but is somewhat less specific (normal is 3.0–4.5 mg/100 ml). A specific radioimmunoassay to detect circulating parathyroid hormone has also been developed; although it has been difficult to standardize, it is proving to be of increasing value. Glucocorticoid administration has also been useful in differentiating the hypercalcemia of hyperparathyroidism from that associated with other diseases. Doses of hydrocortisone given for ten days do not yield the usual lowering of serum calcium levels in hyperparathyroidism.

Neuropsychiatric Features

The association of hyperparathyroidism or hypercalcemia with mental changes has been a relatively recent observation. In the first systematic collection of cases of hyperparathyroidism, Eitinger (1942) noted mental symptoms in 7 of 50 patients. In a review of four large series of patients with this disorder, Agras and Oliveau (1964) found symptoms in 4.2% of 405 cases. In studies in which psychiatric symptoms were specifically sought, the proportion of hyperparathyroid patients experiencing changes in mental status is much higher. Kind (1959) found 50% of his cases to be mentally disturbed. Karpati and Frame (1964) found neuropsychiatric changes in 42%. In 12% of these cases, the manifestations dominated the picture and led to consultation with a psychiatrist or neurologist. In the most thorough study thus far, Petersen (1968), after excluding patients referred primarily because of psychiatric disorders, found a 65% incidence of mental changes in a group of patients with hyperparathyroidism.

The neuropsychiatric changes reported are not specific ones. In the majority of cases, symptoms begin with minor personality changes, usually in the affective sphere. Patients suffer from depressed mood, become listless and apathetic, lose their sense of spontaneity and their initiative, and experience a "loss of drive." Boyd et al. (1929) described this state as "marked lassitude of the body and mind." This is often attributed to physical weakness or fatigue by the patient. These changes are often recognized only retrospectively when surgery has restored the metabolic state to normal. Anderson (1968) found that three quarters of patients reported that they felt better postoperatively, with higher spirits and greater energy than they had had for many years. It is this chronicity which makes it difficult for the patient to appreciate and objectively report mental changes. Noble (1974) reported a case of treatment-resistant depression that responded to antidepressants only after the parathyroid adenoma was removed. In reporting a case of severe depression, Reinfrank (1961) was prompted to suggest adding "mental moan" to the familiar triad of "bone, stone, and abdominal groan" used to remind one of hyperparathyroid symptoms.

In several reports, the patients' mental state was complicated by irritability and by emotional lability (Agras and Oliveau, 1964; Karpati and Frame, 1964). Overt anxiety is less often described. Specific complaints related to cognitive abilities appear relatively rare; problems of this type most frequently noted were impaired concentration and some disturbance of recent memory.

The course of the more minor psychiatric disturbances is usually of an insidious nature over months or even years. When an organic psychosis appears it usually has a sudden onset. The acute organic psychoses are manifested by disorientation, confusion, paranoid ideation, delusions, and hallucinations. They are nonspecific for either hyperparathyroidism or hypercalcemia, although Agras and Oliveau (1964) noted six cases of psychoses from the literature that seemed remarkably similar. All cases presented with clear sensoria but were characterized by severe depression and paranoid delusions, with irritable, boisterous, or violent behavior.

It is not known what percent of patients might present with manifestations of hypercalcemia that are primarily or most conspicuously related to the central nervous system. Cope (1967) concluded that mental changes were diagnostic clues in 3% of 460 patients of internists. Because mental changes are not specific, one must be alert to associated symptoms to provide clues.

Although several associated physical symptoms might be inadvertently attributed to depression, such as anorexia, constipation, sleep disturbance, and fatigue, several other symptoms should encourage suspicion of another underlying disorder. Petersen (1968) points to thirst occurring in conjunction with lack of initiative, depression, and an insidiously developing change of personality, as a helpful diagnostic clue. Headaches of a nonspecific type were found in 50% of the patients of Karpati and Frame (1964), and this symptom is frequently mentioned by others. Muscle weakness is a prominent complaint; it is general in nature, may occur without atrophy, and mainly involves the girdle and/or proximal limb muscles. Stiffness may also occur, and there is one report of a catatonic-like stupor (Cooper and Schapiru, 1973).

Dysken and Halaris (1978) reported a case in which asterixis developed post-ECT in a patient with manic depressive illness, leading to the diagnosis of primary hyperparathyroidism. Seizures, aphonia, hoarseness, deafness, and papilledema have also been reported but do not appear common. The gastrointestinal symptoms of nausea, vomiting, and upper gastric pain should raise suspicions.

Mental changes can be rather closely correlated with the degree of hypercalcemia. Bleuler (1967) points out that the psychiatric disorders of hyperparathyroidism are more constant from person to person, and less dependent on the dynamics of the personality, than are the psychiatric pictures seen with other endocrine disorders. They are not related directly to parathyroid hormone levels, for correction of calcium levels through peritoneal dialysis provides rapid relief of symptoms despite continued elevations of hormone levels (Petersen, 1968). In a review of 60 patients, Petersen found personality changes with affective disorders and disturbances of drive when serum calcium levels were in the 12–16 mg/100 ml range. Acute organic psychosis began at about 16 mg/100 ml. Although another worker reported a lower mean value (15.4 mg/100 ml) for the maximum levels in a series of six psychotic patients (Agras and Oliveau, 1964), calcium levels of 16 to 19 mg% were associated with alterations in consciousness. Hallucinations and paranoid states were common symptoms. Blood levels of over 19 mg% caused somnolence or coma. There are, of course, exceptions. Patients with mental status changes that improved following removal of the parathyroid gland have been reported with calcium levels lower than 12 mg% (Karpati and Frame, 1964; Reinfrank, 1961). At the other extreme, a patient was described as "cheerful and uncomplaining" with a serum calcium level of 20 mg% (Agras and Oliveau, 1964).

Treatment

Most patients regain their former emotional states when parathyroid adenomas are removed and calcium levels return to normal. Recovery time is not related to duration of the disease, severity of illness, or age of the patient. There are no reports of irreversible changes occurring.

There have been a number of reports of psychotic episodes following the removal of parathyroid adenomas in patients with few or no known psychiatric problems prior to surgery. These occurred three to six days after surgery and in the presence of normal serum calcium levels (Karpati and Frame, 1964; Gatewood et al., 1975; Potts and Roberts, 1958; Bergeron et al., 1961; Mikkelsen and Reider, 1979). It has been postulated that the sudden drop in extracellular calcium may precipitate these episodes. Bergeron et al. (1961) and Gatewood et al. (1975) noted depressed serum magnesium levels, and in some cases the abnormal mental behavior improved after administration of magnesium.

Hypoparathyroidism

Hypoparathyroidism is a metabolic abnormality characterized by hypocalcemia and consequent neuromuscular symptoms. The most common form is found secondary to removal or damage of the parathyroid glands, usually following surgery for thyroid disorder or radical neck dissection for cancers. It may also occur secondary to radiation therapy. The symptoms of hypoparathyroidism most frequently develop several days after the trauma, although there may be a delay of months to years.

Idiopathic hypoparathyroidism may also result in a deficiency of parathyroid hormone. Of insidious onset, it is a relatively rare disease and the causes are obscure, although in some forms an autoimmune basis is suspected. Another disorder characterized by signs and symptoms of hypoparathyroidism is pseudohypoparathyroidism, a rare hereditary disorder that causes a diminished end-organ response to the endogenous hormone. Rather than a deficiency of the hormone, there is excessive secretion of parathyroid hormone in response to the resistance at the target tissues—kidney and bone. An even rarer metabolic variant of this disorder is pseudo-pseudohypoparathyroidism, in which a person may have the associated physical traits of pseudohypoparathyroidism but display normal serum calcium and phosphorus levels.

Hypocalcemia, believed to be the cause of most signs and symptoms in hypoparathyroidism, may be caused by other disorders. Lowered serum calcium levels may be found in malabsorption syndromes, osteomalacia secondary to true vitamin D lack or vitamin D resistance, pancreatitis, hypoproteinemia, renal failure, and acute nutritional deficiency with associated hypomagnesemia.

Clinical Features

In milder forms of hypoparathyroidism, patients complain of fatigue, weakness, and tingling sensations. The most prominent symptom is tetany, which may first be experienced as a sensation of numbness or "crawling sensation" in the lips, fingers, or toes. As it becomes more severe, cramps of individual muscles or muscle groups occur. Latent tetany may be diagnosed by the Chvostek sign, a contraction of muscles of the mouth produced by tapping the side of the face just below the zygomatic process or by the Trousseau sign, carpopedal spasm produced by applying a tourniquet around the upper arm.

Generalized seizures are common with severe hypoparathyroidism. In some cases, a typical grand mal seizure appears to be "triggered" by the disorder; in others, an atypical picture is produced (see below). Soft tissue calcification may result in mineral deposits in ectopic sites, and premature closures of epiphyses may lead to multiple skeletal and developmental abnormalities in chronic forms of the disorder. Basal ganglia calcification has been described in up to 50% of patients, and chorea may also be seen (Camp, 1947; Fonseca and Calverley, 1967). Presenile cataracts can be found in the chronic picture.

Laboratory Findings

As in hyperparathyroidism, serum calcium and phosphorus determinations are important. Denko and Kaelbling (1962) used the criteria of at least one serum calcium level below 9 mg% with an elevated serum phosphorus to diagnose hypoparathyroidism for their series. Other workers think that the level of serum phosphorus is most critical in the production of symptoms (Beidelman, 1958). Exact measure of parathyroid hormone by radioimmunoassay is important in the differential diagnosis of hypocalcemia. In 1952, one author recommended routine Sulkowich tests (for calcium in the urine) for all psychiatric patients; however, a series of tests of 2082 patients proved unproductive (Denko and Kaelbling, 1962; Berardinelli, 1951). This test is no longer used, having been supplanted by more direct means of urine calcium measurement.

Neuropsychiatric Features

A clear picture of psychiatric symptomatology is difficult to form, and is nonspecific. In 1962, Denko and Kaelbling collected data from 258 papers and attempted to classify psychiatric disturbances associated with the various types of hypoparathyroidism. Most of these reports were written by nonpsychiatrists and were often incomplete and sketchy.

Secondary hypoparathyroidism (surgically related), the most common form, occurs more frequently in females, partially because thyroid surgery is more frequent in this population. The estimated female/male ratio is eight to one (Denko and Kaelbling, 1962). More than half of the patients of Denko and Kaelbling in this category exhibited some form of mental disturbance. The majority exhibited features of an acute organic brain syndrome (delirium), with disorientation, memory impairment, auditory and/or visual hallucinations, and agitation. In contrast to primary hypoparathyroidism, general intellectual impairment (other than that associated more acutely with the organic brain syndromes) was rare.

Less frequently reported were psychoses, which were thought to have other etiologies, neuroses, and symptoms such as anxiety, irritability, and emotional lability. Affective disorders were occasionally noted, but a consistent severe depressive picture was not described. Most of these symptoms regressed spontaneously or improved with treatment.

Of particular interest to physicians working in general hospitals are the reported cases of postparathyroidectomy psychosis which have been reported. Mikkelsen and Reider (1979) have summarized some of the features from the seven published cases. They postulated that "the sudden drop of extracellular calcium, not always to clearly hypocalcemic levels following the removal of the adenoma, may have been instrumental in precipitating these episodes," Potts and Roberts (1958) attributed the response to a post-parathyroidectomy magnesium deficiency; however, infusion of magnesium did not produce a convincing reversal of symptoms. Bergeron (1961) reported a better response.

In all of these cases in which a drop in calcium level was documented, the clinical picture was that of confusional psychoses with agitation, paranoia, hallucinations, occasional periods of catatonia, irritability, and associated vertigo and weakness. The treatment included returning calcium levels to normal, but the patients either recovered spontaneously or in a manner which did not appear to correspond well with the improved serum calcium levels.

In patients with the more rare primary idiopathic hypoparathyroidism, the most commonly observed problem, general intellectual impairment, was noted in 50 of the 178 patients studied by Denko and Kaelbling (1962). The authors used the term "general intellectual impairment" to refer to functional cognitive level, often interchangeable with IQ. They did not appear to include the more acute changes associated with organic brain syndromes, although 43 patients were also placed in this category. The rest of the patients presented with a spectrum of psychiatric changes, including florid psychoses, neurotic-appearing behaviors, and miscellaneous minor complaints. Most of the latter appeared to improve, although few of those viewed as intellectually impaired responded to treatment. Snowdon et al. (1976) described a paranoid pychosis in a patient with idiopathic hypoparathyroidism. Early in the course of the illness, psychiatric symptoms were most prominent, as the serum calcium was raised toward normal by intravenous calcium lactate, but later they seemed unrelated to considerable fluctuation of the calcium levels.

Intellectual impairment was the most common problem noted with pseudohypoparathyroidism, but there was no clear pattern of psychiatric involvement in this relatively small group. When improvement occurred, it seemed minimal. In the rare condition of pseudo-pseudohypoparathyroidism, 15 of 21 patients were diagnosed as psychiatrically abnormal, with 12 being intellectually impaired and 3 described as neurotic. There were no psychoses, and several patients were found to be of above average or superior intelligence. No improvement following treatment was reported in this group.

Since the mental symptoms related to hypocalcemia are nonspecific, the clinician must be alert to other clues. A mistaken diagnosis of hysteria has often resulted from the early signs of paresthesias, formication (a sensation of insects on the skin), and muscle spasms. These symptoms, in combination with a patient's anxiety and tetanic episodes, may mimic a neurotic or hypochondriacal picture. However, patients do not generally exhibit the "la belle indifference" response of hysteria.

The concept of "partial parathyroid insufficiency" is interesting. Fourman et al. (1963) showed that in a quarter of patients who had undergone thyroidectomy, the plasma calcium was at the lower limits of normal, but could be provoked to fall to definitely subnormal values by calcium deprivation or intravenous administration of edetic acid. Approximately one half of these patients had symptoms in the form of tension and anxiety, panic attacks, depression, and lassitude. In many, there were no other clues as to parathyroid insufficiency. In 1967, Fourman et al. attempted to assess the relevance of such symptoms by a double-blind trial of calcium citrate and placebo, and confirmed that calcium was effective in reducing psychiatric symptoms. The most consistent changes were with regard to depression and diminution of appetite.

A further complicating factor is that alkalosis resulting from hyperventilation may precipitate attacks of tetany. Whether produced by hyperventilation or by other causes, the alkalosis works synergistically with lowered serum calcium to produce overt tetany. Thus, the cycle of excitement, hyperventilation, tetany, and subsequent fear of the attacks, may produce a convincing neurotic picture. An occasional patient may demonstrate severe enough hypocalcemic rigidity as to appear catatonic.

Atypical seizures may also be precipitated by emotional stimuli and resemble grand mal epilepsy. However, they are often found to have no aura, no periods of unconsciousness, no involuntary trauma, and are not accompanied by urinary incontinence (Bronsky, 1958). Raising the serum calcium level is helpful in these patients, whereas the usual antiepileptic medications are not.

In general, there is a lack of correlation between the severity of neuropsychiatric symptoms and the degree of abnormality of serum chemistries, particularly when compared with the relatively good correlation between elevated calcium levels and mental symptoms. It should be remembered that the level of ionized calcium or phosphorus in the tissues seems to be the crucial determinant of symptom production. Especially when rapid changes in calcium occur, serum levels may not reflect the true intracellular or extracellular ionized levels. It has also been shown that the calcium content of cerebrospinal fluid does not necessarily coincide with blood levels (Gregory and Andersch, 1936). Thus, psychiatric symptoms may occur when serum calcium levels are relatively unremarkable.

Denko and Kaelbling (1962) suggest patient groups that might profitably be suspected of hypoparathyroidism include "(1) those with progressive intellectual impairment, (2) acute organic psychoses, and (3) outpatients with a long history of ineffectual treatment, consultations, referrals, and frustration to their physicians." When one of these conditions coexists with epilepsy of nonchildhood origin, paresthesias, spasms, or presenile cataracts, hypocalcemia and hypoparathyroidism should be part of the differential diagnosis.

Treatment

The principal aim of treatment is to restore calcium levels to near-normal by use of supplementary dietary calcium and vitamin D. The response of neuropsychiatric symptoms to treatment is variable. As noted above, the prognosis is best in postsurgical or secondary hypoparathyroidism. There is usually a delay in response of the mental condition of from one to four weeks after the serum calcium reaches normal and another three to four weeks for complete recovery (Greene and Swanson, 1941). Tetany and other neurologic manifestations appear to be more immediately responsive. In patients with more long-term disease, particularly those with primary hypoparathyroidism and pseudohypoparathyroidism, the response is considerably less, suggesting that irreversible changes (dementia) have occurred.

When hypocalcemia occurs in patients with preexisting psychiatric disorders, the response is also variable. Occasionally, treatment of the hypoparathyroidism allows subsequent successful psychiatric treatment of the primary disturbance.

Mechanisms of Neuropsychiatric Symptom Production

The etiology of neuropsychiatric changes related to hypercalcemia is not known. There is no evidence to point to a direct effect of parathyroid hormone on neuromuscular irritability, and, as noted, certain evidence suggests that this is not the case (Petersen, 1968). Speculation has occurred in two other directions. It is commonly noted that an increased concentration of calcium in extracellular fluids has depressive effects on neuromuscular excitability (Karpati and Frame, 1964; Mikkelsen and Reider, 1979). It also promotes the discharge and depletion of norepinephrine and its biosynthetic enzyme, dopamine β-hydroxylase, from nerve granules (Axelrod, 1973). Although the exact means by which calcium ions might have this dampening effect is not known, it is interesting to speculate whether it might in some way relate to the action lithium has on the functioning of the central nervous system.

Another effect that may be significant relates to the metabolic interrelationship of calcium with magnesium. Magnesium deficiency has been noted in hyperparathyroidism and may be as important as the increased calcium levels. Magnesium deficiency in humans has been shown to cause neuromuscular irritability, convulsions, confusion states, and depression (Karpati and Frame, 1964). Neuropsychiatric changes in hyperparathyroidism are in part related to hypomagnesemia.

Much of the speculation about these mechanisms of action for hypo-parathyroid symptoms are the inverse of those previously discussed for hyperparathyroidism. Just as an increased calcium level has a dampening effect on neuromuscular irritability, reduced levels cause increased nerve sensitivity. Some workers feel that the serum phosphorus level may be as important as, or more important than calcium levels, but documentation is lacking. The lack of correlation between severity of psychiatric symptoms and abnormality of serum chemistries implies that other factors are important.

Psychotropic Drugs and Parathyroid Disorders

Lithium

There have been several reports of hypercalcemia and primary hyper-parathyroidism associated with lithium therapy (Garfinkel et al., 1973; Christensson, 1976). In Christensson's report, four of six patients were taken off lithium, with return of the serum calcium to normal levels. When the drug was restarted, calcium levels again became elevated. Following removal of a single parathyroid adenoma, lithium no longer raised the serum calcium levels. It was postulated that in these cases lithium had unmasked a primary hyperparathyroidism.

Two other studies of patients receiving long-term prophylactic lithium therapy demonstrated significant elevations of serum calcium, magnesium, and parathyroid hormone, as well as a decrease in bone mineral content (Christiansen et al., 1976; Groschel et al., 1974). The authors labeled the condition "lithium induced 'primary' hyperparathyroidism," and, as the condition seemed to be without clinical manifestations, did not advise discontinuation of lithium or parathyroid surgery.

Jefferson and Greist (1977) concluded that at present there is insufficient evidence to justify the routine monitoring of serum calcium or parathyroid hormone levels, although further research is clearly indicated. There are also some preliminary reports that long-term lithium therapy may cause major alterations in bone mineral metabolism and possible osteoporosis (Hullen, 1975).

HYPOGLYCEMIC DISORDERS

Hypoglycemia was not described as a clinical entity until 1924, after exogenous insulin came to be used as a treatment for diabetes. Harris (1924) described five nondiabetic patients who complained of symptoms similar to the insulin reactions he had seen in diabetic patients. In 1927, Wilder et al. reported the first case of intractable hypoglycemia resulting from a pancreatic insulin-producing tumor.

As more basic information has become available on the complexity of blood glucose control, numerous causes of pathologic hypoglycemia have been recognized in man. In the past few years, there has been a parallel surge of interest in hypoglycemia among the lay public. Because of a general increased desire to be better informed medically as well as a proliferation of popular beliefs, diets, and literature that relate multiple body dysfunctions to sugar or lack thereof, many patients now complain of symptoms they feel to be secondary to hypoglycemia.

The maintenance of a consistent blood glucose level is an essential part of homeostasis. A blood glucose level below the lower normal limits reflects a deficit in one or both of two kinds of homeostatic processes: (1) those that add glucose to the blood by (a) mobilization of glucose from glycogen stores, (b) formation of carbohydrates from nonglucose sources (gluconeogenesis), and (c) absorption of ingested carbohydrates; and (2) those that remove glucose from the blood through utilization of glucose by liver, adipose tissue, muscle, brain, and other tissue (Fajans, 1977).

A variety of disorders may result in a final pathway or symptom complex called spontaneous hypoglycemia. This is somewhat of a misnomer, for some of the causes can hardly be called spontaneous. A precise classification of disorders leading to hypoglycemia is difficult, since in many instances the exact mechanism is not understood or is multifactorial. The disorders are broadly grouped according to the relationship of the hypoglycemia to the fasting or postabsorptive (fed) state (see Table 6-1).

Clinical Features

The clinical signs and symptoms of hypoglycemia are the same regardless of the underlying cause; those that appear in any given patient will vary according to individual differences in psychological and physiological responses. The symptoms are commonly thought of as falling into two groups, which usually coexist to some degree. The first symptom group is associated with a rapid decline of blood glucose that activates the autonomic nervous system and produces epinephrine release. Commonly seen adrenergic symptoms include palpitations, sweating, anxiety, tremor, weakness, hunger, nausea, and vomiting. A preponderance of these symptoms is usually found with postprandial (reactive) hypoglycemias, and it is these adrenergic symptoms that are most likely to be complained of to the physician.

The second group of symptoms, called neuroglycopenic, usually predominates when a gradual onset of fasting hypoglycemia occurs. They are caused by decreased uptake of glucose and consequent decreased utilization of oxygen by the brain. Although all nerve cells in the central nervous system are affected to some degree, the areas with the highest metabolic rate and energy requirements, particularly the cortex, are first affected.

Early symptoms may be minor; headache, dullness, lightheadedness,

TABLE 6-1. Classification of Spontaneous Hypoglycemia[a]

I. Fasting hypoglycemia
    A. Organic hypoglycemia: recognizable anatomic lesion
        1. Pancreatic islet β-cell disease with hyperinsulinism in the adult[b]
            a. Adenoma, single or multiple
            b. Microadenomatosis, with or without macroscopic islet-cell adenomas
            c. Carcinoma, with metastases
            d. Adenoma(s) or carcinoma, associated with adenomas or hyperplasia of other endocrine glands (familial multiple endocrine adenomatosis)
            e. Hyperplasia (rare)
        2. Pancreatic islet β-cell disease with hyperinsulinism in infancy and childhood[a]
            a. Hyperplasia (leucine-sensitive or -insensitive)
            b. Nesidioblastosis
            c. Adenoma
        3. Nonpancreatic tumors associated with hypoglycemia
        4. Anterior pituitary hypofunction
        5. Adrenocortical hypofunction
        6. Acquired diffuse hepatic disease
        7. Severe congestive heart failure
        8. Severe renal insufficiency in non-insulin-dependent diabetic patients
    B. Hypoglycemia due to specific hepatic enzyme deficiency (infancy and childhood)
        1. Glycogen storage diseases
        2. Glycogen synthase deficiency
        3. Fructose-1,6-diphosphatase deficiency
    C. Functional hypoglycemia: no recognizable or persistent anatomic lesion
        1. Ethanol and poor nutrition
        2. Deficiency of glucagon[c]
        3. Severe inanition
        4. Ketotic hypoglycemia (infancy and childhood)
        5. Transient hypoglycemia in the newborn of low birth weight
        6. Transient hypoinsulinism of the newborn (hyperplasia of pancreatic islet cells reported)
            a. Infant of diabetic mother
            b. Erythroblastosis fetalis
        7. Insulin autoimmunity without previous insulin administration (?)
    D. Exogenous hypoglycemia
        1. Insulin administration
        2. Sulfonylurea administration
        3. Ingestion of ackee fruit (hypoglycin)
        4. Miscellaneous drugs
II. Reactive (postabsorptive) hypoglycemia
    A. Functional hypoglycemia: no recognizable anatomic lesion
        1. Reactive functional: idiopathic
        2. Reactive secondary to mild diabetes
        3. Alimentary hyperinsulinism
    B. Hypoglycemia due to specific hepatic enzyme deficiency
        1. Hereditary fructose intolerence (fructose-1,phosphate aldolase deficiency): infancy and childhood
        2. Galactosemia: infancy and childhood
        3. Familial fructose and galactose intolerance

---

[a] Reprinted with permission from Wintrobe et al. (1977) (in Fajans, 1977).
[b] May manifest also as reactive (postabsorptive) hypoglycemia, which is glucose- or leucine-induced.
[c] May manifest also as reactive (postabsorptive) hypoglycemia, which is amino-acid-induced.

yawning, fatigue, and lethargy may be seen. Relatives of the patient with fasting hypoglycemia often report difficulty arousing the patient in the morning and they may discover that feeding the patient alters his behavior. Early morning seizures are also occasionally noted.

Although information on the frequencies of particular behaviors related to this syndrome is not available, published cases suggest a heightened suspicion of hypoglycemia should ensue when unexplained outbursts of anger, periods of detachment, bizarre fugue-like states, or automatic behaviors occur, or when episodic confusion or amnesic episodes are reported (Boyd and Cleveland, 1967; Berger, 1975; Zivin, 1970; Sparagana and Rubnitz, 1972). In one case, patient was involved in an accident in which her car hit a cyclist and she had no memory of the event. Subsequent police and medical investigation provided persuasive evidence of hypoglycemic condition, resulting in a reduction of culpability (Bovil, 1973). Patients themselves often don't complain of these episodes until they become frequent or severe. Later stage neurologic symptoms include twitching; convulsions; "epilepsy"; bizarre neurologic signs, motor as well as sensory; conjugate deviation of the eyes; positive Babinski signs; and, eventually, coma. Repeated hypoglycemic episodes may lead to permanent loss of intellectual ability. Elderly patients have a lowered threshold to symptom production, and repeated or prolonged episodes are especially likely to result in irreversible brain damage; this may also occur in children.

Laboratory Findings

In interpreting blood glucose values, it is important to remember that a low value is a laboratory finding and not a disorder. Whipple (1944) outlined a triad of diagnostic criteria that must be fulfilled: a typical symptomatic attack, demonstrated coincident hypoglycemia, and relief of symptoms by administration of glucose.

There has been a tendency to consider a patient to have hypoglycemia if the fasting blood glucose is below a certain level, usually around 50 mg%, or if the glucose tolerance test nadir falls below this value (plasma glucose levels are approximately 15% higher than whole blood values). Each laboratory may designate different normal range values. In more recent years, it has become apparent that a significant number of the normal population will occasionally have values below these designated limits; Cahil and Soeldner (1974) reported 23% below 50 mg%, Burns et al. (1965) found 42% below this figure, and Hofeldt (1975), 48%. Moreover, patients may remain asymptomatic while below these levels. In different studies, subjects have been reported to have tolerated blood glucose levels of less than 40 mg% (Hofeldt, 1975) and less than 35 mg% (Cahil and Soeldner, 1974) without symptoms. Levine (1974) reported the possibility of reaching 5–10 mg%

asymptomatically if blood glucose levels are very gradually reduced. These findings highlight the need for clinical correlation.

For patients suspected of having fasting hypoglycemia, an overnight fasting glucose is usually obtained along with plasma insulin levels. The glucose tolerance test is used most often for patients with a history of reactive hypoglycemia, but it is inconsistent in provoking hypoglycemia. When pancreatic islet-cell disease is suspected or must be ruled out, provocative tests of insulin secretion may be necessary in rare cases. Commonly used are the tolbutamide, L-leucine, or glucagon tests. These are accompanied by serial plasma glucose and insulin determinations.

It is important to remember that the syndrome of hypoglycemia cannot be diagnosed or defined biochemically via blood glucose levels. The meaning of these levels must be interpreted in relation to the patient's symptoms.

Fasting Hypoglycemia

Following a fast, the concentration of glucose is maintained at a homeostatic level by glucose production from the liver, which assures a continuing supply for glucose-requiring tissues such as the brain. When production from the liver is impaired by unavailability of gluconeogenic substrate or a liver defect, or is inhibited by excessive insulin production, hypoglycemia and accompanying symptoms may occur. As noted, neuroglycopenic symptoms are most often associated with fasting hypoglycemia.

The most common anatomic lesion causing fasting hypoglycemia is islet-cell tumor of the pancreas, 10% of which are malignant (Fajans, 1977). They usually occur between the third and sixth decade and may secrete hormones other than insulin. Attacks usually occur in the early morning or late afternoon. Patients may learn to avert these episodes by eating, but often gain excessive weight. High fasting insulin levels are found in two thirds of cases.

Over 250 cases of hypoglycemia caused by nonendocrine extrapancreatic tumors have been reported. These tumors are usually massive and occur retroperitoneally or intraperitoneally. It is postulated that the hypoglycemia is produced by over-use of glucose by the tumor, interference with enzymes involved in gluconeogenesis, insulinlike activity in serum or tumor extracts, or the suppression of physiologic insulin antagonists (Leggett and Favazza, 1978).

Hypoglycemia in the fasting state may be found with either hyperpituitarism or hypoadrenocorticalism. The mechanism believed responsible relates to the effect of hormones secreted by these glands on enzymes required for gluconeogenesis and glycolysis.

Liver disease may also lead to hypoglycemia. Tumors, acute necrosis of viral or toxic origin, or severe congestion secondary to heart failure are most commonly involved. Cirrhosis rarely affects blood glucose levels except in terminal stages, but alcohol ingestion in the presence of inadequate diet can precipitate acute symptomatic hypoglycemia. Either chronic inanition or alcohol taken by persons who have been fasting can produce marked symptomatology or even death (Hansten, 1976). In both situations, the inhibition of gluconeogenesis owing to substrate depletion appears responsible.

Another form of fasting hypoglycemia is drug induced. Most of the drugs responsible, such as sulfonylureas (oral antidiabetic drugs) and insulin, are related to the treatment of diabetes mellitus, but other drugs, such as propoxyphene and propranolol, have also been implicated (Leggett and Favazza, 1978). One case of suspected hypoglycemic coma has been attributed to haloperidol (FDA #690101-083-00201).

Increasing numbers of cases of surreptitious drug administration to produce factitious disease have been reported, and this cause should be considered in "unexplained" cases. If the patients are not diabetic themselves, close contact with diabetics or a medical or paramedical background often affords access to medications. In nondiabetics, the discovery of insulin antibodies is helpful in making the diagnosis. Several authors report adding ^{131}I to insulin found in patients' rooms and subsequently confirming its administration with isotope counts (Burman et al., 1973; Whelton et al., 1968.

Reactive Hypoglycemia

In contrast to fasting hypoglycemia, postprandial (reactive or postabsorptive) hypoglycemia occurs several hours after eating, usually in the late morning or mid-afternoon. It is particularly prevalent after a meal rich in carbohydrates. Normally, a rise in plasma glucose occurs following the ingestion of food, triggering insulin release from the pancreatic islet cells. Glucose levels reach a peak when influx from the gut equals uptake by the tissues. As glucose absorption from the gastrointestinal tract subsides, plasma glucose begins to fall and continues to do so, often below fasting levels. This is the so-called hypoglycemic phase of the normal glucose tolerance test, which occurs two to four hours after ingestion of glucose. Falling plasma glucose levels cause insulin secretion to diminish, and trigger release of glucagon, growth hormone, and cortisol (Permutt, 1976). The effect of these hormonal changes is to convert the liver into an organ of net glucose output in preparation for the fasted state. This switch-over from the fed to the fasted state is the critical period during which postprandial hypoglycemia may occur.

As noted above, epinephrine-produced symptoms predominate during this period, although neuroglycopenic symptoms may also be present. In the absence of adrenergic symptoms to warn of the hypoglycemic episode, mental dullness, confusion, and amnesia may go unnoticed by the patient and produce particularly dangerous situations.

In adults, there are three described types of reactive hypoglycemia, all of which are categorized as functional. This term was initially meant to designate forms of hypoglycemia without a known anatomic lesion but with a demonstrable "biochemical lesion" (Merimee, 1977). It is felt that one type represents an early phase of diabetes mellitus. The symptoms are usually mild and transitory, lasting 15–20 min. A family history of diabetes may often be obtained. Unlike patients with some of the other reactive hypoglycemias, which are self-limiting, these patients may progress to insulin deficiency and diabetes mellitus.

A second group, called alimentary hypoglycemia, is usually found among patients who have undergone gastrectomy, gastrojejunostomy, or vagatomy and pyloroplasty. The high incidence of reactive hypoglycemia is due to the rapid passage of carbohydrates into the small intestine and accelerated absorption of glucose, leading to hyperglycemia and consequent excessive insulin secretion. Although most physicians have considered alimentary hypoglycemia a relatively benign disorder, a recent review suggests that significant psychiatric disturbances may result from it (Hafken et al., 1975). Acute confusional states with significant cognitive impairment and recurrent seizures, more chronic states of dementia, and even coma may result. The prevalence of these disorders is unknown, since surgeons do not routinely perform oral glucose tolerance tests (GTT) as a survey for hypoglycemic symptoms postoperatively. The symptoms may follow the surgery by months or years, making diagnosis particularly difficult.

A similar kind of finding has been described among patients with peptic ulcer disease (Zieve et al., 1966; Evensen, 1942; Berry, 1957). The hypoglycemic symptoms are postulated to be produced in a similar manner, that is, through excessive vagal response to ingestion of food, with increased gastric motility and rapid entry of the food (glucose) into the duodenum. Although transient symptoms of hypoglycemia may be produced, more severe and permanent symptoms have not been reported.

Idiopathic Hypoglycemia

This subgroup of reactive hypoglycemia is the most controversial. The variety of labels including, "idiopathic reactive hypoglycemia," "neurogenic hypoglycemia," and "functional hyperinsulinemia," reflects the confusion about this condition. The term functional, originally meaning without a demonstrable anatomic lesion but including a "biochemical lesion," has acquired different connotations. Merimee (1977) noted that it has come to designate a particular variety of hypoglycemia provoked by a relatively modest withholding of food, such as missed breakfast. He went on to argue that hypoglycemia in this sense is not a pathological entity but rather an example of the axiom of false standards (i.e., a standard below which a disorder is defined to exist) creating false diseases. The term functional has also been contaminated by causal and common usage as in "functional" versus "organic," meaning, in the extreme, a psychological condition.

Over a period of years, neurogenic functional hypoglycemia has been set aside as a distinct entity, characterized by postprandial hypoglycemic complaints that are said to be more frequent during periods of emotional or physical tension, favorably influenced by psychotherapy, and abolished entirely in two to three days by institution of low carbohydrate, high protein diets (Fabrykant, 1955a). The concept of neurogenic hypoglycemia rests on the assumption that ingesting food produces an excessive drop in sugar accompanied by the peculiar clinical symptoms in individuals afflicted with disorders of the autonomic nervous system (Fabrykant, 1955b). Two hypotheses have been advanced to explain the mechanism of this hypoglycemia. Wilder (1941) holds that neurogenic stimuli cause a drop in blood sugar to subnormal levels by interfering with hepatic glycogenolysis; Conn (1947) postulates that because of the neurovegetative imbalance (perhaps secondary to conditioning), the pancreatic islet cells respond excessively to physiologic stimuli with insulin production. Although they use slightly different terms, both authors appear to be speaking of the same general disorder.

Verification of these mechanisms is difficult. Most of the reports in the literature are based on observations of patients suspected of having this condition, without a control group. Fabrykant (1955a) was unable to find a uniform response to glucose loading among patients with hypoglycemia ascribed to neurogenic causes. It does appear that particular personality characteristics are found more often in this group. Anthony et al. (1973) found that 27 of 31 reactive hypoglycemic patients had abnormal MMPI profiles resulting from scores on the hypochondrinsis and hysteria scales more than two standard deviations above normal. They speculated about whether prolonged unexplained exposure to such symptoms might result in a utilization of the hysterical defenses of repression and denial that characterized patients with a conversion valley profile. Ford et al. (1976), found similar hysterical characteristics on the MMPI but did not support Anthony's view of etiology, noting that there were no differences in their samples of self-referred "hypoglycemic patients" between those who actually were hypoglycemic and those who were not but believed they were.

The presence of personality disorders does not establish the diagnosis of neurogenic hypoglycemia or shed light on the causal sequence. Fabrykant's (1955b) position seems most plausible when he notes

> in explaining the clinical manifestations of so-called neurogenic hypoglycemia, we must shift the emphasis from psychogenic and neurogenic effects on the islets and on the blood sugar concentration to psychogenic and neurogenic influences on the *response* of body tissues to variations in blood glucose content.

If body tissues are defined in a broad sense, then it is possible that persons with certain personality characteristics are more sensitive to body changes, report them with more frequency and urgency, and more readily attach varying significance to them.

A number of authors have noted a recent tendency to "blame it all on low blood sugar levels"; Yager and Young (1974) entitled an article "Nonhypoglycemia Is An Epidemic Condition." This overdiagnosis by both the patient and physician of functional hypoglycemia, while popular, may not be harmless. Febrykant (1955a) closely examined 50 patients who presented the clinical features of functional hypoglycemia. Thirty-one gave evidence of other clinical entities that could account for the complaints, many of which were treatable. Ford et al. (1976) also warned that incorrect attribution of symptoms to functional hypoglycemia could cause other conditions, especially anxiety and depression, to be overlooked. In an attempt to put this disorder into perspective, Levine (1974) stated, "in reality the syndrome as a cause of disability in the adult is rare, and the proper causal diagnosis can only be made by modern hormonal assays and tests."

Treatment

Early diagnosis, and correction or removal of the underlying problem, when it is known, constitutes optimal management of symptomatic hypoglycemias. With insulinomas this may be lifesaving; however, the frequent presence of multiple tumors, location in inaccessible areas, and the occasional inability to localize a tumor may interfere with this plan. Remission of associated neuropsychiatric symptoms occurs promptly, unless brain damage has occurred as the result of repeated and severe hypoglycemic episodes. In one reported case, a patient who responded favorably to phenothiazines on several occasions, was later diagnosed as having an insulinoma (Boyd and Cleveland, 1967).

Idiopathic functional hypoglycemia, hypoglycemia due to gastric surgery, and that secondary to early diabetes mellitus are best treated by alterations in diet. Recommended diets are usually low in carbohydrate, high in protein, and divided into four to six daily feedings. When dietary change fails to produce symptom relief, anticholinergic drugs have occasionally been found useful. The mechanism of action of these drugs is thought to be secondary to delayed gastric absorption.

Most papers on symptomatic functional hypoglycemia recommend psychotherapy, but there is no controlled evidence of its efficacy. Fabrykant (1955b) notes that psychotherapy is "of no appreciable value by itself," suggesting that in conjunction with other modalities it "may be useful." It should be remembered that functional hypoglycemias are usually self-limiting within several months or years.

REFERENCES

Addison T: *On the Constitutional and Local Effects of Disease of the Supra-renal Capsules.* London, S Highby, 1855.

Agras S, Oliveau DC: Primary hyperparathyroidism and psychosis. *Can Med Assoc J* 91:1366–1367, 1964.

Anderson J: Psychiatric aspects of primary hyperparathyroidism. *Proc R Soc Med* 61:1123–1124, 1968.

Anthony D, Dippe S, Hofeldt FD, et al: Personality disorder and reactive hypoglycemia. *Diabetes* 22:664–675, 1973.

Asher R: Myxedematous madness. *Br Med J* 2:555–562, 1949.

Axelrod J: Neural and endocrine control of catecholamine biosynthesis. *Proc Fourth Int Congr Endocrinol.* Amsterdam, Excerpta Medica, 1973.

Barnes VH, Greenberg AH, Owings J, et al: The effect of chlorodiazepoxide (Librium) on thyroid function and thyrotoxicosis. *Johns Hopkins Med J* 131:298–300, 1972.

Baron JM: Chlorodiazepoxide (Librium) and thyroid function tests. *Br Med J* 1:699, 1967.

Beck HG: The hallucinations of myxedema. *Med Times* 54:201–203, 1926.

Beidelman B: Treatment of chronic hypoparathyroidism with probenecid. *Metabolism* 7:690–698, 1958.

Berardinelli G: Pseudo-hypoparathyroidism with decreased glucose tolerance and diabetes insipidus. *Acta Endocrinol* 7:16–19, 1951.

Berger H: Hypoglycemia: A perspective. *Postgrad Med* 57:81–85, 1975.

Bergeron R, Murphy R, Warren K: Acute pancreatitis, acute hyperparathyroidism and low magnesium syndrome: A case report. *Lahey Clinic Bull* 12:186–190, 1961.

Bernstein IC: A case of hypothyroidism presenting as a psychiatric illness. *Psychosomatics* 6:215–216, 1965.

Berry M: Studies of the unknown factors in duodenal ulcer: Hypoglycemia as a possible etiologic factor. *Am J Gastroenterol* 27:31–34, 1957.

Bessher PD, Gardiner AQ, Hedley AJ, et al: Psychosis after alteration of thyroid status. *Psychol Med* 1:260–262, 1971.

Bleuler M: Endocrinological medicine and psychiatry. *Henry Ford Hosp Med J* 15:309–317, 1967.

Bluestone H: Hyperthyroidism masquerading as functional psychosis. *Am Pract Digest Treat* 8:557–558, 1957.

Blumberg AG, Klein DF: Chlorpromazine-procyclidine and imipramine: Affects on thyroid function in psychiatric patients. *Clin Pharmacol Ther* 10:2350–2355, 1969.

Borman MD, Schmallenberg HC: Suicide following cortisone treatment. *JAMA* 146:337–338, 1951.

The Boston Collaborative Drug Surveillance Program: Acute adverse reactions to prednisone in relation to dosage. *Clin Pharmacol Ther* 13:694–698, 1972.

Bovil D: A case of functional hypoglycemia—a medico–legal problem. *Br J Psychiatry* 123:353–358, 1973.

Boyd IH, Cleveland SE: Psychiatric symptoms masking an insulinoma. *Dis Nerv Syst* 28:457–458, 1967.

Boyd JD, Malgram JE, Stearns G: Clinical hyperparathyroidism. *JAMA* 93:684–688, 1929.

Brewer C: Psychosis due to acute hypothyroidism during the administration of carbimazole. *Br J Psychiatry* 115:1181–1183, 1969.

Bronsky D: Idiopathic hypoparathyroidism and pseudohypoparathyroidism. *Medicine* 37:317–352, 1958.

Browning TB, Atkins RW, Weiner H: Cerebral metabolic disturbances in hypothyroidism. *Arch Intern Med* 93:938–950, 1954.

Brownlie BE, Chambers ST, Sadler WA, et al: Lithium-associated thyroid disease—A report of 14 cases of hypothyroidism and 4 cases of thyrotoxicosis. *Aust NZ J Med* 6:223–229, 1976.

Burch EA, Messervy PW: Psychiatric symptoms in medical illness: Hyperthyroidism revisited. *Psychosomatics* 19:71–75, 1978.

Burman KD, Cunningham EJ, Klachko DM, et al: Factitious hypoglycemia. *Am J Med Sci* 263:23–30, 1973.

Burns TW, Bregand R, van Deenen HJ, et al: Observations on blood glucose concentrations of human subjects during continuous sampling. *Diabetes* 14:186–193, 1965.

Bursten B: Psychoses associated with thyrotoxicosis. *Arch Gen Psychiatry* 4:267–273, 1961.

Cahil GF, Soeldner JS: A non-editorial on nonhypoglycemia. *N Eng J Med* 291:905–906, 1974.

Camp JD: Symmetrical calcification of cerebral basal ganglia. *Radiology* 49:568–577, 1947.

Carmen JC, Wyatt RJ: Use of calcitonin in psychotic agitation or mania. *Arch Gen Psychiatry* 36:72–75, 1979.

Christensson TAT: Lithium, hypercalcaemia, and hyperparathyroidism. *Lancet* 2:144, 1976.

Christiansen C, Baastrup PC, Transbol I: Lithium, hypercalcaemia, hypermagnesaemia, and hyperparathyroidism. *Lancet* 2:969, 1976.

Clark F, Ormston BJ: Diazepam and tests of thyroid function. *Br Med J* 1:585–586, 1971.

Clark LD, Bauer W, Cobb S: Preliminary observations on mental disturbances occurring in patients under therapy with cortisone and ACTH. *N Eng J Med* 256:205–216, 1952.

Clark LD, Quarton GC, Cobb S, et al: Further observations on mental disturbances associated with cortisone and ACTH therapy. *N Eng J Med* 249:178–183, 1953.

Cleghorn RA: Adrenocortical insufficiency: Psychological and neurologic observations. *Can Med Assoc J* 65:449–454, 1951.

Clower CG, Young AJ, Kepas D: Psychotic states resulting from disorders of thyroid function. *Johns Hopkins Med J* 124:305–310, 1969.

Conn JW: Functional hyperinsulinism. A common and well defined clinical entity amendable to medical management. *J. Michigan State Med Soc* 46:451–457, 1947.

Cooper AF, Schapiru K: Case report: Depression, catatonic stupors and EEG changes in hyperparathyroidism. *Psychol Med* 3:509–515, 1973.

Cope O: Hyperparathyroidism. *Am J Surg* 99:394–398, 1967.

Cronin AJ: *The Citadel*. V Gollancz Ltd, London, 1937.

Cushing H: Basophil adenomas of the pituitary body and their clinical manifestations. *Bull John Hopkins Hosp* 50: 137–195, 1932.

Davis PJ: Factors affecting the determination of the serum protein-bound iodine. *Am J Med* 40:918–921, 1966.

Denko J, Kaelbling T: The psychiatric aspects of hypoparathyroidism. *Acta Psychiatr Scand* 38:7–70, 1962.

DeVos JA: Deafness in hypothyroidism. *J Laryngol Otol* 77:390–392, 1963.

Dysken MW, Halaris AE: Post-ECT asterixis associated with primary hyperparathyroidism. *Am J Psychiatry* 135:1237–1238, 1978.

Earle BV: Thyroid hormone and tricyclic anti-depressants in resistant depressions. *Am J Psychiatry* 126:1667–1669, 1970.

Easson WM: Myxedema with psychosis. *Arch Gen Psychiatry* 14:277–283, 1966.

Ebaugh FG, Drake FR: Neuropsychiatric-like symptomatology of Addison's disease: A review. *Am J Med Sci* 234:106–113, 1957.

Eitinger L: Hyperparathyroidism with mental changes. *Nord Med* 14:1581–1585, 1942.

Engle GL, Margolin SG: Neuropsychiatric disturbances in internal disease. *Arch Intern Med* 70:236–259, 1941.

Evensen OK: Alimentary hypoglycemia after stomach operations and influence of gastric emptying on glucose tolerance curve. *Acta Med Scand* 126 (suppl):1–4, 1942.

Fabrykant M: The problem of functional hyperinsulinism or functional hypoglycemia attributed to nervous causes: I. Laboratory and clinical correlations. *Metabolism* 4:469–479, 1955a.

Fabrykant M: The problem of functional hyperinsulinism or functional hypoglycemia attributed to nervous causes: II. Dietary and neurogenic factors. *Metabolism* 4:480–490, 1955b.

Fajans SS: Hyperinsulinism, hypoglycemia, and glucagon secretion, in Thorn G, Adams RD, Braunwald E, et al (eds): *Harrison's Principles of Internal Medicine*, ed 8. New York, McGraw–Hill, 1977, pp 586–595.

Falk WE, Mahnke MW, Poskanzer DC: Lithium prophylaxis of corticotropin-induced psychosis. *JAMA* 241:1011–1012, 1979.

Fawcett JA, Bunney WE: Pituitary adrenal function and depression. *Arch Gen Psychiatry* 16:517–535, 1967.

Federal Drug Administration: Suspected adverse reaction to drugs. #690101-083-00201.

Fonseca OA, Calverley JR: Neurologic manifestations of hypoparathyroidism. *Arch Intern Med* 120:202–206, 1967.

Ford CV, Bray GA, Swerdloff RS: A psychiatric study of patients referred with a diagnosis of hypoglycemia. Am J Psychiatry 133:290–294, 1976.

Fourman P, Davis RH, Jones KH, et al: Parathyroid insufficiency after thyroidectomy: A review of 46 patients with a study of the effects of hypocalcemia on the electroencephalogram. Br J Surg 50:608–619, 1963.

Fourman P, Rawnsley K, Davis RH, et al: Effect of calcium on mental symptoms in partial parathyroid insufficiency. Lancet 2:914–915, 1967.

Freyberg RH, Traeger CH, Patterson M, et al: Problems of prolonged cortisone treatment for rheumatoid arthritis: Further investigations. JAMA 147:1538–1543, 1951.

Garfinkel PE, Ezrin C, Stancer HG: Hypothyroidism and hyperparathyroidism associated with lithium. Lancet 2:331–332, 1973.

Gatewood JW, Organ CH, Meade BT: Mental changes associated with hyperparathyroidism. Am J Psychiatry 132: 129–132, 1975.

Gibson JG: Emotions and the thyroid gland: A critical appraisal. J. Psychosom Res 6:93–116, 1962.

Glaser GH: Psychotic reactions induced by corticotropin (ACTH) and cortisone. Psychosom Med 15:280–291, 1953.

Goldman R: The effect of ACTH on one case of periarteritis nodosa, in Mote JR (ed): Proceedings of the First Clinical ACTH Conference. Philadelphia, Blakiston, 1950, p 437.

Goolker P, Schein J: Psychic effects of ACTH and cortisone. Psychosom Med 15:589–613, 1953.

Greene JA, Swanson LW: Psychosis in hypoparathyroidism: Report of five cases. Ann Intern Med 14:1233–1236, 1941.

Gregory R, Andersch M: The filterable calcium of blood serum. Am J Med Sci 110:263–271, 1936.

Groschel W, Kluge H, Zhalten W, et al: Vergleichende Untersuchungen zum elecktrolytye Rhalten im Serum bei liprophylzne zyklothymer Psychosen. Pharmakopsych-Euro-Psychopharmakol 7:300–306, 1974.

Gull WW: On a cretinoid state supervening in adult life in women. Trans Clin Soc London 7:180–185, 1873.

Gupta VP, Ehrlich GE: Organic brain syndrome in rheumatoid arthritis following corticosteroid withdrawal. Arthritis Rheum 19:1333–1338, 1976.

Hafken L, Leichter S, Reich T: Organic brain dysfunction as a possible consequence of post-gastrectomy hypoglycemia. Am J Psychiatry 132:1321–1324, 1975.

Hall RW, Popkin MK, Kirkpatrick B: Tricyclic exacerbation of steroid psychoses. J Nerv Ment Dis 166:738–742, 1978.

Hamadah K, Teggin AF: Haloperidol, thyrotoxicosis and neurotoxicity. Lancet 2:1019–1020, 1974.

Hansten PD: Drug Interactions. Philadelphia, Lea & Febiger, 1976, p 271.

Harris S: Hyperinsulinism and dysinsulinism. JAMA 83:729–733, 1924.

Hermann HT, Quarton GC: Psychological changes and psychogenesis in thyroid hormone disorders. J Clin Endocrinol 25:327–338, 1965.

Herridge CF, Abey-Wickrama I: Acute iatrogenic hypothyroid psychosis. Br Med J 3:154, 1969.

Hoefer PFA, Glaser GH: Effects of pituitary adrenocorticotrophic hormone (ACTH) therapy. JAMA 143:620–622, 1950.

Hofeldt FD: Reactive hypoglycemia. Metab Clin Exp 24:1193–1208, 1975.

Hoffman WC, Lewis RA, Thorn GW: Electroencephalogram in Addison's disease. John Hopkins Hosp Bull 70:335–361, 1942.

Hoffman WH, Chodoroff G, Piggott LR: Haloperidol and thyroid storm. Am J Psychiatry 135:484–486, 1978.

Hollister LE: Clinical Pharmacology of Psychotherapeutic Drugs. New York, Churchill Livingstone, 1978.

Hullen RP: Magnesium, in Johnson FN (ed): Lithium Research and Therapy. New York, Academic Press, 1975, pp 369–372.

Hurxthal LM, O'Sullivan JB: Cushing's syndrome: Clinical differential diagnosis and complications. Ann Intern Med 51:1–16, 1959.

Ingbar SH, Waeber KA: Diseases of the thyroid, in Thorn G. Adams RD, Braunwald E, et al (eds): *Harrison's Principles of Internal Medicine*, ed 8. New York, McGraw-Hill, 1977, pp 501–508.

Jain VK: A psychiatric study of hypothyroidism. *Psychiatr Clin* 5:121–130, 1972.

Jefferson JW, Greist JH: *Primer of Lithium Therapy*. Baltimore, Williams & Wilkins, 1977.

Josefson AM, MacKeanzie TB: Appearance of manic psychosis following rapid normalization of thyroid status. *Am J Psychiatry* 136:846–847, 1979.

Kales AG, Beall N, Bagor GF, et al: Sleep studies in asthmatic adults: Relationship of attacks to sleep stage and time of night. *J Allergy* 41:164–173, 1968.

Karpati G, Frame B: Neuropsychiatric disorders of primary hyperparathyroidism. *Arch Neurol* 10:387–397, 1964.

Kind H: Psychische Stroungen bei Hyperparathyreoidismus. *Arch Psychiatr Nervenkr* 200:1–11, 1959.

Kleinschmidt HJ, Waxenberg SE, Cuker R: Psychophysiology and psychiatric management of thyrotoxicosis: A two-year follow-up study. *J Mt Sinai Hosp* 23:131–153, 1956.

Krieger DT, Gewirtz GP: Recovery of hypothalmic–pituitary–adrenal function, growth hormone responsiveness and sleep EEG pattern in a patient following removal of an adrenocortical adenoma. *J Clin Endocrinol* 38:1075–1078, 1974.

Lackey FH: Non-activated (apathetic) type of hyperthyroidism. *N Eng J Med* 294:747–748, 1931.

Lake CR, Fann WE: Possible potentiation of haloperidol neurotoxicity in acute hyperthyroidism. *Br J Psychiatry* 123:523–525, 1973.

Leggett J, Favazza AR: Hypoglycemia: An overview. *J Clin Psychiatry* 39:51–57, 1978.

Levine R: Hypoglycemia. *JAMA* 230:462–463, 1974.

Lidz T: Emotional factors in the etiology of hyperthyroidism. *Psychosom Med* 11:2–8, 1949.

Lidz T, Carter JD, Lewis BI, et al: Effects of ACTH and cortisone on mood and mentation. *Psychosom Med* 14:363–377, 1952.

Lindstedt G, Nilsson L, Walinder J, et al: On the prevalence, diagnosis, and management of lithium-induced hypothyroidism in psychiatric patients. *Br J Psychiatry* 130:452–458, 1977.

Logothetis J: Psychotic behavior as the initial indicator of adult myxedema. *J. Nerv Ment Dis* 136:561–568, 1963.

McConnell RJ, Menendez CE, Smith FR, et al: Defects of taste and smell in patients with hypothyroidism. *Am J Med* 59:354–364, 1975.

MacCrimmon DJ, Wallace JE, Goldberg W, et al: Emotional disturbance and cognitive deficits in hyperthyroidism. *Psychosom Med* 41:331–340, 1979.

Malden M: Hypothermic coma in myxedema. *Br Med J* 2:764–765, 1955.

Mazzaferri EL, Skillman EG: Diazepam (Valium) and thyroid function: A double blind, placebo controlled study in normal volunteers showing no drug effect. *Am J Med Sci* 248:129–132, 1964.

Merimee TJ: Spontaneous hypoglycemia in man. *Adv Intern Med* 22:301–317, 1977.

Michael RR, Gibbons JL: Interrelationships between the endocrine system and neuropsychiatry, in Pfeiffer CC, Smythies JR (eds): *International Review of Neurobiology*. New York, Academic Press, 1963, vol 5, pp 243–302.

Mikkelsen EJ, Reider AA: Post-parathyroidectomy psychosis: Clinical and research implications. *J Clin Psychiatry* 40:352–357, 1979.

Mills IH: *Clinical Aspects of Adrenal Function*. Philadelphia, FA Davis, 1964.

Noble P: Depressive illness and hyperparathyroidism. *Proc R Soc Med* 67:1066–1067, 1974.

Olivarus B. de F., Roder E: Reversible psychosis and dementia in myxoedema. *Acta Psychiatr Scand* 46:1–13, 1970.

Park S: Enhancement of anti-psychotic effect of chlorpromazine with L-triiodothyronine, in Prange AJ (ed): *The Thyroid Axis, Drugs and Behavior*. New York, Raven Press, 1974, pp 75–86.

Permutt MA; Postprandial hypoglycemia. *Diabetes* 25:719–733, 1976.

Petersen P: Psychiatric disorders and primary hyperparathyroidism. *J Clin Endocrinol* 28:1491–1495, 1968.

Pitts FN, Guze SB: Psychiatric disorders and myxedema. Am J Psychiatry 118:142–147, 1961.

Post JT: Hypothyroid deafness. A clinical study of sensorineural deafness associated with hypothyroidism. Laryngoscope 74:221–224, 1964.

Potts JT, Roberts B: Significance of magnesium deficiency and its relation to parathyroid disease. Am J Med Sci 235:206–219, 1958.

Prange AJ, Jr, Wilson IC, Knox A, et al: Enhancement of imipramine by thyroid stimulating hormone: Clinical and theoretical implications. Am J Psychiatry 127:191–199, 1970.

Prange AJ, Jr, Wilson IC, Breese GR, et al: Hormonal alteration of imipramine response: A review, in Sacher EJ (ed): Hormones, Behavior, and Psychopathology. New York, Raven Press, 1976, pp 41–67.

Quarton GC, Clark LD, Cobb S, et al: Mental disturbances associated with ACTH and cortisone: A review of explanatory hypotheses. Medicine 34:13–50, 1955.

Reinfrank RF: Primary hyperparathyroidism with depression. Arch Intern Med (Chicago) 108:606–610, 1961.

Reus VI, Gold T, Post R: Lithium-induced thyrotoxicosis. Am J Psychiatry 136:724–725, 1979.

Robbins LR, Vinson DB: Objective psychological assessment of the thyrotoxic patient and the response to treatment: Preliminary report. J Clin Endocrinol 20:120–129, 1960.

Rome HP, Braceland FJ: The psychological response to ACTH, cortisone, hydrocortisone, and related steroid substances. Am J Psychiatry 108:641–651, 1952.

Rosser R: Thyrotoxoicosis and lithium. Br J Psychiatry 128:61–66, 1976.

Sacher EJ: Psychiatric disturbances associated with endocrine disorders, in Arieti S (ed): The American Handbook of Psychiatry, ed 2. New York, Basic Books, 1975, vol 4, pp 300–303.

Sasenbach W, Madison L, Eisenberg S, et al: The cerebral circulation and metabolism in hyperthyroidism and myxedema. J Clin Invest 33:1444–1450, 1954.

Scheinberg, Stead EA, Brannon ES, et al: Correlative observations on cerebral metabolism and cardiac output in myxedema. J Clin Invest 29:1139–1146, 1950.

Schon M, Sutherland AM, Rawson RW: Hormones and neurosis—the psychological effects of thyroid deficiency. Proc Third World Cong Psychiatr 2:835–839, 1961.

Schussler GC: Diazepam competes with thyroxine binding sites. J Pharmacol Exp Ther 178:204–207, 1971.

Selye H, Szabo S: Protection against haloperidol by catatoxic steroids. Psychopharmacol 24:430–434, 1972.

Siegal FP: Lithium for steroid-induced psychosis. N Eng J Med 299:155–156, 1978.

Singer FR, Bethune JE, Massry SG: Hypercalcemia and hypocalcemia. Clin Nephrol 7:154–162, 1977.

Smith CK, Barrish J, Correa J, et al: Psychiatric disturbance in endocrinologic disease. Psychosom Med 34:69–86, 1972.

Snowdon JA, MacFie AC, Pearce JB: Hypocalcaemic myopathy with paranoid psychosis. J Neuro Neurosurg Psychiat 39:448–452, 1976.

Sorkin SZ: Addison's disease. Medicine 28:371–425, 1949.

Sparagana M, Rubnitz ME: Hypoglycemia presenting with neuropsychiatric symptoms. Postgrad Med 51:192–196, 1972.

Spillane JD: Nervous and mental disorders in Cushing's syndrome. Brain 74:72–94, 1951.

Starr AM: Personality changes in Cushing's syndrome. J Clin Endocrinol 12:502–505, 1952.

Thomas FB, Mazzaferri EL, Skillman TG: Apathetic thyrotoxicosis: A distinctive clinical and laboratory entity. Ann Intern Med 72:679–685, 1970.

Tonks CM: Mental illnesses in hypothyroid patients. Br J Psychiatry 110:706–710, 1964.

Treadway CR, Prange Aj, Jr, Doehne EF, et al: Myxedema psychosis: Clinical and biochemical changes during recovery. J Psychiatr Res 5:289–296, 1967.

Trethowan WH, Cobb S: Neuropsychiatric aspects of Cushing's syndrome. Arch Neurol Psychiatry 67:283–309, 1952.

Uitert RV, Russakoff LM: Hyperthyroid chorea mimicking psychiatric disease. Am J Psychiatry 136:1208–1210, 1979.

Von Jauregg JW: Myxedema and cretinism, in Aschaffenburg G (ed): *Handbuch der Psychiatrie.* Leipzig and Vienna, F Deutiche, 1912, vol 2, p 12.

Voth HM, Holzman PS, Kats JB, et al: Thyroid hot spots: Their relationship to life stress. *Psychosom Med* 32:561–580, 1970.

Ward DJ, Rastall ML: Prognosis in "myxedematous madness." *Br J Psychiatry* 113:149–151, 1967.

Weiner MF: Haloperidol, hyperthyroidism, and sudden death. *Am J Psychiatry* 136:717–718, 1979.

Weinberg AD, Katzell TD: Thyroid and adrenal function among psychiatric patients. *Lancet* 1:1104–1105, 1977.

Wheatley D: Potentiation of amitriptyline by thyroid hormone. *Arch Gen Psychiatry* 26:229–231, 1972.

Whelton MJ, Samols E, Williams HS, et al: Factitious hypoglycemia in the diabetic, metabolic studies and diagnosis with radioisotopes. *Metab Clin Exp* 17:923–927, 1968.

Whipple AO: Hyperinsulinism in relation to pancreatic tumor. *Surgery* 16:289–293, 1944.

Whybrow PC, Prange AJ, Treadway CR: Mental changes accompanying thyroid gland dysfunction. *Arch Gen Psychiatry* 20: 48–63, 1969.

Wilder RM: *Clinical Diabetes Mellitus and Hyperinsulinism.* Philadelphia, Saunders, 1941.

Wilder RM, Allan FN, Power MH, et al: Carcinoma and islands of pancreas: Hyperinsulinism and hypoglycemia. *JAMA* 89:348–350, 1927.

Williams GH, Dluhy RG, Thorn GW, et al: Diseases of the adrenal cortex, in Thorn G. Adams RD, Braunwald E, et al (eds): *Harrison's Principles of Internal Medicine,* ed 8. New York, McGraw–Hill, 1977, pp 520–556.

Williams RH: The pancreas, in Williams RH (ed): *Textbook of Endocrinology.* Philadelphia, Saunders, 1968, pp 613–802.

Wilson I, Prange AJ, McClane TK, et al: Thyroid-hormone enhancement of imipramine in nonretarded depressions. *N Eng J Med* 282:1063–1067, 1970.

Wilson WP, Johnson JE, Feist FW: Thyroid hormone and brain function: II. Changes in photically elicited EEG responses following the administration of triiodothyronine to normal subjects. *Electroencephalogr Clin Neurophysiol* 16:329–331, 1964.

Woodbury DM: Relation between the adrenal cortex and the central nervous system. *Pharmacol Rev* 10-275–357, 1958.

Yager J, Young RT: Non-hypoglycemia in an epidemic condition. *N Eng J Med* 291:907–908, 1974.

Yosselson S, Kaplan A: Neurotoxic reaction to haloperidol in a thyrotoxic patient. *N Engl J Med* 293:201, 1975.

Zieve L, Jones DG, Aziz MA: Functional hypoglycemia and peptic ulcer. *Postgrad Med* 40:159–170, 1966.

Zivin I: The neurological and psychiatric aspects of hypoglycemia. *Dis Nerv Syst* 31:604–607, 1970.

7

Fluid–Electrolyte, Acid–Base Disorders

ACID–BASE DISORDERS

General Considerations

Acid is produced as a consequence of normal metabolic processes. Maintaining body pH within a narrow physiologic range depends initially on body buffer systems but ultimately on the kidneys and the lungs.

Levinsky (1977b) defines **acidosis** as "a physiologic disturbance which tends to add acid or remove alkali from body fluids" and **alkalosis** as "any physiologic disturbance which tends to remove acid or add base." If there is a primary increase or decrease in the concentration of carbon dioxide, the terms **respiratory acidosis** and **respiratory alkalosis** are used. If the primary disturbance is in bicarbonate concentration, a **metabolic acidosis** or **metabolic alkalosis** results. Assessing acid–base balance requires consideration not only of the underlying defect but also of the compensatory changes mediated by the kidneys and lungs.

Metabolic Acidosis

Causes

Common causes of metabolic acidosis are (1) renal disease (chronic and acute renal failure and renal tubular acidosis), (2) conditions associated with increased acid production (diabetic and alcoholic ketoacidosis, starvation ketosis, lactic acidosis, and poisoning with drugs such as salicylates, methanol, and ammonium chloride) and (3) conditions associated with alkali loss (diarrhea and ureteroenterostomy) (Levinsky, 1977b).

179

Pathophysiology

In the presence of metabolic acidosis there is a reduction in arterial blood bicarbonate and pH, followed by a compensatory increase in renal excretion of acid and respiratory excretion of CO_2 (hyperventilation). In addition, the intracellular movement of hydrogen ions causes a shift of potassium out of the cells, with resultant hyperkalemia.

Clinical Features

Symptoms of metabolic acidosis are usually difficult to separate from those of the underlying disorder. Under severe acute conditions, hyperventilation occurs, characterized by deep, rapid respirations, often without dyspnea or consciousness of labored breathing (Kussmaul respiration). Other findings may range from fatigue to progressive depression of consciousness and can include vascular collapse. Mental or neurological symptoms may be absent despite severe metabolic acidosis, in which case cerebrospinal fluid pH is likely to be normal or alkalotic. Depressed levels of consciousness and other findings of a metabolic encephalopathy tend to correlate with an acidotic cerebrospinal fluid (Posner and Plum, 1967). Fatigue and anorexia may be found with chronic metabolic acidosis, although the condition may also be without symptoms.

Treatment

Treatment of metabolic acidosis consists of treating the underlying disease and, depending on the severity, the administration of bicarbonate. If the acidosis is corrected too rapidly by bicarbonate infusion, a relative CSF acidosis can occur with associated depression of consciousness and progression to stupor or coma.

Metabolic Alkalosis

Causes

Metabolic alkalosis can occur in association with (1) volume (chloride) depletion (vomiting, gastric drainage, diuretic therapy, and posthypercapneic alkalosis), (2) hyperadrenocorticism, (3) severe potassium depletion, and (4) excessive alkali intake (Levinsky, 1977b).

Pathophysiology

Normally, the kidneys are able to compensate rapidly for alkalotic conditions by the excretion of bicarbonate. Therefore, sustained alkalosis is not likely unless bicarbonate reabsorption is increased or alkali production is maintained at a high rate. Under conditions of volume contraction, increased sodium reabsorption occurs, which, in turn, requires reabsorption of more bicarbonate. Thus, volume depletion will act to maintain a metabolic alkalosis. Arterial blood pH and bicarbonate is increased with a compensatory increase in $PaCO_2$.

Clinical Features

Nonspecific findings may include irritability, neuromuscular hyperexcitability, muscle weakness, apathy, confusion, and stupor. Hypoventilation may also be present, reflecting the compensatory need to retain CO_2.

Treatment

In addition to treating the underlying condition, volume expansion with sodium chloride will usually restore the ability of the kidneys to excrete bicarbonate and correct the alkalosis.

Respiratory Acidosis, Respiratory Alkalosis

These topics are discussed in the chapter on Respiratory Disorders.

SODIUM

General Considerations

Sodium is the predominant extracellular cation, having a serum concentration of about 140 mEq/liter and an intracellular concentration of less than 5 mEq/liter. This distribution across cell membranes is maintained by an active pump mechanism that forces sodium out of the cells against a gradient. Bodily functions dependent on sodium include fluid and acid–base balance, nerve transmission, and muscle contractility.

The intimate relationship between sodium and water metabolism does not allow separation of the two subjects. Serum sodium concentration, for example, is determined more by water metabolism than by total body sodium content. Consequently, hypernatremia or hyponatremia can occur in the presence of an increased, decreased, or normal total body sodium content. If sodium intake is excessive, thirst is stimulated, water intake increases, and increased extracellular volume rather than hypernatremia results. By the same token, if sodium is lost from the body, compensatory mechanisms (including a decrease in antidiuretic hormone secretion) cause a water diuresis as a result of which hyponatremia is corrected at the expense of extracellular volume.

Body sodium content is regulated by a balance between dietary intake and renal excretion. The kidney is quite sensitive to variations in sodium intake, allowing a variation of total body sodium of only about 10% in the face of an intake ranging from 0 to 400 mEq per day (Levinsky, 1977a). A number of intrarenal mechanisms act in concert to regulate sodium excretion in such a way that alteration in one aspect of the system is counterbalanced by changes in the others.

Thirst is a prime determinant of water intake, assuming that water is available and the individual is able to consume it. Factors that moderate thirst include plasma osmolality, extracellular fluid volume, and the renin–angiotensin system.

Antidiuretic hormone (ADH) plays a major role in water excretion. This hormone is synthesized in the supraoptic nuclei of the hypothalamus and transmitted to the posterior pituitary, where it is stored in secretory granules in association with neurophysin, a carrier protein. Its release is regulated by changes in plasma osmolality, which are sensed by osmoreceptors in the hypothalamus. (Other factors such as extracellular volume, emotion, pain, and adrenergic stimuli may also play a role.) ADH is transported in the blood to the kidney, where it activates the enzyme adenylate cyclase, which ultimately leads to an increase in permeability of the collecting duct to water, which, in turn, results in increased water retention and excretion of a more concentrated urine.

Levinsky (1977a) has divided disorders of sodium and water metabolism into three main categories: volume depletion, hypernatremia, and hyponatremia.

Volume Depletion

The term *volume depletion* is used to refer to a deficit in both sodium and water (as opposed to *dehydration* which refers to a water deficit with resultant hypernatremia). The relative proportion of sodium and water lost will determine whether volume depletion is associated with high, low, or normal serum sodium levels.

Causes

Volume depletion can result from extrarenal losses of sodium and water through the gastrointestinal tract (vomiting, diarrhea, and suction), the skin (sweating and burns), and from abdominal sequestation (rapid formation of ascites), or renal losses secondary to renal disease (chronic renal failure, and salt wasting tubular disease), osmotic diuretics, and adrenal insufficiency.

Clinical Features

Findings associated with volume depletion include decreased skin turgor, dry mucus membranes, tachycardia, hypotension, and decreased urine output. Central nervous system symptoms include weakness, lethargy, confusion, and coma.

Treatment

Volume expansion is the treatment for volume depletion. The route and rate of administration and electrolyte composition of the fluid should be determined by the severity of the condition and the patient's electrolyte profile.

Hypernatremia

Causes

In the presence of hypernatremia, a hypertonic condition exists in the body. Usually, hypertonicity leads to thirst and the subsequent restoration of fluid balance. Consequently, severe hypernatremia persists only if access to fluids is restricted. Serum sodium becomes elevated due to pure water loss (body water low, body sodium normal), when water loss exceeds sodium loss (body water low, body sodium low), or when excessive sodium is administered (Friedler et al., 1977). Conditions leading to relatively pure water loss include febrile or hypercatabolic states, and central and nephrogenic diabetes insipidus. Water loss in excess of sodium loss occurs with excessive sweating, vomiting, and diarrhea, and conditions causing an osmotic diuresis (diabetic hyperglycemia and excessive urea). Excessive sodium administration can result from salt poisoning, excessive sodium in dialysate, and administration of sodium bicarbonate (as in the treatment of cardiac arrest).

Clinical Features

Symptoms of hypernatremia are mainly related to the central nervous system, and their appearance and magnitude correlate with the rate and extent of serum sodium increase. The abrupt elevation of plasma osmolality results in an osmotic blood–brain gradient with a subsequent rapid shift of water from the central nervous system. It is felt that this rapid contraction of brain volume could cause tearing of venous sinuses and intracerebral veins with resultant subdural and intracerebral hemorrhage. Both hyperosmolality and hypernatremia cause alterations in CNS function, and it is not possible to separate the relative contributions of each.

In experimental animals, hypernatremia causes lethargy and hyperirritability, followed by tremor and muscle rigidity, hyperreflexia, spasticity, seizures, and coma. In man, similar findings occur, characterized by lethargy, weakness, confusion, stupor, and coma. If the patient is conscious, severe thirst will be present. Illusions and visual hallucinations are common findings in travelers deprived of water by shipwreck or desert travel.

In adults it is often difficult to distinguish symptoms of hypernatremia from those of an underlying medical condition. In otherwise healthy infants with salt poisoning, the most common findings were emesis, fever, and labored respiration but also frequently present were focal neurological abnormalities, seizures, and coma, and often severe irreversible brain damage (Arieff and Guisado, 1976).

The central nervous system abnormalities associated with hypernatremia are in no way diagnostic of the condition but are rather nonspecific manifestations of a metabolic encephalopathy. The electroencephalogram (EEG) of hypernatremic patients may be normal, abnormal with diffuse slowing or, on occasion, abnormal with epileptic activity.

Treatment

Hypernatremia, especially in the very young and very old, is associated with a substantial mortality. Hypotonic fluids are used to correct the condition, the route and rate of administration being determined by the clinical condition and laboratory data. Too rapid correction of the hyperosmolar hypernatremic states, however, can result in cerebral edema, seizures, and even death.

Hyponatremia

Hyponatremia exists when the serum sodium concentration is low, reflecting the presence of proportionately more water than solute. The total body sodium content may be increased, normal, or decreased in the presence of hyponatremia. Under normal conditions, dilution of body fluids is compensated for by water diuresis. Given the rather remarkable ability of the normal kidney to excrete up to 28 liters of dilute urine per day, the presence of hyponatremia almost always implies impairment of renal diluting capacity. Such impairment may occur (1) if ADH secretion is not suppressed, (2) if sodium and fluid delivery to the diluting sites of the nephron is impaired, or (3) if sodium or water transport at the diluting site is abnormal.

Causes

A great number of clinical entities are associated with hyponatremia (Levinsky, 1977a; Friedler et al., 1977; Levin, 1978). **Pseudohyponatremia** occurs in the presence of marked hyperlipidemia or hyperproteinemia. These conditions reduce the percentage of water in plasma, but since the sodium concentration in body fluid remains normal, the condition is asymptomatic. In the presence of an increased plasma concentration of **osmotically active substances**, such as mannitol, or as is the case in hyperglycemia, water shifts from intracellular sites to restore normal osmolality, at the same time producing hyponatremia.

Hyponatremia is usually present in association with **edematous states** (congestive heart failure, hepatic cirrhosis, and nephrotic syndrome), in which water excretion is impaired, resulting in low serum sodium despite increased body sodium. The reduced serum sodium concentration often associated with **volume depletion** has already been discussed. Other hyponatremic conditions include **essential hyponatremia** (rare), **adrenal insufficiency**, **primary dilutional hyponatremia**, and **syndrome of inappropriate ADH secretion** (SIADH). Hyponatremia is often iatrogenically-induced, by administration of large volumes of hypoosmotic fluids to patients with impaired renal diluting capacity.

Psychogenic polydipsia (compulsive water drinking) is a condition in which excessive quantities of water are ingested for a variety of psychiatric reasons, often over long periods of time. Most patients with psychogenic polydipsia have a compensatory excretion of large volumes of dilute urine and do not develop hyponatremia or symptoms of water intoxication. An impairment of the kidneys' ability to generate solute-free water, however, may quickly result in severe and sometimes fatal water intoxication (Noonan and Ananth, 1977; Rendell et al., 1978). A survey of state mental hospital patients found that 6.6% had a history consistent with compulsive water drinking and 3.3% had symptoms of water intoxication (Jose and Perez-Cruet, 1979).

The **syndrome of inappropriate ADH secretion** is characterized by:

1. Hyponatremia and hypoosmolality of extracellular fluids
2. Persistence of urinary sodium despite hyponatremia
3. Absence of signs of dehydration
4. Normal renal function
5. Normal adrenal function

Conditions which have been associated with SIADH include malignancies (especially bronchiogenic), pulmonary disease, CNS conditions (trauma, encephalitis, tumors, and aneurysm), certain drugs (including thiothixene, thioridazine, haloperidol, fluphenazine, and amitriptyline), and a number of miscellaneous conditions (De Troyer and DeManet, 1976; Friedler et al., 1977). Acute psychosis, per se, has been suggested as a possible cause of SIADH (Dubovsky et al., 1973).

Clinical Features

Symptoms associated with hyponatremia are related to the etiology, the acuteness of onset, and the severity of the condition. Arieff and Guisado

(1976) summarize several studies of gradually induced, sustained hyponatremia (caused by a combination of sodium depletion and water ingestion). Table 7-1 is a composite listing of characteristic findings from a number of reports. In general, there is a correlation between severity of symptoms and the magnitude of hyponatremia (Figure 7-1). The subacute and chronic conditions are of gradual onset, with lethargy and sleepiness being common presentations.

The production of sodium deficiency in normal volunteers by a combination of salt-free diet and sweating, caused a number of subjective manifestations (McCance, 1936). These included a loss of sense of flavor and taste; widespread, variable, and only mildly painful muscle cramps (one subject noted "constant mild cramps of the fingers and thumb when using forceps at the balance"); breathlessness, fatigue, and exhaustion with mild exertion (one subject's arms got tired when shaving and jaw got tired when eating); and apathy and mental dullness. Restoration of sodium balance was associated with prompt recovery.

**TABLE 7-1.   Clinical
Manifestations of Sustained
Hyponatremia**

Serum sodium 131 mEq/liter average
    Thirst
    Impaired taste sensation
    Anorexia
    Muscle cramps
    General exhaustion
    Dyspnea on exertion
    Dulled sensorium

Serum sodium 120–130 mEq/liter
    Nausea
    Vomiting
    Abdominal cramps

Serum sodium below 115 mEq/liter
    Weakness
    Lethargy
    Restlessness
    Confusion
    Delirium
    Impaired respiration

Additional findings
    Muscle twitching
    Convulsions
    Focal weakness
    Hemiparesis
    Ataxia

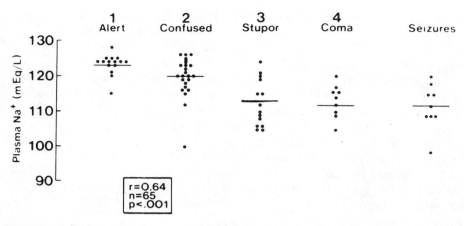

FIGURE 7-1. Relationship between plasma sodium concentration and depression of sensorium in 65 patients with plasma sodium of 128 mEq/liter or less. [From Arieff et al. (1976) with permission of author and publisher.]

Weiner and Epstein (1972) make two clinically useful points. First they stress that hyponatremia may be associated with *focal* as well as diffuse neurological manifestations, and they caution against assuming the presence of a localized lesion unless the findings persist after correction of the deficit. They also mention that chronic headache may be the only symptom of persistent hyponatremia.

With hyponatremia of rapid onset (acute water intoxication), neurological findings appear as the serum sodium drops below 125 mEq/liter and include headache, nausea, vomiting, muscle twitching, asterixis, grand mal seizures, and coma (Table 7-2). Water intoxication that lowers serum sodium to less than 125 mEq/liter in less than 24 hr is associated with a 50% mortality and permanent brain damage in a substantial number of survivors (Arieff and Guisado, 1976).

Animal studies also support the correlation of acuteness of onset with

TABLE 7-2.   Clinical Manifestations of Acute Hyponatremia (Water Intoxication)

Headache	Cramps
Nausea	Asterixis
Vomiting	Delirium
Confusion	Stupor
Dysphasia	Coma
Incoordination	Seizures—
Lethargy	myoclonic,
Agitation	focal,
Muscle weakness	generalized

severity of symptoms (Arieff et al., 1976). When serum sodium was lowered to 120 mEq/liter over a 2-hr period, seizures and coma were common findings. When such a reduction was produced over two or three days, most animals remained asymptomatic.

Psychogenic Polydipsia.   Since psychogenic polydipsia usually occurs in patients with pre-existing psychiatric impairment, the clinical manifestations may be both atypical and misleading. Noonan and Ananth (1977) described a 32-year-old woman with symptoms that included visual and auditory hallucinations, compulsive hand washing, agitation, and dizzy spells. Severe hyponatremia (serum sodium 110 mEq/liter) was diagnosed and treated, and the patient recovered rapidly. After several relapses into a semicomatose state, it was discovered that the patient would lie in the bathtub with her mouth to the faucet and ingest water in such a way that she could not be heard.

Two fatalities associated with compulsive water drinking were reported by Rendell et al. (1978). Prior to relapse, one of their patients presented with bizarre behavior and posturing, limited attention span, echolalia, loose associations, poor concentration, impaired judgment and memory, and auditory hallucinations. With correction of the electrolyte imbalance, there was marked improvement, with only a blunt affect and an underlying thought disorder remaining.

Another patient was admitted to a *psychiatric ward* because of the "sudden onset of irrational and agitated behavior" (Swanson and Iseri, 1958). Although aware of his surroundings, he was hyperactive, with a short attention span and rambling, irrational, and neologistic speech. Associated neurological findings, vomiting, and incontinence prompted a metabolic evaluation and lead to the diagnosis of water intoxication secondary to excessive water ingestion and tap water enemas.

The interrelationship between psychosis and hyponatremia may be difficult to determine. Raskind et al. (1975) described three women with agitated, psychotic depressions, excessive water drinking, and inappropriate ADH secretion whose overall psychiatric symptoms did not correlate with the serum sodium level. Nonetheless, in two of them, a superimposed delirium did resolve with restoration of electrolyte balance (including paranoid ideation and agitation in one of them). The authors postulated an underlying limbic system–hypothalamic dysfunction to account for the triad of psychosis, increased water ingestion, and inappropriate ADH secretion.

Electroencephalogram.   As with other types of encephalopathy, the EEG findings in hyponatremia consist of nonspecific slow wave activity that correlates with the severity of the condition and usually normalizes with restoration of electrolyte balance.

Pathophysiology

The neurological abnormalities associated with acute hyponatremia may be related to brain edema with increased intracranial pressure. Under

conditions of more prolonged hyponatremia, sodium and potassium depletion limits the increased brain water content. Sodium depletion, however,
may interfere with neurotransmitter transport and inhibit brain energy metabolism and be responsible for the symptoms that occur under subacute
and chronic conditions (Arieff and Guisado, 1976).

Treatment

If possible, the underlying cause of the hyponatremia should be corrected. Mild to moderate hyponatremia associated with edema is usually
asymptomatic, and specific efforts need not be made to elevate the serum
sodium. When associated with volume depletion, hyponatremia will respond to appropriate volume replacement. Conditions due to water overload
are treated by restricting free water intake, but if the acuteness and severity
of the situation constitute a medical emergency, hypertonic sodium chloride
may be administered. Since both severe hyponatremia and rapid infusion
of hypertonic sodium chloride can cause irreversible brain damage, treatment must be artfully pursued. In certain cases of chronic SIADH, the use
of demeclocycline has been promising.

POTASSIUM

General Considerations

About 98% of body potassium is located in cells, making it the main
intracellular cation. It plays a major role in determining cell volume and
body-fluid osmolality, acts as a cofactor in metabolic processes, and is intimately involved in neuromuscular function. Potassium balance is controlled by the kidney and the GI tract, and factors altering these functions
can result in excess or deficiency of the ion.

Under conditions of negative potassium balance, plasma level initially
decreases by about 1 mEq/liter for each 100- to 200-mEq loss. Once plasma
level falls below 2 mEq/liter, however, the plasma potassium concentration
does not correlate well with total body loss, which can range from moderate
to very severe. A positive potassium balance is corrected by compensatory
measures which include increased renal excretion and increased intracellular transfer (Levinsky, 1977a).

Hyperkalemia

Causes

Hyperkalemia can be caused by (1) excessive intake (oral or intravenous
supplementation with potassium chloride, administration of potassium-con-
taining drugs such as large amounts of potassium penicillin, and transfusion

of stored blood) (2) impaired renal excretion (renal failure, potassium-sparing diuretics, and mineralocorticoid deficiency), (3) potassium shift from intracellular sites (trauma, acidosis, drugs such as succinylcholine and digitalis, hyperkalemic periodic paralysis and hyperosmolality), and (4) pseudohyperkalemia (an artifactual elevation of serum potassium caused by potassium leakage from platelets, leukocytes, or red blood cells during in vitro clotting, or by local potassium release from forearm vessels during fist clenching in preparation for venipuncture) (Kunau and Stein, 1977).

Pathophysiology

Hyperkalemia lowers resting membrane potential which may lead to a depolarization block and paralysis, or to partial depolarization and neuromuscular hyperexcitability (Weiner and Epstein, 1972).

Clinical Features

Potassium toxicity has a major effect on the heart, causing electrocardiographic changes (tall, peaked T waves, increased PR interval and QRS widening) and arrhythmias, which include supraventricular tachycardia, atrial fibrillation, sinus arrest, heart block, and ventricular fibrillation. The greatest danger from hyperkalemia is death due to cardiac arrest.

The neuromuscular effects of hyperkalemia are nonspecific and consist of weakness, hyporeflexia, paresthesias of the extremities, and deficits in sensory perception. In more severe cases, a flaccid ascending paralysis may occur, which, at times, can involve the muscles of speech and respiration (Weiner and Epstein, 1972).

Treatment

Serum potassium levels can be lowered by minimizing potassium intake, promoting redistribution to intracellular sites (using hypertonic glucose or sodium bicarbonate), and by increasing rate of excretion (using oral or rectal cation exchange resins or by dialysis). The adverse effect of excess potassium on neuromuscular membranes may be counteracted by calcium infusion. The particular treatment or combination of treatments used is determined by the severity of the condition.

Hypokalemia

Causes

Levinsky (1977a) lists causes of hypokalemia as (1) gastrointestinal (decreased intake and loss from vomiting, diarrhea, fistulas, etc.), (2) renal (diuretics, mineralocorticoid excess, osmotic diruesis, and renal tubular disease), and (3) intracellular shift (alkalosis, hypokalemic periodic paralysis, barium poisoning, and insulin administration).

Pathophysiology

Hypokalemia alters neuromuscular excitability by increasing the resting membrane potential, rendering the tissue less excitable. In addition, depletion of intracellular potassium may interfere with cellular function by altering intracellular enzymes (Weiner and Epstein, 1972).

Clinical Features

Hypokalemic symptoms appear as serum levels drop below 3 mEq/liter but vary with the acuteness of onset and the presence or absence of acidosis. Neuromuscular findings predominate, especially in younger individuals. These include skeletal muscle weakness, lassitude, lethargy, hyporeflexia, drowsiness, irritability, and confusion.

The muscular weakness induced by hypokalemia is characteristically most prominent in the legs, especially in the quadriceps, with lesser involvement of the upper extremities, and sparing of the muscles innervated by the cranial nerves. With more severe potassium loss, the weakness becomes generalized, and death may result from respiratory muscle paralysis. A flaccid, ascending paralysis, similar to that seen with hyperkalemia may also occur.

Muscle pain and paresthesias may be a presenting complaint that overshadows weakness to the extent that a musculoskeletal misdiagnosis may be made (Weiner and Epstein, 1972). Finally, positive Chvostek and Trousseau signs indicative of latent tetany may occur with hypokalemia in the presence of normal magnesium and calcium levels.

In addition to neuromuscular abnormalities, electrocardiographic changes are common, and consist of T-wave depression and a prominent U wave. Less commonly, arrhythmias may occur. Potassium deficiency may impair renal function, leading to a concentrating defect and associated polyuria and polydipsia.

Treatment

In milder cases, removal of the offending condition is often sufficient to allow restoration of potassium balance. If supplementary potassium is required, the oral route is preferred, since it is safer and better tolerated. If the oral route is unavailable or if rapid correction of the deficit is necessary, intravenous potassium should be cautiously administered.

MAGNESIUM

General Considerations

Most magnesium in the body is located within cells, with about 2,000 mEq being equally distributed between bone and soft tissues. Plasma and interstitial fluid contain only about 20 mEq. About 30% of blood magnesium is protein bound, with the remainder being in a diffusible form. Under normal conditions, magnesium is readily absorbed from the GI tract and excreted by the kidney, with blood levels remaining in a narrow range between 1.5 and 2.0 mEq/liter (normal range will vary from laboratory to laboratory). Because most magnesium is intracellular, blood levels may not be a reliable measure of magnesium excess or deficiency but generally are a useful clinical guideline.

Magnesium plays a vital role in the body, being essential for normal growth and development and necessary for the activation of numerous enzymatic reactions.

Hypermagnesemia

Causes

Massry and Seelig (1977) state that hypermagnesemia can be found in association with the following:

1. Renal failure, acute and chronic
2. Administration of pharmacologic doses of magnesium
3. Use of magnesium-containing oral purgatives or rectal enemas
4. In newborns whose mothers had been treated with magnesium for eclampsia
5. Adrenal insufficiency

Clinical Features

Magnesium excesses are reflected in neurological and cardiovascular alterations. Randell et al. (1964) studied the effect of hypermagnesemia in patients with renal failure who had been given magnesium-containing antacids or laxatives, and in both normal and renal failure patients who experimentally ingested or received intravenous infusions of magnesium. They concluded:

> The manifestations in all of these patients were quite similar; they included nausea, vomiting, malaise, hypotension, drowsiness, difficulty in voiding and defecating, dysarthria, ataxia of gait, decreased reflexes and respirations, coma, electrocardiographic changes, carotid sinus sensitivity, and cardiac arrest.

As shown in Figure 7-2, the severity of clinical manifestations correlates with the degree of elevation of serum magnesium. Since respiratory depression does not occur until after the deep tendon reflexes have disappeared, the presence of a patellar reflex indicates that magnesium levels are not life-threatening.

As hypermagnesemia is most commonly found in association with renal failure, it is often difficult to distinguish symptoms due to magnesium excess from those of the underlying disease.

Treatment

The intravenous administration of calcium is usually effective in reversing the manifestations of hypermagnesemia although in refractory or chronic situations dialysis may be necessary.

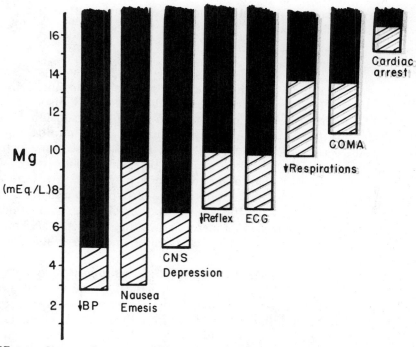

FIGURE 7-2. Signs and symptoms of hypermagnesemia. The hatched areas represent the variable serum concentrations at which the toxic phenomena may occur during the infusion of magnesium, and the solid areas imply uniform occurrence of the phenomena at the concentrations represented. The relationships portrayed represent generalizations rather than precise observations. Since studies in man, especially at the higher serum concentrations, have been few, many of the observations are from animal experiments. [From Randall et al. (1964) with permission of author and publisher.]

Hypomagnesemia

Causes

The extensive listing of causes of hypomagnesemia by Massry and Seelig (1977) include the following:

1. Impaired dietary intake (kwashiorkor, starvation, prolonged intravenous feeding)
2. Impaired intestinal absorption (malabsorption syndromes, massive resection of small intestine)
3. Prolonged or severe body fluid loss (nasogastric suction, fistulas, severe diarrhea)
4. Excessive urinary loss (diuretics, primary aldosteronism, hypercalcemic conditions, diabetic acidosis, hyperthyroidism, chronic alcoholism)
5. Miscellaneous causes (idiopathic, acute intermittent porphyria with inappropriate antidiuretic hormone secretion, multiple transfusions with citrated blood).

Clinical Features

Signs and symptoms specifically attributable to magnesium deficiency are often difficult to separate from those of the underlying disorder. In addition, the frequent association of hypokalemia and hypocalcemia with hypomagnesemia further complicates clear definition of the clinical manifestations. In fact, Yendt (1972) points out that in the absence of other electrolyte abnormalities, severe hypomagnesemia may be asymptomatic and that correction of an associated electrolyte imbalance may lead to resolution of clinical abnormalities despite the persistence of hypomagnesemia. Finally, resolution of symptoms with the administration of magnesium does not necessarily confirm a causal relationship, since the response may be due to the nonspecific depressant effect magnesium has on neuromuscular excitability.

Nonetheless, both animal and human studies support the concept of a magnesium deficiency syndrome. In cattle, a naturally occurring magnesium deficiency syndrome known as kopziekte, grass tetany or staggers results in restlessness, poor appetite, grazing away from the herd, muscle twitching, unsteady gait, gnashing of teeth, and a wild and anxious look, which may be followed by convulsions and coma (Flink et al., 1954). In experiments with rats, a magnesium deficient diet led to intensive peripheral vasodilation, growth disturbance, seizures, cachexia, and death.

Experimental magnesium deficiency was produced in man by omission of dietary magnesium (Shils, 1964; 1969). In all patients who became consistently symptomatic, hypocalcemia and hypokalemia were also present, leading to the conclusion that magnesium is essential for normal calcium and potassium metabolism and that "there is no specific magnesium deficiency 'syndrome,' but rather the spectrum of nonspecific neurologic and gastrointestinal manifestations related in part to secondary changes in calcium and potassium metabolism" (Shils, 1969).

In the seven patients studied (Shils, 1969), findings included Trousseau sign (five), Chvostek sign (two), muscle fibrillations (two), tremor (three), areflexia (two), lethargy and generalized weakness (four), personality change (five) and anorexia, nausea, and vomiting (five). All abnormalities were reversed when magnesium was replaced.

Personality changes in two subjects with experimentally induced magnesium deficiency were described as follows (Shils, 1964):

1. The subject began to stay in bed much of the time, in marked contrast to his usual activity on the ward, and he changed from a friendly, outgoing and cooperative person to one who was apathetic, surly and uncooperative most of the time.

2. Although there were no gross neurological changes, the patient developed a less cooperative almost belligerent attitude during the terminal phase of the magnesium depletion period; this gave way to a more cooperative attitude following reinstitution of this ion.

In 1975, Seelig et al. introduced into the English literature a syndrome that had been known in Europe for many years as *cryptotetany* or *spasmophilia*. These patients have a marginal magnesium deficit, latent tetany, anxiety, and a variety of "psychosomatic" complaints. Apparently, electromyographic abnormalities can be brought out by hyperventilation and muscle ischemia. Although patients with this condition have been reported to respond favorably to treatment with parenteral magnesium or thyroxine, rigorously controlled studies remain to be done.

Signs and symptoms attributed to hypomagnesemia have been summarized by Hall and Joffe (1973) (Table 7-3). Similar findings have been reported by others (Flink et al., 1957; Randall et al., 1959; Fishman, 1965; Snively and Becker, 1968). It should be stressed that there is no diagnostic clinical syndrome, and that some of these findings may be more closely related to the underlying illness or associated electrolyte disturbances. The role of magnesium in mental illness was recently summarized by Ananth and Yassa (1979).

Treatment

Magnesium deficiency is treated by correcting the underlying abnormality (if possible) and by replacement therapy. Both the route of administration and rate of replacement are determined by the magnitude of the deficiency and severity of the manifestations. Because of difficulty in accurately estimating total body magnesium stores from serum magnesium levels, replacement therapy is to a large extent empirical. Both the hypokalemia and hypocalcemia which occur in association with magnesium deficiency tend to be corrected by magnesium replacement alone.

TABLE 7-3.   Signs and Symptoms of Hypomagnesemia[a]

Neurological	
Convulsions (grand mal or multifocal)	Pronounced startle response
Hyperreflexia	Muscular weakness
Positive Babinsky sign	Psychiatric
Tremor (coarse)	Depression
Coma	Marked agitation
Athetoid or choreiform movements, or both	Disorientation
Myoclonic jerks	Confusion
Ataxia	Hallucinations (auditory or visual seen in
Nystagmus	50% of cases)
Clonus	Irritability
Positive Chvostek sign	Restlessness
Trousseau sign absent	Cardiovascular
Carpopedal spasm	Low voltage (nonspecific T-wave depression)
Fasciculations	Tachycardia
Vertigo	Arrhythmias (premature ventricular
Paresthesias	contractions and ventricular tachycardia)
Tetany	Hypertension
EEG disturbances	Vasomotor changes
Auditory hyperacusis	Other
Gait disturbances	Painful, cold hands and feet
	Increased perspiration

[a] From Hall and Joffe (1973) with permission of authors and publisher. Copyright 1973, American Medical Association.

CALCIUM

Disordered calcium metabolism is discussed in the chapter on Endocrine Disorders (hyperparathyroidism and hypoparathyroidism).

PHOSPHORUS

General Considerations

Although 85% of body phosphorus is in bone, it is abundantly present in all tissues and is involved in most metabolic processes. Phosphorus is necessary for cellular integrity, as a regulator of enzymatic activity, for fuel storage and energy transformation, for oxygen transport, and for all synthetic and catabolic processes (Knochel, 1977b). While serum phosphorus levels in adults range between 3.0 and 4.5 mg%, they tend to be higher in children and in postmenopausal women and are also susceptible to variations in dietary intake and renal excretion.

Hyperphosphatemia

Definite clinical manifestations have not been attributed to hyperphosphatemia.

Hypophosphatemia

Causes

Severe hypophosphatemia can occur secondary to (1) pharmacologic phosphate binding in the gut (by antacids such as aluminum hydroxide, aluminum carbonate, and magnesium hydroxide), (2) severe burns, (3) hyperalimentation, (4) nutritional recovery syndrome, (5) respiratory alkalosis, (6) diabetic ketoacidosis, and (7) alcohol withdrawal (Knochel, 1977a; Knochel, 1977b). A more extensive listing of causes of hypophosphatemia (usually of less severity) is given by Fitzgerald (1978) and Juan and Elrazak (1979).

Pathophysiology

Although severe hypophosphatemia clearly seems to cause an encephalopathy (it does not occur if hyperalimentation contains adequate phosphorus), neither the structural nor biological abnormalities have been defined. A deficiency in adenosine triphosphate (ATP) and/or 2,3-diphosphoglyceric acid (2,3-DPG) may play a role, since ATP is vital to cellular energy resources and 2,3-DPG is necessary for oxygen delivery to the tissues (Kreisberg, 1977).

Clinical Features

Although hypophosphatemia is quite common, it is usually mild and without consequence. Lotz et al. (1968), in a metabolic balance study of antacid-induced phosphorus depletion, found that relatively mild hypophosphatemia was associated with weakness, malaise, anorexia, intention tremor, bone pain, and joint stiffness.

Severe hypophosphatemia is felt to cause (1) dysfunction of red cells, leukocytes, and platelets; (2) dysfunction of the central nervous system; (3) rhabdomyolysis, and (4) possibly to contribute to hepatic and renal dysfunction and alcoholic ketoacidosis (Knochel, 1977a; Knochel, 1977b).

Central nervous system findings associated with severe hypophosphatemia may include "irritability, apprehension, muscular weakness, numbness, paresthesias, dysarthria, confusion, obtundation, convulsive seizures, and coma" (Knochel, 1977b). When occurring in association with alcohol withdrawal, this constellation, except for the absence of hallucinations, may resemble delirium tremens.

Kreisberg (1977) goes as far as to state "except for the absence of hallucinations, the signs and symptoms of phosphorus deficiency and hypophosphatemia can mimic those observed in almost every important neurologic and psychiatric disorder." While research and clinical observations have not yet substantiated this claim, the recent reawakening of interest in the subject should lead to better definition of the syndrome.

Of eight patients treated with hyperalimentation lacking phosphorus supplementation, five developed severe hypophosphatemia (mean serum phosphorus 0.50 mg%). Three of them had circumoral and peripheral paresthesias, hyperventilation, and obtundation, with two also having associated slowing of the electroencephalogram (Travis et al., 1971). Three additional cases of hyperalimentation-induced hypophosphatemia showed the following progression (Silvis and Paragas, 1972): Case 1—mild drowsiness and mild tingling of hands, feet, and periorbital areas → grand mal seizures, disorientation, unresponsiveness, and flaccid paralysis; Case 2—tingling of hands and feet → increased tingling and numbness → anesthesia of distal extremities, hyporeflexia, marked weakness, diplopia; Case 3—weakness, sleepiness, fatigue, muscle ache, and nausea → lethargy, restlessness, confusion → tremors, grand mal seizure, disorientation, and twitching.

Persistent severe hypophosphatemia has also been associated with a syndrome of anorexia, dizziness, bone pain, proximal muscle weakness, and waddling gait (Krane and Potts, 1977).

Treatment

Depending on the circumstances, phosphate can be administered intraveneously, by mouth (skim or low-fat milk), or by rectum (Fleet enema). Intake must be monitored, since excessive use of phosphate salts can lead to hyperphosphatemia and metastatic deposition of calcium and phosphate.

PSYCHIATRIC-DRUG-INDUCED FLUID–ELECTROLYTE DISORDERS

The dry mouth caused by the anticholinergic activity of many psychiatric drugs (antipsychotics, tricyclic antidepressants, and antiparkinson agents) may induce excessive fluid intake. Although it is highly unlikely that this alone could lead to water intoxication, it could well be an aggravating factor.

Lithium-induced nephrogenic diabetes insipidus results in the excretion of a large volume of dilute urine. If a patient is unable to compensate for the loss with an appropriate intake, dehydration with hypernatremia will occur.

The syndrome of inappropriate ADH secretion (SIADH) has been described in conjunction with the use of several psychiatric drugs (amitriptyline, thiothixene, thioridazine, haloperidol, and fluphenazine), but in these case reports a cause and effect relationship was not well established (Ajlouni et al., 1974; Moses and Miller, 1974; Luzecky et al., 1974; De Rivera, 1975; Vincent and Emery, 1978; Beckstrom et al., 1979). It was suggested that "when patients taking psychotherapeutic drugs show deterioration of their behavior, with irritability, personality changes, or progressive alteration of sensorium, SIADH must be considered in the differential diagnosis" (Matuk and Kalyanaraman, 1977).

REFERENCES

Ajlouni K, Kern MW, Tures JF, et al: Thiothixene-induced hyponatremia. *Arch Intern Med* 134:1103–1105, 1974.

Ananth J, Yassa R: Magnesium in mental illness. *Compr Psychiatry* 20:475–482, 1979.

Arieff AI, Guisado R: Effects on the central nervous system of hypernatremic and hyponatremic states. *Kidney Int* 10:104–116, 1976.

Arieff AI, Llack F, Massry SG: Neurological manifestations and morbidity.of hyponatremia: Correlation with brain and water electrolytes. *Medicine* 55:121–129, 1976.

Beckstrom D, Reding R, Cerletty J: Syndrome of inappropriate antidiuretic hormone secretion associated with amitriptyline administration. *JAMA* 241:133, 1979.

De Rivera JLG: Inappropriate secretion of antidiuretic hormone from fluphenazine therapy. *Ann Intern Med* 82:811–812, 1975.

De Troyer A, DeManet JC: Clinical, biological and pathological features of the syndrome of inappropriate secretion of antidiuretic hormone. *Quart J Med* 45:521–531, 1976.

Dubovsky SL, Grabon S, Berl T, et al: Syndrome of inappropriate secretion of antidiuretic hormone with exacerbated psychosis. *Ann Intern Med* 79:551–554, 1973.

Fishman RA: Neurological aspects of magnesium metabolism. *Arch Neurol* 12:562–569, 1965.

Fitzgerald F: Clinical hypophosphatemia. *Ann Rev Med* 29:177–189, 1978.

Flink EB, McCollister R, Prasad AS, et al: Evidences for clinical magnesium deficiency. *Ann Intern Med* 47:956–968, 1957.

Flink EB, Stutzman FL, Anderson AR, et al: Magnesium deficiency after prolonged parenteral fluid administration and after chronic alcoholism complicated by delirium tremens. *J Lab Clin Med* 43:169–183, 1954.

Friedler RM, Koffler A, Kurokawa K: Hyponatremia and hypernatremia. *Clin Nephrol* 7:163–172, 1977.

Hall RCW, Joffe JR: Hypomagnesemia, physical and psychiatric symptoms. *JAMA* 224:1749–1751, 1973.

Jose CJ, Perez-Cruet J: Incidence and morbidity of self-induced water intoxication in state mental hospital. *Am J Psychiatry* 136:221–222, 1979.

Juan D, Elrazak MA: Hypophosphatemia in hospitalized patients. *JAMA* 242:163–164, 1979.

Knochel JP: Hypophosphatemia. *Clin Nephrol* 7:131–137, 1977a.

Knochel JP: The pathophysiology and clinical characteristics of severe hypophosphatemia. *Arch Intern Med* 137:203–220, 1977b.

Krane SM, Potts JT: Disorders of bone and bone mineral metabolism, in Thorn GW, Adams RD, Braunwald E, et al (eds): *Harrison's Principles of Internal Medicine*, ed 8. New York, McGraw–Hill, 1977, pp 2005–2014.

Kreisberg RA: Phosphorus deficiency and hypophosphatemia. *Hosp Pract* 12:121–128, 1977.

Kunau RT, Stein JH: Disorders of hypo- and hyperkalemia. *Clin Nephrol* 7:173–190, 1977.

Levin ML: Hyponatremic syndromes. *Med Clin North Am* 62:1257–1272, 1978.

Levinsky NG: Fluids and electrolytes, in Thorn GW, Adams RD, Braunwald E, et al (eds): *Harrison's Principles of Internal Medicine*, ed 8. New York, McGraw–Hill, 1977a, pp 364–375.

Levinsky NG: Acidosis and alkalosis, in Thorn GW, Adams RD, Braunwald E, et al (eds): *Harrison's Principles of Internal Medicine*, ed 8. New York, McGraw–Hill, 1977b, pp 375–382.

Lotz M, Zisman E, Bartter FC: Evidence for a phosphorus-depletion syndrome in man. *N Eng J Med* 278:409–415, 1968.

Luzecky MH, Burman KD, Schultz ER: The syndrome of inappropriate secretion of antidiuretic hormone associated with amitriptyline administration. *South Med J* 67:495–497, 1974.

McCance RA: Experimental sodium chloride deficiency in man. *Proc R Soc Med* 119:245–268, 1936.

Massry SG, Seelig MS: Hypomagnesemia and hypermagnesemia. *Clin Nephrol* 7:147–153, 1977.

Matuk F, Kalyanaraman K: Syndrome of inappropriate secretion of antidiuretic hormone in patients treated with psychotherapeutic drugs. *Arch Neurol* 34:374–375, 1977.

Moses AM, Miller M: Drug-induced dilutional hyponatremia. *N Eng J Med* 291:1234–1238, 1974.

Noonan JPA, Ananth J: Compulsive water drinking and water intoxication. *Compr Psychiatry* 18:183–187, 1977.

Posner JB, Plum F: Spinal-fluid pH and neurological symptoms in systemic acidosis. *N Eng J Med* 277:605–613, 1967.

Randall RE, Rossmeisl EC, Bleifer KH: Magnesium depletion in man. *Ann Intern Med* 50:257–287, 1959.

Randall RE, Cohen MD, Spray CC, et al: Hypermagnesemia in renal failure. *Ann Intern Med* 61:73–88, 1964.

Raskind MA, Orenstein H, Christopher TG: Acute psychosis, increased water ingestion, and inappropriate antidiuretic hormone secretion. *Am J Psychiatry* 132:907–910, 1975.

Rendell M, McGrane D, Cuesta M: Fatal compulsive water drinking. *JAMA* 240:2557–2559, 1978.

Seelig MS, Berger AR, Spielholz N: Latent tetany and anxiety, marginal magnesium deficit, and normocalcemia. *Dis Nerv Syst* 36:461–465, 1975.

Shils ME: Experimental human magnesium depletion: I. Clinical observations and blood chemistry alterations. *Am J Clin Nutr* 15:133–143, 1964.

Shils ME: Experimental human magnesium depletion. *Medicine* 48:61–85, 1969.

Silvis SE, Paragas PD: Paresthesias, weakness, seizures, and hypophosphatemia in patients receiving hyperalimentation. *Gastroenterology* 62:513–520, 1972.

Snively WD, Becker B: Body fluids and neuro-psychologic disturbances. *Psychosomatics* 9:295–305, 1968.

Swanson AG, Iseri OA: Acute encephalopathy due to water intoxication. *N Eng J Med* 258:831–834, 1958.

Travis S, Sugerman HJ, Ruberg RL, et al: Alterations of red-cell glycolytic intermediates and oxygen transport as a consequence of hypophosphatemia in patients receiving intravenous hyperalimentation. *N Eng J Med* 285:763–768, 1971.

Vincent FM, Emery S: Antidiuretic hormone and thioridazine. *Ann Intern Med* 89:147–148, 1978.

Weiner MW, Epstein FH: Signs and symptoms of electrolyte disorders, in Maxwell MH, Kleeman CR (eds): *Clinical Disorders of Fluid and Electrolyte Metabolism*. New York, McGraw–Hill, 1972, pp 629–661.

Yendt ER: Disorders of calcium, phosphorus, and magnesium metabolism, in Maxwell MH, Kleeman CR (eds): *Clinical Disorders and Electrolyte Metabolism*. New York, McGraw–Hill, 1972, pp 460–487.

8

Metabolic Disorders

PORPHYRIA

The term porphyria refers to a group of diseases, each with characteristic manifestations, that have in common excessive excretion of one or more porphyrins, porphyrinogens, and/or porphyrin precursors in the urine and/or feces. The term porphyrinuria refers to porphyrins appearing in the urine and is thus a sign rather than a disease. Classification of these disorders is not entirely satisfactory, but most commonly they are separated into two general groups. The first is erythropoietic porphyria, a blood disorder in which excessive quantities of porphyrins are accumulated in the normoblasts and erythrocytes, the blood forming tissues. The second group is that of the hepatic porphyrias, which includes porphyria variegata, porphyria cutanea tarda, hereditary coproporphyria, and acute intermittent porphyria. It is this latter syndrome that has the most important psychiatric implications and, consequently, is the one most often described in the psychiatric literature.

Clinical Features

Acute intermittent porphyria is an inborn error of metabolism in which there is a genetic defect in the enzymic biosynthesis of porphyrins. It is characterized by the excretion in the urine, both during the acute attack and often during remission, of large amounts of porphobilinogen together with its precursor Δ-aminolevulinic acid (ALA).The disease is an uncommon one. It is found slightly more often in women, and usually occurs between the ages of 20 and 25, being extremely rare below age 15 or after age 60. Familial occurrence of the disease is strong, with transmission probably as a mendelian dominant characteristic. The mortality rate is high.

From a clinical standpoint, porphyria is a deceptive and often misdiagnosed condition. Because of its rarity, extreme variability, and common initial presentation without physical signs, it is uncommon for the diagnosis to be considered at an early stage. Cartwright (1977a) lists four major characteristics: (1) periodic attacks of intense abdominal colic, usually accompanied by nausea and vomiting(2) obstinate constipation; (3) neurotic or even psychotic behavior; and (4) neuromuscular disturbances. Although the sequence of symptom onset may be altered or reversed, in the most common progression abdominal pain occurs first, followed by psychic changes; neurological symptoms develop in the latter stages of the disease. The earlier symptoms continue as later ones develop.

The most fiequent presenting complaint is colic-like abdominal pain, accompanied by nausea, vomiting, and severe constipation. The pain may be extremely severe and is generally without localizing signs or abdominal rigidity. Though not usual, fever, leukocytosis, and tachycardia may be found. These findings may lead to the diagnosis of renal colic, acute appendicitis, or pancreatitis, although the absence of diarrhea tends to rule out gastrointestinal infections. It is not uncommon for patients with porphyria to have multiple surgical scars on their abdomens.

In temporal association with the abdominal pain, the physician may become aware of particular personality features about the patient, such as demanding behavior, irritability, and marked anxiety. These features may proceed to a psychotic state, with both organic and schizophrenia-like symptoms as part of the clinical picture.

Neurologic symptoms are common and include peripheral neuropathy with neurotic extremity pain, hypesthesias, paresthesias, and foot or wrist drop. A gradually increasing paresis may begin in the arms and legs, occasionally being mistaken for a "toxic" paralysis, poliomyelitis, or the Guillain–Barré syndrome. There may be a temporary loss of vision. Often these findings are vague and sound "neurotic." During the later stages, convulsions and/or a complete flaccid quadriplegia may occur. Bulbar paralysis is the major cause of death in acute porphyria. Even at these advanced stages, however, complete neuronal recovery has been reported (Ebaugh and Holt, 1963).

The course of the disease is quite variable. Recurrent abdominal crises may be present for years, with the patient completely asymptomatic between attacks. In general, psychotic and neurological symptoms are late manifestations, portending a grave prognosis.

Often following the diagnosis of porphyria in a relative, some patients may be found who are asymptomatic but have increased amounts of porphobilinogen, the diagnostic feature of porphyria, in their urine. This condition is called latent porphyria. How it is converted to the manifest disease is unknown. Acute attacks may be precipitated by exposure to many different drugs—barbiturates and sulfonamides have been most commonly implicated. Factors such as low carbohydrate intake, pregnancy, menstruation, infections, and alcohol have been precipitating factors for other patients. In many attacks, no precipitating agents can be discovered.

Laboratory Findings

All routine laboratory examinations may be found to be entirely normal. The most likely abnormality is to be seen in the color of the urine. Freshly voided urine may be normal in color but upon standing in the sunlight turns to a burgundy wine or even black color. This color change can be hastened by adding a small amount of acid to the urine or by heating it.

The most common qualitative determination of porphobilinogen in the urine is by the Watson–Schwartz modification of the Ehrlich reaction. This is a simple screening test for the diagnosis of symptomatic patients with porphyria, but is unreliable in asymptomatic patients. Quantitative measures of $\triangle$-aminolevulinic acid and porphobilinogen in the urine can be done by chromatographic methods. For the diagnosis of porphyria in the latent stage, a more reliable and specific method is the measurement of the activity of uroporphobilinogen I synthetase in erythrocytes. The metabolic defect associated with acute intermittent porphyria results in a deficiency of this enzyme.

Neuropsychiatric Features

Psychiatric phenomena have been an integral part of the description of porphyria since it was first reported. As is true of most metabolic diseases, the literature describing neuropsychiatric components of porphyria is conflicting. Many of the claims are made on the basis of few cases, and often the sample is biased by studying only patients admitted to a psychiatry unit, who are usually incompletely diagnosed or described. For discussion purposes, three phases of porphyria may be considered: (1) premorbid personality, (2) mental status associated with the acute attacks, and (3) the clinical picture after impairment of brain tissue has occurred.

Many early writers felt that the premorbid personality of porphyric patients was distinctive. They described patients as being "highly neurotic" (Copeman, 1891) or as having "nervous constitutions" (Gunther, 1936). In 1945, Roth described 10 patients, noting that "the disease occurs with special frequency, if not exclusively amongst people with severe neurotic personality disorders." He felt that most porphyric patients had an underlying hysterical character. Subsequent reports have quoted Roth and also noted hysterical features in patients' personalities (Schneck, 1946; Olmstead, 1953).

There has been the suggestion that emotional events tended to precipitate acute attacks. Eldahl (1938) described a case of porphyria that developed after the patient was upset by another patient dying in the same ward. (The patient, however, had been receiving barbiturates.) Gunther (1936) noted that "psychoneurosis plays an important part in the genesis of the disease and in determining the time of onset of the acute attack." Vischer and Aldrich (1954) added to this line of reasoning by correlating urine coproporphyrin levels with the patients' emotional state over a period of months, presenting evidence that the psychic factors apparently did play a role in the course of their patients' illness. Ackner et al. (1962) noted, however, that most workers do not consider the level of urinary coproporphyrin as significant in acute intermittent porphyria.

Others, particularly more recent observers, have disagreed. Waldenstrom (1937) felt that the patients did not manifest neurotic traits between acute attacks. Cross (1956), reporting two cases in which psychiatric symptoms were prominent, stated that "sweeping assertions about the importance of psychogenic factors, especially in diseases of metabolism, are open to the charge of belonging to the post-hoc, ergo propter hoc category." Subsequent authors, while noting the presence of "nervous features," felt that the features were more likely to be consequences of the vicissitudes of the illness or of the stress placed upon the patients as the result of having a serious and unpredictable illness (Whittaker and Whitehead, 1956; Duret-Cosyns and Duret, 1959; Eilenberg and Scobie, 1960; Cashman, 1961). Later, more careful studies using normal controls and some studies utilizing psychological testing found no support for the importance of emotional disturbance in precipitating acute attacks of porphyria or for the claim of premorbid neurosis among porphyric patients (Ackner et al., 1962; Luby et al., 1959; Wetterberg and Osterberg, 1969). In 1968, Roth published an unconvincing reiteration of his stance.

The symptoms that occur in connection with acute attacks are quite variable and reportedly have often led to hospitalization in psychiatric units. One study (McEwin et al., 1972), however, which used urine screening tests on 1774 psychiatric patients, yielded only 7 patients considered to have acute intermittent porphyria and 2 others diagnosed as porphyria cutanea tarda. This finding suggests that these diseases are indeed rare even among patients on acute psychiatric wards which, it might be argued, should be fruitful catchment areas.

There is no specificity to the acute porphyric attack. Psychiatric phenomena appear to be present in 50–70% of the cases (Ackner et al., 1962). Often, patients become anxious, irritable, or restless shortly before the onset of abdominal pain or other features, but these symptoms may precede other signs and symptoms by weeks. During the acute attack, patients may be described as histrionic, irascible, emotionally labile, or displaying inappropriate and bizarre behavior. As the syndrome progresses, the clinical picture may come to look more like schizophrenia, with paranoia, auditory hallucinations, occasional catatonic states, and excited violence. One report describes a patient committing homicide during a fatal fulminant attack of acute intermittent porphyria (Trafford, 1976). It is interesting to note that the "insanity" of King George III, which had been felt by some to be manic-depressive disease, is much more likely to have been a classic case of porphyria (Macalpine and Hunter, 1966).

In later stages, usually when other neurologic signs such as paralysis and atrophy are prominent, the mental status looks more like a typical acute organic brain syndrome. Descriptive terms that have been used for this phase include toxic-confusional state, delirium, and early dementia. Progressively more severe disorientation and confusion may terminate in coma. Vivid visual hallucinations have been described, in one case consisting of peculiar colored geometric forms (Keeler, 1962). Prognostic studies are not available, but it appears that even apparently terminal states may occasionally reverse, depending on the general course of the underlying disease. EEG changes during this period do not appear to be specific or consistent. If present, changes are described as consisting of varying amounts of diffuse, intermittent, slow activity. There is not a good correlation between the EEG abnormality and the clinical state of the disease process (Ackner, 1962).

Features such as emotional lability, histrionic behavior, neurologic symptoms without definitive signs, intermittent abdominal pain without localization, and vague multiple system complaints are indeed a deceptive group of symptoms. However, alertness to the clinical pictures of severe abdominal pain with unexplained psychiatric symptoms, and limb weakness, paralysis, and/or wasting should alert one to a possible diagnosis of porphyria. A history of dark urine and ingestion of sulfonamides or barbiturates is additionally confirmatory. Although porphyria is rare and thus may seem a remote possibility, its early diagnosis may prevent unnecessary surgery and psychiatric treatment, unnecessary admissions to psychiatric hospitals, and administration of drugs that might precipitate attacks, and may save the patient's life.

Treatment

There are several approaches to the management of the acute porphyric attack. In the first, based upon an original observation by Rose et al. (1961), a high intake of glucose is provided either orally or intravenously. This high carbohydrate intake suppresses induction of ALA synthetase, hopefully leading to remission. Although this form of therapy is widely used and advocated, the clinical response has been variable and has often proved inadequate (Becker and Kramer, 1977).

A second form of therapy currently under investigation is the administration of heme in the form of hematin. Several studies have shown that intravenous hematin therapy profoundly reduces ALA production in patients suffering acute attacks and that this is followed by remission of clinical symptoms and a rapid recovery.

Symptomatic treatment for pain and constipation may be effected with opiates and neostigmine. Chlorpromazine has been described in several reports as particularly successful in treating the psychotic symptoms and violent behavior associated with porphyria (Carney, 1972; Broomfield, 1962). It is not clear why chlorpromazine is effective. Although Melby et al. (1956) and Monaco et al. (1957) suggested that a peripheral neuromuscular blocking action may be important, chlorpromazine has not been shown to have this property. Experiences with other antipsychotic drugs have not been reported. Paraldehyde has also been used for symptom control.

Prevention of acute attacks is most critical. Barbiturates are notorious in provoking attacks and must be assiduously avoided. Even though they are being replaced by antianxiety agents for treatment of more minor psychiatric conditions, there are several areas of use that might be overlooked. Intravenous infusion of barbiturates is occasionally used for patients thought to be catatonic or hysterical to aid in rapid mobilization. In one case, a patient with porphyria who was thought to have a hysterical paralysis was given sodium pentothal diagnostically and later died (Hirsch and Dunsworth, 1955). Acute crises have also been provoked by barbiturates given in association with electroconvulsive therapy (Mann, 1961).

WILSON DISEASE (HEPATOLENTICULAR DEGENERATION)

Wilson disease is a rare inborn error of copper metabolism, with excessive copper deposition in tissues leading to degenerative changes in the central nervous system, liver, kidney, and bone. It is inherited as an autosomal recessive trait.

Clinical Features

Wilson disease occurs in about one in 200,000 persons, and since only one in 200 in the general population is heterozygous for the gene, most cases are the result of consanguinous marriages (Cartwright, 1977b).

The onset of clinical manifestations usually occurs between the ages of 6 and 20 although findings can first appear as late as the fifth decade. Usually the diagnosis is made somewhere between late childhood and early adulthood. Sex distribution is equal.

The disease has a number of modes of presentation (Scheinberg and Sternlieb, 1965; Dobyns et al., 1979).

Liver Disease

Liver disease usually appears between ages 6 and 15 and resembles chronic active hepatitis, fulminant hepatitis, or postnecrotic cirrhosis. Cartwright (1978) stresses that "the diagnosis of Wilson's disease should always be considered in patients below the age of 30 years with antigen-negative viral hepatitis, chronic active hepatitis, juvenile cirrhosis and crytogenic cirrhosis." Although greater than 98% of such patients will not have Wilson disease, diagnosing those that do is quite important, since a specific and effective therapy is available. Diagnosis at this stage may be particularly difficult, since the characteristic Kayser–Fleischer corneal rings and neurological disease may not be present.

Hemolytic Anemia

A Coombs negative hemolytic anemia may precede other symptoms by several years,and if the hemolysis is severe, the associated transient jaundice may be mistaken for liver disease. The hemolytic episodes may be recurrent but tend to be transient and self-limited.

Bone and Joint Disease

A number of bone abnormalities, which are usually of minor clinical significance, have been found in association with Wilson disease. These noninflammatory destructive and degenerative processes include osteoporosis, osteomalacia, osteoarthritis, bone fragmentation, chondromalacia patellae, and osteochondritis (Strickland and Leu, 1975).

Renal Disease

While not a major feature of Wilson disease, renal abnormalities are common and may, at times, be the presenting manifestations. Impaired proximal tubular reabsorption can lead to aminoaciduria, peptiduria, glucosuria, uricosuria, and phosphaturia (Cartwright, 1978). Other findings may include a reduced glomerular filtration rate, mild azotemia and proteinuria.

Neurological Disease

Neurological manifestations are an integral part of Wilson disease and a most common form of presentation. Occurring somewhat later than hepatic disease and hemolytic anemia, neurological findings tend to appear between 12 and 32 years of age. Strickland and Leu (1975) evaluated 40 Chinese patients with Wilson disease and found the neurological signs and symptoms shown in Table 8-1. Similarities to both parkinsonism and multiple sclerosis are common.

Early neurological symptoms include incoordination, tremor, dysarthria, excessive salivation, dysphagia, masklike facies, and deterioration of school performance. Denny-Brown (1964) commented on two different neurological syndromes: pseudosclerosis and progressive lenticular degeneration. The former is characterized by onset occurring between ages 19 and

**TABLE 8-1. Neurological
Symptoms and Signs in 40 Patients
with Wilson Disease**[a]

Poor coordination	28
Psychological impairment	27
Tremor	26
Dysarthria	26
Dysphagia	26
Masked-facies	25
Disturbed walking	25
Rigidity	24
Dementia	23
Dystonia and hypertonia	23
Drooling	22
Choreoathetosis	12
Coma	12
Blurred vision	6
Headache	5
Convulsions	3

[a] Reproduced by permission of publisher and
author from Strickland and Leu (1975).

35 years (adult form), a slowly progressive course of tremor (flapping at the wrist and wingbeating at the shoulders), and dysarthria, with a good response to treatment. The latter appears between ages 7 and 15 (juvenile form), with dystonia (abnormal posture of the limbs when outstretched or walking), a set expression, open mouth and facile smile, and a rapid tremor of the fingers. The course tends to be irregular, with sudden severe relapses and a poor response to treatment.

The neurological manifestations at onset may be quite subtle and not recognized until the disease has progressed. In the Chinese population, **poor coordination** was first noted as difficulty eating with chopsticks or writing Chinese characters (Strickland and Leu, 1975). Cartwright (1978) observed that the earliest neurological manifestation is often **incoordination** involving fine movements such as writing, typing, and piano playing. He described several graphic examples:

1. A young pianist who had been appropriately progressing from lesson to lesson began to repeatedly strike the same cord.
2. Over a four-month period, an outstanding high school basketball player was demoted from first to second to third team and finally dropped altogether.
3. A young man who was responsible for watering the horses was repeatedly reprimanded by his father because he could not reach the corral with a full bucket.

Tremor is a common finding and is aggravated by excitement or by attention being drawn to it. It may be localized to one hand or more generalized, involving extremities, head, and trunk. The tremor may be fine, slow and coarse, or choreoathetoid.

Difficulty speaking may have a subtle onset, apparent at first only with words like "Methodist–Episcopal" but progressing to a more generalized slurring and, at times, to microphonia and aphonia. Cartwright (1978) noted that "in many patients a most unusual and characteristic laugh develops in which most of the sound is produced during inspiration."

Deterioration of school performance is a common occurrence and may be attributed to problems with writing, speaking, and walking, and embarrassment due to drooling, clumsiness, and poor coordination. Patients may withdraw both academically and socially.

If the disease progresses without treatment, increasingly greater neurological deterioration occurs, with the patients becoming bedridden and totally incapacited by uncontrollable tremors, a dystonic posturing, and rigidity.

> In the terminal stage, the muscles become set in a stiff vacuous smile, permanent contractures and deformities are prominent, the neck and trunk become rigid, the upper extremities are held rigidly in flexion at the elbow, wrist and metacarpal joints, and the lower extremities are held in a position of extension (Cartwright, 1977b).

Psychiatric Manifestations

A patient with Wilson disease is more likely to be initially referred to a psychiatrist than to a neurologist, internist, or pediatrician (Cartwright, 1978). The literature is replete with examples of psychiatric misdiagnosis that have resulted in inappropriate, needless, and deleterious treatment, and have greatly delayed accurate diagnosis and proper treatment.

Wilson (1912), in his classic article, noted that two of his patients were initially thought to be hysterical and were treated accordingly. In one "the earliest symptoms were that the patient became rather untidy in her dress, failed to obtain the same number of marks at school as formerly, later developed transient delusions, became emotional and was easily provoked to laughter."

To further illustrate the deceptiveness of the illness and the hazards of misdiagnosis, two cases reported by Cartwright (1978) will be described. A 17-year-old girl with nervousness, emotional lability, and deteriorating school performance was first diagnosed as having adolescent adjustment problems. Despite treatment by a psychiatrist with chlorpromazine, she became more withdrawn, with increasing tremor and incoordination. Abnormal liver function tests and extrapyramidal dysfunction were attributed to the chlorpromazine by an internist and neurologist. A second psychiatrist diagnosed a schizoaffective disorder and treated her with amitriptyline, but she continued to deteriorate. She was referred to a third psychiatrist, who reaffirmed the diagnosis and hospitalized her for electroshock therapy. At this time, a consultant noticed the following: pancytopenia, drooling, mask-

like facies, dysphagia, microphonia, spider angiomas, splenomegaly, choreoathetoid movements, dystonia, severe spasticity, and easily visible Kayser–Fleischer rings and, *22 months* after the initial manifestations, correctly
diagnosed Wilson disease.

The second patient was a 24-year-old woman initially diagnosed as
having "nervous exhaustion" and treated with tranquilizers. She became
depressed, attempted suicide, and was admitted to a psychiatric hospital,
where she remained for a month receiving supportive therapy. A second
psychiatrist treated her with imipramine and then chlorpromazine without
benefit. She became psychotic and was rehospitalized, at which time she
received three electroshock treatments. Additional medication, followed by
eight more shock treatments did not prevent the progression of her illness,
but physical symptoms were interpreted as "your way of showing resent-
ment toward your husband" (Francone, 1976). In spite of further physical
symptoms, a neurologist concluded that the problem was psychological and
referred her to another psychiatrist, who explained her hand tremor as a
suppressed desire to hit her husband. Because of dehydration, she was again
hospitalized but put on a psychiatric ward because of a diagnosis of severe
conversion hysteria. She was then transferred to a county mental hospital
where she remained six weeks, receiving psychotherapy three times a week.
Finally, *32 months* after the onset of symptoms, the correct diagnosis of
Wilson disease was made.

The patient described by Scheinberg (1975) consulted five neurologists
and psychiatrists, who made diagnoses of (1) manic-depressive psychosis,
(2) minimal cerebral dysfunction, (3) obsessive compulsive personality, (4)
anxiety, (5) tremors of undiagnosed origin, and (6) hyperactivity, before the
sixth physician, an ophthalmologist, saw the Kayser–Fleischer rings and
made the correct diagnosis.

There is no characteristic psychiatric syndrome associated with Wilson
disease, and patients have been misdiagnosed as having mania, depression,
schizophrenia, schizoaffective disorder, hysteria, conversion reaction, adolescent adjustment reaction, anxiety, toxic psychosis, confusional state,
and psychoneurosis (Goldstein et al., 1968). The use of psychiatric drugs
can further frustrate proper diagnosis since the liver, blood, and neurological
findings of Wilson disease can be confused with drug side effects.

If the possibility of Wilson disease is entertained in patients presenting
with psychiatric manifestations, the correct diagnosis need not be delayed,
since associated neurological findings and Kayser–Fleischer rings are usually
present. Cartwright (1978) goes so far as to suggest routine ceruloplasmin
screening in all psychiatric patients under 30 years of age.

Pathogenesis

Wilson disease is a copper storage disease in which dietary copper
intake and copper absorption are normal, but a decreased biliary copper

excretion results in progressive copper accumulation in the body. It is postulated that an abnormality exists in hepatic lysosomal enzymes that are involved in copper excretion (Strickland and Leu, 1975). From birth, copper accumulates, at first in the liver, but after a number of years hepatic cells are destroyed and copper is released into the serum, reaching other tissues in excessive amounts. Copper deposition in red blood cells, kidney, and central nervous system can cause tissue destruction with the already mentioned clinical manifestations. Deposition in the cornea results in a greenish-brown ring of pigment at the periphery of Descemet's membrane—the Kayser–Fleischer ring.

Under normal conditions, most serum copper is bound to the enzyme ceruloplasmin. In Wilson disease, ceruloplasmin levels are markedly reduced and, consequently, there is an increased binding of copper to albumin. Because this binding is not tight, an increased amount of copper is excreted in the urine (hypercupriuria). Because of the relatively greater reduction in serum ceruloplasmin, total serum copper levels are usually reduced (Cartwright, 1977b).

Diagnosis

Clinical

The classic triad of Wilson disease is **Kayser–Fleischer corneal rings, liver disease,** and **neurological dysfunction**. The presence of Kayser–Fleischer rings alone has been considered pathognomonic of Wilson disease although they may be absent, especially early in the course of the disease (recently, pigmented corneal rings have been reported in primary biliary cirrhosis and chronic aggressive hepatitis [Fleming et al., 1977].) Thus, an eye examination should be an essential part of evaluating a patient with unexplained hepatic, neurologic, or psychiatric disease. The rings are often visible to the naked eye, but slip-lamp examination by an experienced observer may be necessary to detect them. In patients with *neurological* abnormalities suggestive of Wilson disease, the *confirmed absence* of Kayser–Fleischer rings is considered sufficient to rule out the diagnosis. The rings may be absent, however, in younger patients with active hepatic disease or hemolytic anemia.

Laboratory

The altered copper metabolism in Wilson disease produces:

1. Decreased serum copper
2. Decreased serum ceruloplasmin
3. Increased urine copper
4. Increased liver copper

This constellation of findings, however, is not always present in Wilson disease and, alternatively, other diseases can cause abnormalities in copper metabolism (Strickland and Leu, 1975; Werlin, et al., 1978). Therefore, in questionable cases, the physicians must perform multiple tests and integrate the results with clinical findings to arrive at a proper diagnosis. Tracer studies utilizing orally and intravenously administered radioactive cooper have also been of diagnostic value. According to Cartwright (1978) a low serum urate level can be a helpful diagnostic clue.

These laboratory tests are also employed to screen the relatives of symptomatic patients with Wilson disease. If the diagnosis can be established in asymptomatic individuals, treatment can be instituted before the disease becomes clinically apparent.

Treatment

In both asymptomatic and symptomatic patients, therapy is directed at removing copper from the body. The copper chelating agent, D-penicillamine, is the treatment of choice and is given over the lifetime of the patient. In the asymptomatic patient, this is a most effective form of preventive medicine. In the symptomatic patient, results can be striking. With time, the Kayser–Fleischer rings are likely to fade, the neurological abnormalities resolve and the liver function abnormalities normalize.

Sternlieb and Scheinberg (1964) described four patients who "were bedridden and completely incapacitated by uncontrollable tremors, rigidity, and dystonic posturing" and who were unable to feed, wash, or dress themselves. With treatment, they all improved dramatically, and while one died from liver failure, the other three returned to essentially normal lives (one attending school and two working). Not all treatment is so dramatically successful, however, and disability may be permanent, especially if treatment is delayed.

When Strickland et al. (1973) did follow up studies, they found that 35 of 36 patients who did not get penicillamine were *dead* while 31 of 35 who were treated were *alive*, and 18 had become asymptomatic.

With such an undisputably effective treatment available for a disease that is otherwise progressively debilitating and ultimately fatal, the need for acurate early diagnosis cannot be overstressed. As already discussed, initial and often continued misdiagnosis appears to be the rule rather than the exception. This is doubly unfortunate, since the patient is further exposed to the ravages of disease, and the likelihood of optimal response to treatment is diminished.

A preliminary study with oral zinc sulphate suggests that this treatment may reduce copper absorption and perhaps reduce copper stores (Hoogenraad et al., 1978). The role of zinc in the therapy of Wilson disease requires further definition.

Neuropsychiatric Manifestations of Drugs Used to Treat Wilson Disease

Several cases of a penicillamine-induced myasthenia gravis-like syndrome have been reported (Atcheson and Ward, 1978).

Use of Psychotropic Drugs in Patients with Wilson Disease

There is no evidence that any psychotropic drug has a favorable or adverse effect on the clinical progression of Wilson disease or on the underlying abnormalities of copper metabolism. The use of psychotropic drugs in such patients should be governed by the problem requiring treatment and the extent of organ function impairment. For example, advanced liver involvement or renal disease secondary to Wilson disease would compromise metabolism and excretion of drugs handled by those particular organs.

REFERENCES

Ackner B, Cooper JE, Gray CH, et al: Acute porphyria: A neuropsychiatric and biochemical study. *J Psychosom Res* 6:1–24, 1962.

Atcheson SG, Ward JR: Ptosis and weakness after start of D-penicillamine therapy. *Ann Intern Med* 89:939–940, 1978.

Becker DM, Kramer S: The neurological manifestations of porphyria: A review. *Medicine* 56:411–422, 1977.

Broomfield B: Acute intermittent porphyria treated with chlorpromazine. *Proc R Soc Med* 55:799–800, 1962.

Carney MP: Hepatic porphyria with mental symptoms. *Lancet* 2:100–101, 1972.

Cartwright GE: Disorders of porphyrin metabolism, in Thorn GW, Adams RD, Braunwald E, et al (eds): *Harrison's Principals of Internal Medicine*, ed 8. New York, McGraw–Hill, 1977a, pp 655–661.

Cartwright GE: Hepatolenticular degeneration (Wilson's disease), in Thorn GW, Adams RD, Braunwald E, et al (eds): *Harrison's Principals of Internal Medicine* ed 8. New York, McGraw–Hill, 1977b, pp 661–664.

Cartwright GE: Diagnosis of treatable Wilson's disease. *N Engl J Med* 298:1347–1350, 1978.

Cashman MD: Psychiatric aspects of acute porphyria. *Lancet* 1:115–116, 1961.

Copeman SM: In Proceedings of the Pathological Society of London. *Lancet* 1:197–200, 1891.

Cross TN: Porphyria—A deceptive syndrome. *Am J Psychiatry* 112:1010–1014, 1956.

Denny-Brown D: Hepatolenticular degeneration (Wilson's disease), two different components. *N Engl J Med* 270:1149–1156, 1964.

Dobyns WB, Goldstein NP, Gordon H: Clinical spectrum of Wilson's disease (hepatolenticular degeneration). *Mayo Clin Proc* 54:35–42, 1979.

Duret-Cosyns S, Duret RL: Etudy psychiatrique de la porphyrie essentielle. *Ann Med-Psychol* 2:193–197, 1959.

Ebaugh FG, Holt JW: Porphyria and neuronal dysfunction. *Am J Med Sci* 245:95–108, 1963.

Eilenberg MD, Scobie BA: Prolonged neuropsychiatric disability and cardio-myopathy in acute intermittent porphyria. *Lancet* 1:858–860, 1960.

Eldahl A: A case of acute porphyria developing during hospitalization. *Acta Med Scand* 97:415–417, 1938.

Fleming CR, Dickson ER, Wahner HW, et al: Pigmented corneal rings in non-Wilsonian liver disease. *Ann Intern Med* 86:285–288, 1977.

Francone CA: "My battle against Wilson's disease." *Am J Nurs* 76:247–249, 1976.

Goldstein NP, Ewert JC, Randall RV, et al: Psychiatric aspects of Wilson's disease (hepatolenticular degeneration): Results of psychometric tests during long-term therapy. *Am J Psychiatry* 124:1555–1561, 1968.

Gunther H: Porphyrie (Hamatoporphyrie). *Neue Dtsch Klin* 14:256–260, 1936.

Hirsch S, Dunsworth FA: An interesting case of porphyria. *Am J Psychiatry* 111:703, 1955.

Hoogenraad TU, Vanden Hammer CJA, Koevoet R, et al: Oral zinc in Wilson's disease. *Lancet* 2:1262, 1978.

Keeler MH: A case of acute intermittent porphyria with hallucinations of geometric forms. *J Nerv Ment Dis* 134:572–574, 1962.

Luby ED, Ware JG, Senf R, et al: Stress and the precipitation of acute intermittent porphyria. *Psychosom Med* 21:34, 1959.

Macalpine I, Hunter R: The "insanity" of King George III: A classic case of porphyria. *Br Med J* 1:65–71, 1966.

McEwin R, Lawn J, Jonas CT: Survey of porphyria among psychiatric patients. *Med J Aust* 2:303–306, August 1972.

Mann J: Acute porphyria provoked by barbiturates given with electroshock therapy. *Am J Psychiatry* 118:509–511, 1961.

Melby JD, Street JP, Watson CJ: Chlorpromazine in the treatment of porphyria. *JAMA* 162:174–178, 1956.

Monaco RN, Tuper RD, Robbins JJ, et al: Intermittent acute porphyria: Treatment with chlorpromazine. *N Engl J Med* 256:309–311, 1957.

Olmstead EG: The neuropsychiatric aspects of abnormal porphyrin metabolism. *J Nerv Ment Dis* 117:300—302, 1953.

Rose JA, Hellman ES, Tschudy DP: Effective diet on the induction of experimental prophyria. *Metabolism* 10:514–518, 1961.

Roth N: The neuropsychiatric aspects of porphyria. *Psychosom Med* 7:291–301, 1945.

Roth N: The psychiatric syndromes of porphyria. *Int J Neuropsychiatry* 4:32–44, 1968.

Scheinberg IH: A psychogenetic anecdote. *Psychosom Med* 37:368–371, 1975.

Scheinberg IH, Sternlieb I: Wilson's disease. *Annu Rev Med* 16:119–134, 1965.

Schneck JM: Porphyria: Neuropsychiatric aspects in the case of a Negro. *J Nerv Ment Dis* 104:432–434, 1946.

Sternlieb IS, Scheinberg IH: Penicillamine therapy for hepatolenticular degeneration. *JAMA* 189:748–754, 1964.

Strickland GT, Frommer D, Leu M-L, et al: Wilson's disease in the United Kingdom and Taiwan. *Quart J Med* 42:619–638, 1973.

Strickland GT, Leu M-L: Wilson's disease: Clinical and laboratory manifestations in 40 patients. *Medicine* (Baltimore) 54:113–137, 1975.

Trafford PA: Homicide in acute porphyria. *Forensic Sci* 7:113–120, 1976.

Vischer JS, Aldrich CK: Acute intermittent porphyria: A case study. *Psychosom Med* 16:163–168, 1954.

Waldenstrom J: Studien uber porphyrie. *Acta Med Scand*, supp 82, 1937.

Werlin SL, Grand RJ, Perman JA, et al: Diagnostic dilemmas of Wilson's disease: Diagnosis and treatment. *Pediatrics* 62:47–51, 1978.

Wetterberg L, Osterberg E: Acute intermittent porphyria: A psychometric study of 25 patients. *J Psychosom Res* 13:91–93, 1969.

Whittaker SRF, Whitehead TP: Acute and latent porphyria. *Lancet* 1:547–551, 1956.

Wilson SAK: Progressive lenticular degeneration: A familial nervous disease associated with cirrhosis of the liver. *Brain* 34:296–509, 1912.

Connective Tissue Disorder (Systemic Lupus Erythematosus)

Systemic lupus erythematosus (SLE) is a disseminated disease of multiform character and unknown cause. Current evidence shows that immunologic mechanisms of tissue injury are important in its pathogenesis. Roles for genetic predisposition and viral infection are also hypothesized (Mannik and Gilliland, 1977). The serum of patients with SLE contains many antibodies, collectively called antinuclear antibodies (ANA). The complexes formed by the combining of ANA with specific antigens appear to contribute to the inflammatory process and to formation of fibrinoid deposits that are commonly found in blood vessels, among collagen fibers, and on serosal surfaces. The widespread nature of these changes accounts for the multitude of clinical manifestations. Demonstration of the presence of ANA is essential for the diagnosis.

CLINICAL FEATURES

The prevalence of SLE is two to three per 100,000 persons; it occurs predominantly among women, in a nine-to-one sex ratio. The mean age of onset is about 30 years of age, although it may first occur in the second through the seventh decade (Feinglass et al., 1976). Recent estimates indicate that 77% of patients with SLE survive for five years.

SLE is characterized by multisystem involvement and is subject to remissions and exacerbations in one or more systems. Arthritis and arthralgias are the most frequent presenting complaints and the most common symptoms during the course of the illness (occurring in approximately 90% of patients) (Feinglass et al., 1976; Dubois and Tuffanelli, 1964; Johnson and Richardson, 1968). Fever, malaise, anorexia, and weight loss are commonly seen. A variety of skin changes occurs, the most characteristic of which is the butterfly rash over the cheeks and bridge of the nose.

Renal involvement is one of the most serious manifestations and the

215

most likely to result in death. Detectable abnormalities occur in about half of SLE patients, ranging from mild proteinuria to total renal failure. Cardiopulmonary abnormalities are moderately frequent. Pericarditis, myocarditis, pleural involvement, or parenchymal infiltrates may be found. Other, less common signs or symptoms include lymph-node enlargement and hepatomegaly.

LABORATORY FINDINGS

A mild normochromic, normocytic anemia is common. In over half of the patients, this is accompanied by leukopenia. Infrequently, clotting defects due to antibodies may be found and present potentially serious problems.

Urinalysis may show microscopic hematuria and/or mild proteinuria. With extensive involvement, this proteinuria becomes significant. The serum albumin:globulin ratio may be reversed, with an elevation of gamma-globulin noted with serum electrophoresis. The erythrocyte sedimentation rate (ESR) also tends to be high.

The most characteristic laboratory findings are the autoantibodies. Although the presence of ANA is almost a sine qua non for diagnosis of active SLE, it should be noted that antinuclear antibodies may be found in other diseases. The lupus erythematosus test (LE cell test) is positive less frequently, approximately 60–80% of the time. Decreased total serum hemolytic complement is found in most patients during flare-ups of the disease. Approximately 20% of patients demonstrate positive tests for rheumatoid factor.

There are no specific diagnostic tests for CNS involvement in SLE. Certain tests may be unremarkable in the presence of demonstrable neurologic deficits and, conversely, may be abnormal without associated clinical signs. Several tests, however, can provide collaborative data.

Cerebrospinal fluid is abnormal somewhere in the range of 32–48% of the time in patients with clinical neurologic findings (Feinglass et al., 1976; Johnson and Richardson, 1968; Guze, 1967; Small et al., 1977). Usually, there is a significant elevation of protein and a mild lymphocytic pleocytosis.

Electroencephalographic data have been of little diagnostic or localizing value (Johnson and Richardson, 1968). Abnormalities may be found in 71–80% of SLE patients who show clinical neurologic signs. The usual picture is bilateral diffuse slowing, but focal signs may be seen if seizures are present.

Some clinicians feel that brain scans may be a sensitive tool in the diagnosis of cerebral lupus. Bennahum et al. (1974), found 11 of 12 scans done during symptomatic episodes to be abnormal. Others feel this technique is less reliable (Feinglass et al., 1976).

NEUROPSYCHIATRIC FEATURES

During the past three decades, much has been written about the frequency and clinical appearance of neuropsychiatric features in SLE. Reports clearly point to a relationship between SLE and psychiatric symptoms. However, because the studies vary in method and quality, it is difficult to arrive at representative figures for frequency of occurrence of neuropsychiatric manifestations and to gain a clinical picture of them. Gurland et al. (1972) have critically reviewed these problems.

Estimates of the frequency of psychiatric disorders in lupus patients range from 3% to 65%, with a mean of approximately 21% (Gurland et al., 1972). Estes and Christian's survey (1971) of 150 patients followed closely over several years, determined that 42% showed disorders of mental function. In general, studies that report the higher incidences employed psychiatric interviews of individual patients rather than medically oriented interviews or reviews of records. The higher figures are not surprising, in the light of the acute episodes of fever and malaise that mark the disease and its chronic disabling effects, which are certain to have a marked impact on mental functioning.

Although it is well known that neuropsychiatric manifestations are prominent late in SLE, it is not generally appreciated that they may also be an early feature. One study reported that neuropsychiatric involvement either preceded the diagnosis or occurred within the first year following diagnosis (Siekert and Clark, 1955; Feinglass et al., 1976). In over half of reported cases these features are found in the first three years (Gurland et al., 1972). Psychiatric symptoms occur in episodes that rarely last longer than six months and more commonly last less than six weeks. Despite the shortness of these episodes, some studies report that cerebral complications are second only to renal as a cause of mortality (MacNeil et al., 1976).

Psychiatric symptoms associated with lupus are not distinctive. Because most of the neuropsychiatric changes are secondary to vasculitis, any form of disturbance may be seen. Psychosis is one of the most common central nervous system manifestations (referred to in some studies as "major psychiatric symptoms"). Estimates of the incidence of psychosis vary from 12% to 52% in one group of reports on patients who had had one or more psychiatric episodes (Johnson and Richardson, 1968). Several good studies find a mean incidence of approximately 29% for psychoses (Gurland et al., 1972).

Most investigators appear to use the term psychosis to describe organic brain syndromes. Common clinical presentations include disorientation, disturbances of attention, difficulties with calculation, delusions, often of a paranoid type, and hallucinations that are frequently visual and often bizarre (Lief and Silverman, 1960; Guze, 1967; O'Connor, 1959; Stern and Robbins, 1960). Excessive motor activity has also been described but is not the rule. Less commonly, there is chronic dementia associated with general disturbances of intellectual function and failing memory. Milder forms of intellectual deterioration may occur. Clark and Bailey (1956) found memory deficits in many patients, often associated with changes of personality, anxiety, and emotional lability. Dubois (1964) emphasized the management problems presented by patients with slight organic brain damage resulting in personality difficulties and impaired judgment. It is often quite difficult to decide how much is attributable to brain damage and how much is a result of a chronic illness and physical deterioration.

Also described are "functional" psychoses that have been called schizophreniform because they are characterized by a relatively clear sensorium, and hallucinations and delusions suggestive of schizophrenia. Organic features may be present but minor. It has been noted that the mental picture tends to clear as the lupus goes into remission, which would seem unlikely to occur if the underlying process was truly schizophrenia. This diagnosis is made less frequently in more recent studies. Kronfol et al. (1977) reported a case of "pure" catatonia with no other signs of organic or functional psychoses felt to be secondary to SLE.

Depending on their severity and the method of classification, depressive reactions are either included among the psychoses or reported separately. Some authors consider depression to be the most common mental change; it has been reported in from 10% to 35% of SLE patients (Shearn and Pirofsky, 1953; Andrew, 1975). The diagnosis of depression is highly related to the criteria used and the thoroughness of observation. Manic behavior has been described but is not particularly frequent. Other diagnoses include the entire clinical spectrum of personality disorders, neurotic reactions, psychophysiologic reactions, and other anxiety-related symptoms. The anxiety and acute neurotic reactions appear to fluctuate and be intermittent. Some patients complain of overwhelming feelings of impending disaster, quite unwarranted by the state of their disease (Clark and Bailey, 1956).

Despite the attention focused on psychiatric symptoms in SLE, only one study compares these symptoms to those found in other medical illnesses. Ganz et al., (1972), using structured interviews, compared 68 SLE patients with 36 rheumatoid arthritis patients attending the same clinics. They found that the SLE groups clearly demonstrated more psychiatric symptoms, but there were no overall differences in the kind of symptoms shown. Both groups showed exactly the same proportion of organic symptoms (22%) and nearly equal high proportions of depressive symptoms (51% and 47%, respectively).

Neurological Features

Neurologic signs and symptoms may occur separately or concurrently with psychiatric manifestations. Seizures are most frequently reported, occurring in 7–57% of SLE patients (Johnson and Richardson, 1968). Seizures most commonly occur in the terminal phases of SLE, often secondary to uremia, hypertension, or steroid treatment, but they are also found as a primary manifestation. They may be transient or recurrent, and occur in all forms, with grand mal seizures being most common.

Cranial nerve dysfunction secondary to lesions at any central or peripheral location may occur. Abnormalities related to extraocular movement and pupillary abnormalities are very common (Macrae and O'Reilly, 1957). Other reports list facial weakness, ptosis, sensory deficits, optic neuritis, vertigo, and dysarthria as high frequency findings (Clark and Bailey, 1956). Hemiplegia, quadriplegia, chorea, evidence of peripheral neuropathy, parkinsonian symptoms, and a myasthenia gravis-like picture have also been observed. Cerebellar signs may result in significant ataxia.

TREATMENT

Steroids are commonly used in the nonspecific treatment of SLE. The role of steroids in the production of neuropsychiatric manifestations is controversial, for it is well known that many patients receiving steroids or ACTH for whatever reason develop psychosis and other psychiatric symptoms. These drugs also lower seizure thresholds. It might therefore be argued that both seizures and psychoses are complications of therapy. However, the majority of reported neuropsychiatric episodes began or occurred while patients were receiving low doses or no steroids (Feinglass et al., 1976). The overall impression is that most psychoses are due not to steroid treatment but to the underlying disease. Some workers feel otherwise. Sergent et al. (1975) described patients with SLE whose psychoses they felt were secondary to treatment with corticosteroids. The presence of neurologic signs or systemic disease activity may help separate these cases.

The conflicting opinions concerning steroids make practical decisions about their use in the treatment of psychiatric manifestations in SLE difficult. There are many reports of favorable responses to corticosteroids. Some authors suggest that augmentation of corticosteroids, often to high doses, is probably a safer therapeutic approach than steroid reduction in patients already receiving steroids (Dubois, 1964; Feinglass et al., 1976). Others have been less impressed with the efficacy of these agents, and challenge both the efficacy and safety of large-dose therapy (Bennahum et al., 1974; Gibson and Myers, 1976). Thus, useful generalizations regarding steroid use, either in the presence of, or as treatment for neuropsychiatric symptoms, cannot be made. Only by relating improvement or deterioration of mental status to steroid doses in the individual patient can treatment strategies be delineated. Medical indications based on the entire clinical status of the patient often must receive considerations over the psychiatric picture alone.

Beyond the use of steroids, treatment is dictated by the clinical picture. No treatment appears to be specific. The treatment of psychiatric disturbances associated with SLE is largely symptomatic, and the use of the entire range of psychiatric modalities has been described. Antipsychotic medications are useful to control psychotic symptoms, and the usual psychosocial interventions have adjunctive value.

REFERENCES

Andrew WF, Jr: Psychiatric illness associated with systemic lupus erythematosus. *South Med J* 68:1207–1210, 1975.

Bennahum DA, Messner RP, Shoop JD: Brain scan findings in central nervous system involvement by lupus erythematosus. *Ann Intern Med* 81:763–765, 1974.

Clark EC, Bailey AA: Neurologic and psychiatric signs associated with systemic lupus erythematosus. *JAMA* 160:455–457, 1956.

Dubois ED, Tuffanelli DL: Clinical manifestation of systemic lupus erythematosus. *JAMA* 190:112–119, 1964.

Estes D, Christian CL: The natural history of systemic lupus erythematosus by prospective analysis. *Medicine* 50:85–95, 1971.

Feinglass EJ, Arnett FC, Dorsch CA, et al: Neuropsychiatric manifestations of systemic lupus erythematosus: Diagnosis, clinical spectrum and relationship to other features of the disease. *Medicine* 55:323–339, 1976.

Ganz VF, Gurland BJ, Demming E, et al: The study of the psychiatric symptoms of systemic lupus erythematosus: A biometric study. *Psychosom Med* 34:207–219, 1972.

Gibson T, Myers AR: Nervous system involvement in systemic lupus erythematosus. *Ann Rheum Dis* 35:398–406, 1976.

Gurland BJ, Ganz VF, Fleiss JL, et al: The study of the psychiatric symptoms of systemic lupus erythematosus. *Psychosom Med* 34:199–206, 1972.

Guze SB: The occurrence of psychiatric illness and systemic lupus erythematosus. *Am J Psychiatry* 123:1562–1570, 1967.

Johnson RT, Richardson EP: The neurologic manifestations of systemic lupus erythematosus. *Medicine* 47:337–369, 1968.

Kronfol Z, Schlesser M, Gsuang MT: Catatonia and systemic lupus erythematosus. *Dis Nerv Syst* 38:729–731, 1977.

Lief VF, Silverman T: Psychosis associated with lupus erythematosus disseminatus. *Arch Gen Psychiat* 3:608–611, 1960.

MacNeil A, Grennan DMO, Ward D, et al: Psychiatric problems in systemic lupus erythematosus. *Br J Psychiatry* 128:442–445, 1976.

Macrae D, O'Reilly S: On some neuro–oto–ophthalmological manifestations of systemic lupus erythematosus and peri arteritis nodosa. *Eye Ear Nose Throat* 36:721–724, 1957.

Mannik M, Gilliland BC: Systemic lupus erythematosus, in Thorn GW, Adams RD, Braunwald E (eds): *Harrison's Principles of Internal Medicine*, ed 8. New York, McGraw-Hill, 1977, pp 426–430.

O'Connor JF: Psychoses associated with systemic lupus erythematosus. *Ann Intern Med* 51:526–536, 1959.

Sergent JS, Lockshin MD, Klempner NS, et al: Central nervous system disease in systemic lupus erythematosus: Therapy and prognosis. *Am J Med* 58:644–655, 1975.

Shearn M, Pirofsky B: Disseminated lupus erythematosus: Analysis of thirty-four cases. *Arch Intern Med* 9:790–796, 1953.

Siekert RG, Clark EC: Neurologic signs and symptoms as early manifestations of systemic lupus erythematosus. *Neurology* 5:84–88, 1955.

Small P, Mas MF, Kohler PF, Harback RJ: Central nervous system involvement in SLE. *Arthritis Rheum* 20:869–878, 1977.

Stern M, Robbins ES: Psychoses in systemic lupus erythematosus. *Arch Gen Psychiatry* 3:205–210, 1960.

Striated Muscle Disorder (Myasthenia Gravis)

DEFINITION

Myasthenia gravis is a neuromuscular disease characterized by voluntary muscle weakness and fatigability which increases with use of the involved muscles and improves with rest.

CLINICAL FEATURES

The incidence of myasthenia gravis has been estimated at 1:20,000 with a bimodally distributed age of onset. The major peak occurs in the third decade, with females outnumbering males 4.5 to 1, while a later peak in the fifth decade has an equal sex distribution (Osserman and Genkins, 1971). In a series of 33 patients, however, 45% were first diagnosed between ages 60 and 82 (Herishanu et al., 1976). The time between the onset of symptoms and the diagnosis is quite variable; in Hokkanen's (1969) report, the interval ranged from a few weeks to 28 years with 84% being diagnosed in the first 5 years. The onset of the illness can range from insidious to abrupt, and its course can be quite variable. Grob (1958) reported that of 300 patients with generalized myasthenia gravis who had been followed for an average of 10 years, 30% died, with 70% of the deaths occurring within one year of onset and 85% within three years. Death is usually a result of respiratory failure or aspiration. Spontaneous remissions of 6 or more months occur in up to 25% of patients, but most experience a "gradual extension of the involved areas leading to a relatively steady state of weakness which remained unchanged for many years, with the exception of moderate fluctuations in severity" (Grob, 1958).

Exacerbations

Exacerbations of the disease may occur spontaneously but are often associated with upper respiratory infection, other infections, emotional

221

events, fatigue, high carbohydrate meals, alcohol, certain medications, and the premenstrual period, and occasionally with parturition, and physical exercise.

Initial Manifestations

In a series of 300 patients, Grob (1958) found the following initial manifestations:

Ptosis	26%	Difficulty chewing	4%
Diplopia	24%	Weakness of arms	3%
Blurred vision	3%	Hands	3%
Weakness of legs	13%	Neck	3%
Generalized fatigue	6%	Face	3%
Difficulty swallowing	6%	Trunk	1%
Slurred and nasal speech	5%	Shortness of breath	1%

Drooping of the eyelids (ptosis) occurs in 90% of cases and may initially be unilateral. Ptosis which shifts from one eye to the other is considered almost pathognomonic of myasthenia gravis (Osserman and Genkins, 1971).

Typical Features

A composite patient with myasthenia gravis would have a characteristically sleepy appearance due to ptosis, often with a compensatory wrinkling of the forehead. Ptosis is often accompanied by diplopia and blurred vision. Facial muscle weakness results in an apathetic expression with a "myasthenic vertical snarl" appearing with attempted smiling or when asked to show teeth (owing to weakness of the orbicularis oris). Chewing becomes more difficult as a meal progresses, and masseter weakness can also result in sagging of the jaw (hanging-jaw sign). Palatal muscle weakness can lead to nasal regurgitation of food during swallowing; choking or aspiration of food may also occur. Myasthenic speech, which may be clear at the start and later decrease in volume and clarity, has been described as having a feeble, mushy, nasal quality. The tongue may be weak and may occasionally be bilaterally longitudinally furrowed (the "trident tongue"). Neck muscle weakness is also common, and the patient may have to support his head.

Proximal muscles tend to be involved before distal, which may lead to early difficulties with shaving or combing the hair. Although respiratory distress may be a presenting manifestation, it is more common for respiratory muscle involvement to occur in the latter stages of the disease. Diaphragm weakness tends to result in inspiratory dyspnea, while intercostal and abdominal muscle involvement can lead to expiratory dyspnea.

Since weakness becomes worse with repeated muscle use, it is characteristic for a patient to be at his best on awakening and weakest in the evening. Even with a rest, however, most patients have some persistent weakness.

Sensory complaints are present in about 15% of patients, with complaints of pain in both involved and uninvolved muscles (more severe as the day progresses), headache, ocular pain, and paresthesias.

CLINICAL CLASSIFICATION

Based on the study of over 1200 patients, the following classification was devised and has been accepted in many clinical centers (Osserman and Genkins, 1971).

A. Pediatric
  1. Neonatal—self-limited and occurring only in infants of myasthenic mothers.
  2. Juvenile—may occur any time from birth to puberty, is permanent, and is not associated with a myasthenic mother.
B. Adult
  1. Ocular myasthenia (Group I)—localized form, may be limited to only one eye, characterized by ptosis and diplopia, excellent prognosis.
  2. Mild generalized (Group IIA)—slow onset, gradual spread to skeletal and bulbar muscles, good response to drugs, respiratory muscles spared, very low mortality.
  3. Moderate generalized (Group IIB)—gradual onset with ocular presentation common, progression to more severe and generalized involvement of skeletal and bulbar muscles but sparing of respiratory muscles, activities restricted, drug response less adequate, mortality low.
  4. Acute fulminating (Group III)—rapid onset of severe bulbar and skeletal weakness with early respiratory involvement, progression usually complete in 6 months, drug response poor, mortality high, highest percentage of thymomas.
  5. Late severe (Group IV)—severe findings develop at least two years after onset of Group I or II symptoms, sudden or gradual progression, poor drug response and prognosis.

NEUROPSYCHIATRIC FEATURES

Although myasthenia gravis in its classic form is not difficult to diagnose, milder or atypical presentations are commonly misdiagnosed as psychiatric illness. Because of the frequent association of emotional upset with precipitation or exacerbation of the disease, appropriate diagnosis can be considerably delayed. Muscle weakness that is both dramatic and reversible can be mistaken for hysteria.

Most commonly, myasthenia gravis is confused with weakness and fatigability of "emotional" origin. A careful history will usually lead to the proper diagnosis, although confirmation with appropriate drug testing is necessary (see below). Myasthenic weakness characteristically gets worse with continued use of the involved muscles while a "neurasthenic" patient may complain of weakness, yet not show objective deterioration of strength. For example, over time, a myasthenic's speech may become soft and barely intelligible, in contrast to the "psychoneurotic patient who also complains of weakness but can talk interminably without change in voice or enunciation" (Adams, 1977). According to Grob (1958), myasthenic weakness is likely to increase in the premenstrual period, as opposed to neurasthenic weakness which is likely to be more pronounced during the menses.

The distinction between myasthenic and "functional" weakness is not always readily apparent, and misdiagnoses can be made in either direction. Grob (1958) reported that 20% of females and a lesser percent of males referred to the Johns Hopkins Myasthenia Gravis Clinic with a diagnosis of myasthenia gravis actually had "weakness of emotional origin."

As early as 1887, hysteria was considered to have a possible relationship to myasthenia gravis, and more recently Ball and Lloyd (1971) stated (without substantiation): "It has long been known that myasthenics are prone to develop hysterical symptoms and other forms of psychiatric illness."

When a more formal psychiatric evaluation was performed on 25 patients selected at random from myasthenia gravis patients at the Mayo Clinic, the following was found (MacKenzie et al.,1969):

1. There was no typical personality profile.
2. There was no increase in the incidence of emotional difficulties prior to the onset of the illness.
3. Forty-four percent (mostly in the early onset group) had difficulty adapting to the illness.
4. In 28%, onset of the illness was at the time of distinct psychological stress.
5. Forty-eight percent experienced substantial exacerbation of weakness following emotional upset (especially anger).
6. In 16% (4 patients) periods of emotional stress were associated with prolonged exacerbation of symptoms (the authors suggest that a deteriorating clinical course should prompt a careful search for emotional factors).

Three teenage girls were noted to have an increase in myasthenic weakness just prior to a date—a situation that might easily be attributed only to "nerves."

An episode of weakness following a refreshing summer drink could also be mistaken for psychological fatigue unless one is aware that the quinine in tonic water is sufficient to decompensate a person with myasthenia gravis.

A striking example of myasthenic misdiagnosis was a 16-year-old girl with recurrent aphonia and decreased energy that was later compounded by difficulty swallowing and aspiration pneumonia (Ball and Lloyd, 1971). A psychiatric consultant diagnosed her illness as hysterical but also said that "my impression has been that she suffers from a severe disturbance of personality, with schizoid features and is liable to psychotic episodes." Following admission to a psychiatric inpatient unit, medical and neurological evaluation led to the diagnosis of myasthenia gravis and appropriate treatment was instituted. Two years later she was described as "an attractive, active, outgoing girl with a wide range of interests quite suitable for a girl her age."

When myasthenic symptoms occur for the first time in the geriatric age group, the possibility of misdiagnosis is high. This is due, in part, to a tendency to consider myasthenia gravis a disease of young adulthood and middle age and not to appreciate that a substantial number of patients are over the age of 60 when they first develop the illness. Diagnosis is further complicated by an increased number of coexisting conditions in the geriatric age group that have symptoms similar to those of myasthenia or that impair the ability of the patient to give a reliable history. For example, a 76-year-old woman with double vision was initially diagnosed as having basilar artery disease, and a 69-year-old man with episodes of nocturnal dyspnea was, at first, thought to have heart disease (Herishanu et al., 1976).

PATHOGENESIS

The neurotransmitter, acetylcholine, is synthesized in motor nerve terminals, stored in vesicles, and released to interact with acetylcholine receptors, causing increased sodium–potassium permeability, which results in electrical depolarization. The amplitude of depolarization depends on the number of receptors activated. Normally, the number of interactions is well in excess of that necessary to trigger an action potential. If the number of interactions is reduced below a certain critical margin, neuromuscular transmission will not occur.

The basic defect in myasthenia gravis is "a reduction of available acetylcholine receptors at neuromuscular junctions, brought about by an autoimmune attack" (Drachman, 1978a). Antiacetylcholine receptor antibodies have been found in up to 87% of patients with myasthenia gravis, and these humorally mediated antibodies appear to accelerate degradation of acetylcholine receptors and also to block active sites on the receptor molecule. Cell-mediated immune responses may also be involved.

Although the thymus appears to play an important role in the disease, its exact function is not known. Abnormalities of the thymus are present in about 75% of myasthenic patients, with 85% of these showing germinal center formation and the remainder either gross or microscopic thymomas. A thymoma, while histologically benign, can behave malignantly by being locally invasive.

DIAGNOSIS

A thorough history is the framework upon which the diagnosis is built. Characteristically, the myasthenia gravis patient experiences neuromuscular fatigue and is unable to sustain or repeat muscular contractions. If three or more muscles are tested electromyographically, a decremental response will be found in 95% of myasthenic patients (Drachman, 1978b).

If a small dose of the neuromuscular blocking agent curare (d-tubocurarine) is given to a normal person it will not block enough acetylcholine receptors to impede neuromuscular transmission, while in the myasthenic patient a clinically apparent increase in weakness will occur.

A most useful procedure in the diagnosis of myasthenia gravis is the edrophonium (Tensilon) test. This drug is an anticholinesterase agent which inhibits the breakdown of acetylcholine, allowing an increased number of acetylcholine–receptor interactions. A positive test will result in both subjective and objective improvement in muscle strength, which does not occur with administration of a placebo.

Differential Diagnosis

Other conditions that can cause episodic muscle weakness include (1) the Eaton–Lambert syndrome, (2) episodic kalemic paralysis, and (3) myasthenic syndrome associated with antibiotics.

The Eaton–Lambert syndrome is a myasthenic–myopathic condition usually found in association with malignant tumors, which is apparently due to a defect in acetylcholine release. As opposed to myasthenia gravis, ocular and bulbar involvement is rare, weakness is usually confined to the trunk and extremities, initial movements are weak with strength *improving* with repeated contractions (rapid rates of nerve stimulation cause a diagnostic *increment* in action potential amplitude), and response to anticholinesterase drugs is variable, while guanidine is an effective therapeutic agent.

The episodic kalemic paralyses consist of at least four syndromes of recurrent muscle weakness in each of which "the patient may develop over a period of a few hours a disorder of skeletal muscles which may vary from weakness of the trunk and limb muscles to total paralysis, and which subsides and disappears completely after a few hours or days" (Adams, 1977).

These syndromes include:

1. Familial periodic paralysis
2. Hyperthyroidism with periodic paralysis
3. Congenital paramyotonia and hyperkalemic paralysis of von Eulenberg
4. Hereditary periodic adynamia

A myasthenic syndrome can develop in association with the use of certain antibiotics (neomycin, streptomycin, dihydrostreptomycin, kanamycin, polymyxin B, bacitracin, lincomycin, colistin, and gentamicin). This syndrome usually occurs after surgery, and appears to be caused by antibiotic-induced impairment of acetylcholine release. The clinical picture usually involves generalized weakness with respiratory involvement, and differs from naturally occurring myasthenia gravis in that paralysis of parasympathetic functions also occurs (dilated pupils, atonic bladder). The weakness is most responsive to calcium infusion (Fenichel, 1978).

TREATMENT

Modern treatment of myasthenia gravis allows most patients to lead useful, productive lives (Drachman, 1978b).

Anticholinesterase Drugs

The preferred treatment for most patients with myasthenia gravis is the administration of the anticholinesterase agents (neostigmine, pyridostigmine, ambenonium). Careful regulation of size and timing of dose is necessary to avoid fluctuations of strength, to anticipate periods of need, and to avoid drug side effects. Havard (1977) stresses that "myasthenic patients, like other individuals, are subjected to the fatigue of mental and physical strain, and the temptation to increase the dose of medication to counter such physiological fatigue must be resisted." Excessive amounts of these drugs can actually cause *increased* weakness, respiratory insufficiency, and signs of cholinergic excess such as salivation, sweating, nausea, abdominal cramps, diarrhea, bradycardia, and miosis.

Steroids

In patients whose response to anticholinesterase drugs is less than satisfactory, steroids are often quite beneficial.

Thymectomy

Surgical removal of the thymus gland has been associated with remission in 20–36% of patients, and improvement in 57–86% (Drachman, 1978b). Opinions vary widely as to the indications for thymectomy (in the absence of tumor) and to the preferred surgical technique.

Other

Less well established treatment approaches include the use of immunosuppressive drugs, as well as serum antibody depleting techniques such as thoracic duct drainage, plasmapheresis, and plasma exchange.

NEUROPSYCHIATRIC EFFECTS OF ANTIMYASTHENIC DRUGS

Since the anticholinesterase drugs used to treat myasthenia gravis do not easily cross the blood–brain barrier, toxic psychoses are not anticipated. Another anticholinesterase, physostigmine, does readily enter the brain, has been used quite effectively to treat anticholinergic delirium, and has an intrinsic mood depressing effect. It is possible, therefore, that if enough of the poorly penetrating drugs do reach the brain that neuropsychiatric side effects could occur.

Steroids can have quite pronounced central nervous system effects, and the myasthenic patient appears no more or less susceptible to them.

THE USE OF PSYCHOTROPIC DRUGS IN PATIENTS WITH MYASTHENIA GRAVIS

Psychotropic drug use in the myasthenic patient has been best addressed by Martin and Flegenheimer (1971) who temper theoretical considerations with practical experience. They state that although **chlorpromazine** intensifies the effects of d-tubocurarine and gallamine, it has been used safely in doses over 800 mg per day. Antipsychotic drugs would not appear contraindicated in patients with myasthenia gravis, although caution should be exercised in their use.

These authors have also used **imipramine** and **amitriptyline** in doses over 200 mg/day without difficulty, but they have found tricyclic antidepressants to be of only occasional value in treating depressed myasthenics.

They have also used antianxiety drugs such as **meprobamate, barbiturates, diazepam**, and **chlordiazepoxide** in their usual dosage without untoward effect.

When **lithium** was used to treat a manic-depressive patient, symptoms of myasthenia gravis emerged on four occasions and improved or disappeared when the drug was reduced or discontinued (Neil et al., 1976). A parallel was drawn between this observation and the ability of lithium to prolong the duration of action of neuromuscular blocking agents such as succinylcholine and pancuronium. Finally, Martin and Flegenheimer (1971) mentioned, without elaborating, that ECT has been used in patients with myasthenia gravis, and suggest that under such circumstances succinylcholine should be avoided.

REFERENCES

Adams RD: Myasthenia gravis and episodic muscular weakness, in Thorn GW, Adams RD, Braunwald E, et al (eds): *Harrison's Principles of Internal Medicine*, ed 8. New York, McGraw-Hill, 1977, pp 1996–2001.

Ball JRB, Lloyd JH: Myasthenia gravis as hysteria or sounds of silence. *Med J Aust* 1:1018–1020, 1971.

Drachman DB: Myasthenia gravis. *N Engl J Med* 298:136–142, 1978a.

Drachman DB: Myasthenia gravis. *N Engl J Med* 298:186–193, 1978b.

Fenichel GM: Clinical syndromes of myasthenia in infancy and childhood. *Arch Neurol* 35:97–103, 1978.

Grob D: Myasthenia gravis: Current status of pathogenesis, clinical manifestations, and management. *J Chr Dis* 8:536–566, 1958.

Havard CWH: Progress in myasthenia gravis. *Br Med J* 2:1008–1011, 1977.

Herishanu Y, Abramsky O, Feldman S: Myasthenia gravis in the elderly. *J Am Geriatr Soc* 24:228–231, 1976.

Hokkanen E: Myasthenia gravis. *Ann Clin Res* 1:94–108, 1969.

MacKenzie KR, Martin MJ, Howard FM: Myasthenia gravis: Psychiatric concomitants. *Can Med Assoc J* 100:988–991, 1969.

Martin RD, Flegenheimer WV: Psychiatric aspects of the management of the myasthenic patient. *Mt Sinai J Med* 38:594–601, 1971.

Neil JF, Himmelhoch JM, Licata SM: Emergence of myasthenia gravis during treatment with lithium carbonate. *Arch Gen Psychiatry* 33:1090–1092, 1976.

Osserman KE, Genkins G: Studies in myasthenia gravis: Review of a twenty-year experience in over 1200 patients. *Mt Sinai J Med* 38:497–537, 1971.

11

Vitamin Disorders

HYPERVITAMINOSIS A

General Considerations

Vitamin A (retinol) is a fat-soluble vitamin necessary in the body for epithelial integrity, formation of photoreceptor pigments in the retina, and stability of lysosomes. Foods plentiful in vitamin A include fish liver oil, eggs, butter, and green leafy and yellow vegetables. The minimum daily adult requirement for vitamin A is 5000 IU, while the usual therapeutic dose is 25,000–50,000 IU/day. Toxicity from ingestion of excessive amounts of vitamin A can be either acute or chronic.

Clinical Features

Acute Hypervitaminosis A

Acute vitamin A intoxication, although not recognized as such, was first described in 1856 in arctic explorers after they ate polar-bear liver, which contains several million units of the vitamin. Several hours after intake, the following transient symptoms may appear: severe headache, vertigo, nausea, vomiting, drowsiness, irritability, and blurred and double vision (Feldman and Schlezinger, 1970; Van Itallie and Follis, 1974b). These findings have been associated with increased cerebrospinal fluid pressure.

Chronic Hypervitaminosis A

High doses of vitamin A taken over a period of months to years can produce a wide range of abnormalities involving the liver, skin, and nervous system. Table 11-1 summarizes findings from 17 cases (Muenter et al, 1971). Nonspecific complaints such as weakness, fatigue, anorexia, headache, muscle stiffness, and sleep disturbance could easily give the impression of a functional psychiatric disorder. In these cases, the duration of intake ranged

**TABLE 11-1.   Symptoms and Signs in Seventeen Cases
of Chronic Vitamin A Intoxication in Adults and
Adolescents**[a]

Symptom or sign	Number of cases
Skin (dryness, maculopapular rash, fissures, desquamation, pigmentation, pruritis)	17
Hair loss	14
Generalized weakness and fatigue	14
Pain in bones and joints	13
Marked tenderness of bones to palpation	11
Anorexia	9
Headache	9
Hepatomegaly	8
Muscle stiffness	7
Endocrine (absent or decreased menorrhea)	7
Papilledema	6
Diplopia	6
Weight loss	6
Splenomegaly	6
Polyuria, polydipsia, urinary frequency	6
Psychiatric symptoms	6
Edema of lower extremities	6
Insomnia	5
Bleeding (nose and lips)	5
Brittle nails	4
Somnolence	3
Exophthalmus	2
Yellow discoloration of skin	2
Other neurologic symptoms	2
Gingivitis	1
Lymphadenopathy	1

[a] From Meunter et al. (1971) with permission of authors and publisher.

from two months to nine years, and the daily dose of vitamin A from 41,000 to 600,000 IU.

Hypervitaminosis A is one of a number of possible causes of the syndrome of benign intracranial hypertension (pseudotumor cerebri). The condition is characterized by headache, papilledema, increased intracranial pressure, occasional sixth nerve palsies, and visual field defects occurring in an otherwise healthy and alert person (Feldman and Schlezinger, 1970; Mikkelsen et al, 1974; Vollbracht and Gilroy, 1976). One patient who complained of balance difficulty and the sensation of "being pushed forward by some unknown force" was initially thought to have a brain tumor (Vollbracht and Gilroy, 1976). Although for over two years he had been taking only 10,000–20,000 IU/day of vitamin A, discontinuation of the vitamin led to resolution of the symptoms.

Other psychiatric manifestations described in association with vitamin A intoxication include irritability, social isolation, and depression. DiBenedetto (1967) described a 51-year-old woman admitted to a psychiatric ward complaining of severe depression with additional complaints and physical abnormalities consistent with a long history of excessive vitamin A intake. This was confirmed by an elevated fasting serum vitamin A level. Discontinuation of the supplementary vitamin was followed by improvement in both psychological and physical symptoms. Although a causal relationship to depression could not be firmly established, it is likely that symptoms of hypervitaminosis A did lead to the psychiatric hospitalization. If a history of high vitamin A intake is not given, the confusing and, at times, unusual symptoms may be quite misleading.

Diagnosis

Diagnosis is best established by a history of excessive vitamin A ingestion and resolution of symptoms following withdrawal of the vitamin. While the serum level of vitamin A tends to be increased in cases of intoxication, there is not a good correlation between serum level and severity of symptoms.

Treatment

Intake of supplementary vitamin A should be discontinued. Elevated serum vitamin A levels will initially fall abruptly but may not return to normal for several weeks. Relief of nonspecific symptoms should occur within weeks, while liver enlargement and alopecia may resolve more slowly. If symptoms resulting from intracranial hypertension are severe, the short-term use of steroids will generally provide relief.

THIAMINE (VITAMIN B$_1$) DEFICIENCY

General Considerations

Thiamine (vitamin B$_1$) is a water-soluble vitamin that plays a role in carbohydrate metabolism and in the pentose monophosphate pathway for glucose metabolism and is essential for central and peripheral nerve cell and myocardial function. Because the vitamin is not stored in the body to any appreciable extent, a constant dietary supply is necessary. Foods rich in thiamine include dried yeast, whole grains, meat, enriched cereal products, nuts, legumes, and potatoes. The usual therapeutic dose is 5–30 mg/day.

Under clinical conditions, thiamine deficiency states are never "pure" but occur in association with deficiencies of calories, protein, and other vitamins. This is true for Oriental beriberi, despite its historical relation to thiamine deficiency and despite the fact that many of its manifestations do respond favorably to thiamine administration.

Wernicke encephalopathy and Korsakoff syndrome (Wernicke–Korsakoff syndrome) are also related to thiamine deficiency but do not occur in Orientals with beriberi. Instead, these syndromes are found in Occidentals suffering from malnutrition, usually in association with alcoholism. While multiple deficiencies are likely to be present, the administration of thiamine alone under clinical experimental conditions has been shown to improve the ophthalmoplegia, nystagmus, and ataxia of Wernicke syndrome (Victor et al., 1971).

"Pure" thiamine deficiency states have been produced experimentally in both animal and man by eliminating or greatly reducing the thiamine content in otherwise balanced diets. Under the best of experimental conditions, synthetic diets were carefully prepared to insure the presence of all essential vitamins and minerals except thiamine.

Clinical Features

Experimental Thiamine Deficiency

When multiple episodes of thiamine deficiency were induced in rhesus monkeys, the neurologic signs produced were consistent with most aspects of Wernicke syndrome and some aspects of beriberi (Mesulam et al., 1977). Clinical deterioration was maximal between 39 and 105 days, with anorexia appearing first, followed several days later by apathy and a characteristic lower extremity weakness. More advanced findings included nystagmus, sixth-nerve weakness, ataxia, dysmetria, and congestive heart failure. Edema and peripheral neuropathy were not noted. Administration of thiamine resulted in prompt resolution of most of the abnormalities.

Spillane (1974a) summarized several experimental thiamine deficiency studies in man. Characteristically, subjects complained of "mental and physical inefficiency" which was present for weeks or months before the appearance of more substantial findings. In one study, the "surreptitious" administration of thiamine reversed symptoms, which included "nausea, vomiting, depression, irritability, quarrelsomeness, general weakness, inefficiency, failing memory, and confusion of thought." Symptoms that appeared consistently in a number of studies include anorexia, apathy, fatigue, weight loss, and calf tenderness. During experimental thiamine deprivation, deterioration was noted on the "psychoneurotic" scales (Hypochondriasis, Depression, and Hysteria) of the Minnesota Multiphasic Personality Inventory (MMPI) which later normalized with thiamine supplementation (Brozek, 1957). Clearly, neuropsychiatric symptoms can be produced by thiamine deficiency.

Beriberi

In the Orient, three main types of beriberi have been described. The most common, **subacute beriberi** (wet beriberi) is characterized by edema of the legs, which may generalize to involve other areas of the body, together with appetite loss, paresthesias, muscle cramps, altered deep tendon reflexes, and cardiac abnormalities. **Acute fulminating beriberi** develops abruptly, often without premonitory symptoms, is characterized by heart failure, and is often fatal. The third type, **dry beriberi**, develops in an insidious fashion, and is characterized by peripheral neurological disturbances including paresthesias and pain in the feet, heaviness and tiredness of the legs, cramping and tenderness of the calf muscles, abnormal deep tendon reflexes, and abnormal vibration and position sense. Involvement is maximal in the lower extremities, and there is some similarity to the peripheral neuropathy found in alcoholics. For reasons yet unknown, central nervous system manifestations (including those of the Wernicke–Korsakoff syndrome) tend to be absent in Oriental beriberi (Van Itallie and Follis; 1974a).

Wernicke–Korsakoff Syndrome (Cerebral Beriberi)

Wernicke encephalopathy is best known by the triad of ocular palsies, nystagmus, and ataxia, although 90% of patients have mental symptoms and 80% have polyneuropathy (Victor et al., 1971).

In the early stages, the most common mental function abnormality is a quiet delirium, which Victor et al., (1971) called a "global confusional state" and described as consisting of "general fatigue and apathy, an impairment of awareness and responsiveness, disorientation and confusion, inattention and failure of concentration, and derangements of perception and memory." Most patients showed signs of severe physical and mental exhaustion, tiring after the mildest exertion, having difficulty performing the simplest tasks, and drifting off to sleep while being examined. Because of drowsiness, inattentiveness, and disinterest in the initial stage of the illness, accurate assessment of the degree of memory impairment is often not possible. As the memory defect is less responsive to treatment with thiamine, it tends to become more apparent as the other manifestations respond to the vitamin.

Less commonly, Wernicke syndrome will present as an agitated, delusional–hallucinatory state characteristic of delirium tremens. Finally, 10% of the 229 carefully evaluated patients with Wernicke syndrome had no evidence of mental abnormality (Victor et al., 1971).

Korsakoff syndrome (psychosis) is felt to represent a different aspect of the same disease process responsible for Wernicke syndrome. It is characterized by a gross defect in memory (especially for recent events) and an impaired ability to form new memories. Additional findings may include mild impairment of perceptual and conceptual function and a lack of spontaneity and initiative. Confabulation, while commonly found in Korsakoff syndrome, is not consistently present and may also occur in association with other neurological conditions.

Confabulation is more likely to occur in the earlier stages of Korsakoff syndrome (amnesic–confabulatory psychosis) and be absent in the later stages (chronic nonconfabulatory amnesic states).

Diagnosis

Clinical manifestations and dietary history are important aspects in the diagnosis of beriberi and Wernicke–Korsakoff syndrome. Laboratory tests such as urinary thiamine levels and red blood cell transketolase activity can be helpful in confirming the diagnosis, but are often unnecessary, since treatment is usually initiated on clinical grounds alone, is safe and inexpensive, and is helpful in confirming a tentative diagnosis. It is important to realize that Wernicke encephalopathy can occur in association with disorders other than chronic alcoholism. These include gastrointestinal cancer, thyrotoxicosis, hyperemesis gravidarum, and chronic hemodialysis (Anonymous, 1979).

Treatment

Central to the effective treatment of experimental thiamine deficiency, Oriental beriberi, and Wernicke–Korskoff syndrome is the administration of adequate amounts of thiamine. The dose, duration of treatment, and route of administration are determined by the severity of the illness. Acute cardiovascular beriberi, for example, is considered a medical emergency, which, quite fortunately, often responds dramatically to intravenous thiamine. The more chronic the condition, the less likely there is to be a complete response to thiamine, as exemplified by chronic Korsakoff syndrome and dry beriberi.

In clinical situations, other nutritional deficiencies always coexist with thiamine deficiency, so that it is important to provide a diet complete in all essential requirements. Finally, there is some recent evidence that the memory defect in Korsakoff syndrome may be improved by treatment with vasopressin (LeBoeuf et al., 1978).

NIACIN (NICOTINIC ACID) DEFICIENCY

General Considerations

Niacin (nicotinic acid, nicotinamide, vitamin B_3), a water-soluble vitamin, plays an important role in oxidation–reduction reactions and carbohydrate and tryptophan metabolism. The main sources of niacin are liver, lean meat, fish, poultry, yeast, legumes, and whole grain-enriched cereal products. Since there are no appreciable stores of niacin in the body, requirements must be met either by ingestion of the vitamin or by synthesis from dietary tryptophan. By a complex biosynthetic pathway requiring the presence of thiamine, riboflavin, pyridoxine, and nicotine-adenine dinucleotide phosphate, 1 mg of niacin can be generated from about 60 mg of dietary tryptophan (Spivak and Jackson, 1977). The usual therapeutic dose of nicotinamide is 100–1000 mg/day.

Although the first description of pellagra appeared in northern Spain and Italy during the early 18th century, it was not until the 20th century that it was correctly identified as a deficiency disease. A variety of socioeconomic factors, especially changes in the processing of corn, led to pellagra becoming endemic in the United States between 1900 and World War II. In 1928, 1929, and 1930 reported deaths from pellagra exceeded 7000, and there were estimated to be greater than 200,000 pellagrins in this country.

Despite the identification of nicotinic acid in 1937 and its demonstrated effectiveness against "black tongue" in dogs and pellagra in man, 2000 people died in this country from the disease in 1940. It was not until the social upheaval of World War II elevated standards of living and altered dietary habits that the disease ceased to be endemic. According to Sydenstricker (1958):

> Since 1945, pellagra has been a clinical curiosity seen only in the occasional food-fadist, senile recluse or chronic alcoholic. In fact, it requires considerable ingenuity at the present time to develop the disease, what with the flour and meal and grits and rice all expensively enriched with the things the mills have carefully removed.

In addition to dietary deficiency, pellagra can sometimes be found in association with other conditions which include (1) Hartnup disease, a rare hereditary condition in which tryptophan and other amino acid absorption and excretion is abnormal; (2) carcinoid tumor in which tryptophan is diverted to form serotonin; and (3) the use of drugs such as isoniazid, ethionamide, and 6-mercaptopurine, which interfere with vitamin metabolism.

Although pellagra is most closely associated with niacin deficiency, it has been repeatedly demonstrated that niacin therapy alone does not reverse all manifestations of the disease and that the disease should more properly be considered a multiple deficiency illness. Other factors likely to be deficient include protein, thiamine, riboflavin (vitamin B_2) and folic acid. The term "pellagra sine pellagra" refers to the disease in the absence of dermatitis. This is generally felt to represent an atypical presentation of niacin deficiency, although some authorities feel that riboflavin deficiency is actually responsible for the dermatitis of pellagra.

Clinical Features

General

Classic pellagra is known by the tetrad of the four D's: Dermatitis, Diarrhea, Dementia, and Death (Follis and Van Itallie, 1974a).

Skin lesions tend to be symmetric and more prominent over exposed areas. Initially they may resemble the erythema of sunburn, followed by vesiculation and peeling. Chronic findings include (1) a rough, scaly hypertrophy, in which the skin is thick, inelastic, and deeply pigmented over pressure points, and (2) atrophic areas of dry, scaly, inelastic skin.

Gastrointestinal manifestations include stomatitis and glossitis, with burning of the mouth, pharynx, and esophagus, anorexia, abdominal discomfort, nausea, vomiting, and diarrhea.

In the series of 18 patients reported by Spivak and Jackson (1977), the triad of dermatitis, diarrhea, and dementia was present in only 20%. All patients had dermatitis, since the authors required its presence for inclusion in the study. Additional findings included neuropathy 56%, edema 56%, dementia 50%, glossitis 39%, diarrhea 39%, and stomatitis 11%.

Neuropsychiatric

Early in the course of the disease, neuropsychiatric findings in pellagra may be nonspecific and misleading. Symptoms such as nervousness, irritability, insomnia, and depression are apt to be mistaken for psychoneurosis or "neurasthenia."

Frostig and Spies (1940) describe at length the initial symptoms found in 60 cases of subclinical and mild pellagra (associated deficiencies in thiamine and riboflavin were also often present). They summarize their findings as follows:

> The symptoms of the initial nervous syndrome associated with pellagra are: a, hyperesthesia to all forms of sensation; b, increased psycho-motor drive; c, increased emotional drive with a definite trend toward depression and apprehension; d, weariness and increased fatigability; e, headache; and f, sleeplessness. In general, these patients appear to have anxiety states with depressive features.

The mood changes they described were those of an apprehensive depression, with a gloomy and pessimistic outlook and the constant anticipation of imminent danger. They state that "men previously strong, courageous, and enduring, become shaky, weary, and apprehensive even before the usually recognized clinical signs of pellagra develop."

Spillane (1947b) reviewed in detail the neurological and mental manifestations of pellagra and stressed the ease with which early symptoms could be mistaken for psychoneuroses. He quoted one author as saying, "When neurasthenic symptoms have lasted for several years without obvious cause, the physician should suspect pellagra." Early symptoms can include fatigue, lassitude, anorexia, anxiety, fears, emotional instability, restlessness, insomnia, depression, impaired memory, distractibility, palpitations, and headache (Spies et al., 1938).

As the disease progresses, its neuropsychiatric symptoms become more severe. While the older literature described almost every type of major psychiatric syndrome (acute confusional psychosis, acute mania, melancholia, dementia, catatonia, and dementia praecox), detailed mental status examinations were not described. It is generally felt that these conditions were actually variations of an organic brain syndrome. Careful evaluation will *usually* detect defects in orientation, memory, and cognitive function consistent with organic impairment.

A recent report (Spivak and Jackson, 1977) did mention a patient with manic behavior without impaired orientation, yet a more detailed mental status evaluation was not presented. These authors also stressed the value of the electroencephalogram in detecting central nervous system involvement (diffuse slow wave activity) but did not mention whether it was normal or abnormal in the manic patient.

Whether niacin deficiency can occasionally present as a functional psychosis has been suggested in reports of schizophrenic patients who improve dramatically when treated with niacin (and other vitamins). Whether this represents a niacin deficiency state, a pharmacologic non-deficiency-related response to vitamin therapy, or merely coincidence is difficult to resolve. It does seem clear that the typical central nervous system manifestations of pellagra are consistent with an organic brain syndrome (encephalopathy) rather than schizophrenia, and that there is no constellation of findings that is diagnostic or even strongly suggestive of the disease.

Diagnosis

Spillane (1947) states:

> Fatigue, loss of weight and depression are usually present and the facies may be diagnostic with its characteristic ruddy complexion and dull, listless stare, so that experienced physicians may recognize the pellagrin at a glance.

Since then, pellagra has become a rarity and, consequently, so have physicians experienced in dealing with the illness, so that diagnosis on clinical grounds along is not as easily made. A history of an appropriately deficient diet together with the characteristic skin lesions is quite helpful in directing one toward the proper diagnosis.

Although there is no simple confirmatory laboratory test, low plasma tryptophan levels are suggestive (but not specific) and low urinary N-methylnicotinamide and N-methyl-2-pyridone-5-carboxamide levels may be of supportive value.

Finally, clinical response to treatment with niacin is an important aspect of establishing a diagnosis.

Treatment

Pellagra must be treated as a multiple-deficiency disease. While the administration of niacinamide is central to treatment, a balanced diet and adequate supplementation with other vitamins is essential. In fact, the rapid replacement of a single vitamin may actually produce an imbalance that will aggravate other deficiencies. With prompt treatment, the prognosis for pellagra is excellent, whereas undue delay can result in irreversible brain damage.

VITAMIN B$_6$ DEFICIENCY

General Considerations

Three naturally occurring pyridines—pyridoxine, pyridoxal, and pyridoxamine—are collectively referred to as vitamin B$_6$. Food sources rich in the vitamin include dry yeast, liver, organ meats, whole grain cereals, fish, and legumes. Because of its wide distribution, primary dietary deficiency of vitamin B$_6$ is generally felt to be rare. On the other hand, a survey of male and female students and students using oral contraceptives found not only large differences in vitamin B$_6$ requirements but evidence of subclinical deficiencies in many of the subjects (Driskell et al., 1976). Whether these observations are confirmed and whether they are of any clinical importance remains to be determined.

In the body, phosphorylated forms of the vitamin function as coenzymes in a large number of reactions involving decarboxylases, transaminases, and deaminases. Vitamin B$_6$ is required for the activity of the enzyme tryptophan decarboxylase, which is involved in the synthesis of the neurotransmitter serotonin. The vitamin also plays a role in the metabolism of niacin, methionine, and fatty acids.

Vitamin B$_6$ disorders are divided into dependency states (inborn errors of metabolism in which vitamin levels are normal but utilization is impaired) and deficiency states. The former disorders include (1) infantile convulsive disorder, (2) familial pyridoxine-responsive anemia, (3) cystathionuria, (4) homocystinuria, and (5) xanthurenic aciduria (Lipton and Kane, 1972). Functional deficiency states are most commonly induced by interactions with drugs such as isoniazid, cycloserine, hydralazine, penicillamine, and oral contraceptives (Lipton and Kane, 1972; Rose et al., 1972; Brown et al., 1975; Van Itallie, 1977).

Clinical Features

General

Vitamin B$_6$ deficiency can affect the blood (microcytic, hypochromic anemia), skin (seborrhea, cheilosis) and nervous system (see below) but none of these findings is diagnostically specific.

Neuropsychiatric

In infancy, vitamin B_6 dependency or deficiency can be associated with seizures and mental retardation. Early diagnosis is important to prevent irreversible damage.

In adults, drug-induced functional deficiencies of vitamin B_6 have been implicated in causing organic brain syndromes and depression. Isoniazid use has been associated with convulsions, peripheral neuropathy, and toxic psychoses, and cycloserine use with convulsions, drowsiness, headache, tremor, dysarthria, confusion, disorientation, hyperirritability, paresthesias, aggressive behavior, and toxic psychoses. How often such abnormalities are due to vitamin B_6 deficiency as opposed to other actions of the drug or unrelated factors is not clear. At times, a prompt response to vitamin administration lends support to a causal relationship.

Much has been written about depression, oral contraceptives, and vitamin B_6 deficiency. Many women taking oral contraceptives have abnormalities of tryptophan metabolism indicative of a relative or absolute deficiency of vitamin B_6 which can be corrected by the daily administration of 20–30 mg of the vitamin (Wynn, 1975; Brown et al., 1975). It has been postulated that deranged tryptophan metabolism leads to depletion of central nervous system serotonin, which is then manifested clinically as depression. The depression associated with oral contraceptive use has been described as follows: "Crying spells, pessimism, self-depreciation, and changes in sex desire are predominant whereas sleep disturbance and appetite disorder are not common" (Malek-Ahmadi and Behrmann, 1976).

In a double-blind, placebo controlled, crossover study of the effect of vitamin B_6 on depression associated with the use of oral contraceptives, those women who had biochemical evidence of absolute vitamin B_6 deficiency showed a statistically significant improvement in mood when treated with pyridoxine (40 mg/day) (Adams et al., 1974). There was no significant improvement in either the group with placebo or in the non-vitamin-B_6-deficient group given pyridoxine. When the data were examined by Fisher's exact test to adjust for the small number of subjects, the beneficial effect of pyridoxine was present only when the vitamin was given as first treatment. The difference in response to pyridoxine in the two groups of women was not statistically significant when vitamin administration followed two months of placebo use.

Although the value of pyridoxine in treating oral contraceptive-associated depression has also been suggested in anecdotal reports (Baumblatt and Winston, 1970; Winston, 1973), there is a need for more rigorously controlled studies to establish its true worth. Meanwhile, an empirical trial of pyridoxine (25–100 mg/day) seems reasonable in appropriate cases.

On a broader level, the issue of whether depression is pharmacologically induced by oral contraceptives is not fully resolved. Sheehan and Sheehan

(1976) reviewed the area and concluded:

> After carefully reviewing the many studies on this subject, we are forced to the
> inevitable conclusion that there is an inverse relationship between the quality and
> rigor of the experimental design of the study and the real incidence of depression

While they acknowledge that oral contraceptives can cause vitamin B_6 deficiency, they question whether the deficiency is causally related to the depression. In support of this position, they mention a number of "well-controlled" studies that found no significant difference in the incidence of depression between birth-control-pill users and controls.

When a group of depressed patients was screened, only 1 out of 23 had evidence of B_6 deficiency, while suggestive evidence was present in another three (Nobbs, 1974). Although the author felt that vitamin B_6 deficiency was not an important factor in the pathogenesis of depression in the patients studied, lack of information as to clinical characteristics of the study population (including sex and oral contraceptive status), and response to treatment with vitamin B_6, and the small number of subjects allows no closure on the issue of vitamin-B_6-deficiency depression. It seems reasonable to assume that vitamin B_6 deficiency may be associated with a depressive syndrome that can be corrected by vitamin supplementation but that this syndrome is uncommon.

A possible role for pyridoxine has also been suggested in the treatment of premenstrual depression that is not associated with oral contraceptive use (Winston, 1973). A controlled study, however, found that only 1 of 13 women improved with pyridoxine, and since 1 also got worse, it is unlikely that vitamin B_6 deficiency plays a major role in this syndrome (Stokes and Mendels, 1972).

Diagnosis

A number of biochemical tests have been used to evaluate vitamin B_6 status (Nobbs, 1974; Driskell et al., 1976; Van Itallie, 1977). These include:

1. Direct assay of pyridoxal phosphate in plasma.
2. Xanthurenic acid excretion following a tryptophan load.
3. Urinary 4-pyridoxic acid levels.
4. In vitro stimulation of erythrocyte glutamic-oxaloacetic transaminase activity by pyridoxal phosphate.
5. Measurement of erythrocyte alanine aminotransferase activity with coenzyme stimulation.

Treatment

Although the recommended adult daily intake of vitamin B_6 is about 2 mg, treatment of deficiency or dependency states usually requires much higher doses. Deficiencies usually respond to 50–100 mg/day while dependency states may require several hundred milligrams daily. Given the complexities of the biochemical tests used to diagnose deficiency, an empirical trial of vitamin B_6 therapy is a realistic alternative if there is clinical support for a deficiency state. This does not mean that all, or even most, depressed patients should be treated with, or be expected to respond to, vitamins.

VITAMIN B_{12} AND FOLIC ACID DEFICIENCIES

General Considerations

Vitamin B_{12}

Vitamin B_{12} is an essential vitamin which cannot be manufactured by the body and, consequently, must be supplied in the diet. In the body it exists mainly in two forms: Methylcobalamin and adenosylcobalamin, while the widely used vitamin preparation is cyanocobalamin, which must be coverted to the active form before it can be utilized.

Vitamin B_{12} acts as a coenzyme in the formation of succinyl coenzyme A which is involved in the citric acid cycle, gluconeogenesis, and the biosynthesis of myelin. In addition, vitamin B_{12} is required for the methylation of homocysteine to form methionine, a process which also involves 5-methyltetrahydrofolate; thus intimately linking the metabolism of vitamin B_{12} and folic acid.

Under normal conditions at least 2 mg of vitamin B_{12} are stored in the liver and another 2 mg elsewhere in the body. Since the minimum daily requirement for the vitamin is only about 2.5 mcg, it would take several years for a deficiency state to develop even if vitamin B_{12} intake were totally curtailed.

Dietary sources of vitamin B_{12} include meats (especially liver, beef, and pork) and dairy products. Plants do not synthesize the vitamin, but it is formed by microorganisms in leguminal nodules, this providing a source for strict vegetarians.

Dietary vitamin B_{12} forms a stable complex with intrinsic factor, a glycoprotein formed by gastic parietal cells. In the terminal ileum, the B_{12}–intrinsic factor complex is bound to mucosal receptors, and the vitamin is absorbed. Following absorption, it is bound to transcobalamin II, a transport protein, and distributed for use and storage.

Vitamin B_{12} deficiency has a number of causes, which have been classified under inadequate intake, malabsorption, and transcobalamin II deficiency (Bunn et al., 1977). Only in strict vegetarians is inadequate intake likely to result in deficiency. The most common cause is malabsorption, which may be due to (1) inadequate production of intrinsic factor (as in pernicious anemia, postgastrectomy states, and congenital absence of intrinsic factor); (2) terminal ileum abnormalities (such as sprue, regional enteritis, malignancy, surgical resection, and selective vitamin B_{12} malabsorption); (3) competition for vitamin B_{12} (because of fish tapeworm or blind loop syndrome); and (4) drugs (such as para-amino salicylic acid, colchicine, neomycin, and ethanol).

Folic Acid

Folic acid, or pteroylglutamic acid, is a water-soluble vitamin that functions as a coenzyme in the synthesis of DNA, is required for methionine synthesis, and is apparently a coenzyme in norepinephrine and serotonin biosynthesis (Thornton and Thornton, 1978). Proposed nervous system functions for folic acid include nucleoprotein synthesis, methylation processes, and monoamine metabolism (Anonymous, 1976).

Under normal conditions, at least 5–10 mg of folic acid is stored in the body, with the liver being the main storage site. Since the usual requirement for folic acid is about 50 mcg per day, body stores can be depleted after only several months of dietary deprivation and, hence, deficiency states are common (Bunn et al., 1977).

Dietary sources of folic acid include green leafy vegetables, fruits, and liver. Both cooking and canning may destroy a portion of dietary folic acid. Absorption occurs in the proximal jejunum and, unlike vitamin B_{12}, folic acid does not have a specific binding protein. Dihydrofolate reductase is an enzyme which catalyzes the conversion of folic acid to tetrahydrofolate, its biologically active form. Inhibition of the enzyme can result in megaloblastic anemia.

Folic acid deficiency can be caused by (1) inadequate intake (owing to poor diet, as commonly occurs in chronic alcoholics, the indigent, and the elderly); (2) inadequate absorption (owing to malabsorption syndromes, blind loops, and certain drugs, such as phenytoin, barbiturates, and ethanol); (3) inadequate utilization (because of the presence of folic acid antagonists, such as methotrexate, pyrimethamine, triamterene, pentamidine, and trimethoprim; enzyme deficiency; vitamin B_{12} deficiency; or scurvy); and (4) increased requirement (as in pregnancy, infancy, malignancy, and active hematopoiesis).

The relation between drugs, toxins, and dietary amino acids and vitamin B_{12} and folic acid absorption and utilization have been summarized by Waxman et al. (1970).

Interrelationship Between B_{12} and Folic Acid

The complexities of vitamin B_{12} and folic acid metabolism are not well understood. It is known that large doses of folic acid can at least partially correct the hematological abnormalities caused by vitamin B_{12} deficiency. The conversion of homocysteine to methionine requires methylcobalamin as a cofactor, the latter being regenerated by the transfer of a methyl group from methyltetrahydrofolic acid. It is possible that a deficiency of vitamin B_{12} can lead to a "functional" deficiency of folate. Also, it has been shown that folic acid can correct impaired vitamin B_{12} absorption owing to anti-convulsant drugs.

Clinical Features

General Features—Vitamin B_{12} Deficiency

The clinical onset of vitamin B_{12} deficiency is insidious. The classic symptom triad of pernicious anemia—weakness, sore tongue, and numbness and tingling of the extremities—is not always present, or may be masked by more prominent complaints. In general, the clinical manifestations are determined by the degree of anemia and neurological involvement. Gastrointestinal symptoms may include burning of the tongue, anorexia, diarrhea and constipation, vague abdominal pain, and weight loss. Cardiovascular symptoms may include dyspnea, palpitations, chest pain, and congestive heart failure. Physical findings may include pallor, a lemon-yellow skin color, rapid pulse, an enlarged spleen and liver, and a wide variety of neurological findings. The neurological manifestations of peripheral neuropathy, subacute combined degeneration, and cerebral dysfunction are discussed below.

General Features—Folic Acid Deficiency

Folic acid deficiency results in anemia, and clinical manifestations are related to the severity of the anemia.

Neuropsychiatric Features—Vitamin B_{12} Deficiency

It cannot be overstressed that neurological findings can be present in the **absence of anemia** (Strachan and Henderson, 1965; Reynolds, 1976a; Roos, 1978). **Thus, a normal blood picture and even a normal bone marrow does not exclude the possibility of a vitamin-B_{12}-deficiency neuropathy.** However, while the hematological and neurological complications do not correlate closely, it is often only a question of time before the manifestation that appears first is no longer an isolated finding.

In addition, when anemia is present, the characteristic megaloblastic picture may be lacking and mislead one from suspecting a vitamin-B_{12}-deficiency neuropathy. For example, the presence of an adequate supply of folic acid can correct the megaloblastosis. Also, if iron deficiency is superimposed on vitamin B_{12} deficiency, the appearance of megaloblastic red blood cells may be masked.

Roos (1978) extensively reviewed the neurological manifestions of vitamin B_{12} deficiency dividing them into peripheral neuropathy, myelopathy (subacute combined degeneration), and encephalopathy.

Peripheral Neuropathy. The peripheral neuropathy of vitamin B_{12} deficiency usually develops in an insidious fashion, with the most common presenting complaint being paresthesias, often in the absence of objective findings. These may consist of tingling, pins and needles, or burning sensations, commonly involving the extremeties in a symmetrical fashion (lower greater than upper).

More advanced findings suggestive of a polyneuropathy include reduced or absent deep-tendon reflexes, tender peripheral-nerve trunks, localized weakness and wasting, and altered touch and pain sensation. Clinically, it is often difficult to differentiate the peripheral neuropathy from the myelopathy.

Myelopathy (Subacute Combined Degeneration). According to Roos (1978), "A patient has myelopathy if he has ataxia of the upper and lower limbs, spasticity of the lower limbs, extensor plantar reflexes, or a positive Romberg's sign." Complete loss of vibration sense distal to the anterior-superior-iliac spine has also been equated with the presence of a myelopathy. Certain authors, however, have stricter criteria and require the presence of a pyramidal tract lesion to make the diagnosis. Involvement of the spinal cord tends to be symmetrical, so that persistent asymmetrical sensory or motor abnormalities should suggest another diagnosis. Impaired vibration sense in the lower extremities is a common finding.

Encephalopathy (Cerebral or Psychiatric Findings). When Thomas Addison described pernicious anemia in the mid-1800's, he noted that "the mind occasionally wanders." The wide spectrum of mental abnormalities that has been reported in association with vitamin B_{12} deficiency ranges from apathy and irritability to dementia, confusional states, paranoid states, and schizophreniform psychoses (Holmes, 1956; Hällström, 1969; Hart and McCurdy, 1971; Lipton and Kane, 1972; Shulman, 1972; Geagea and Ananth, 1975; Roos, 1978). The incidence of abnormal mental states varies from series to series, but overall 4–16% of patients can be considered psychotic, while less severe symptoms have been reported in as high as 75%. In her series of postgastrectomy vitamin-B_{12}-deficient patients, Roos (1978) felt that "depression (suicidal attempts in 20%), emotional lability and lack of initiative, combined with impairment of memory and powers of abstraction" was a fairly uniform constellation of mental changes.

Whether depression is a symptom that can be directly attributed to vitamin B_{12} deficiency has been questioned by Shulman (1967; 1972). He observed that the incidence of depression in pernicious anemia was no higher than in other disabling illnesses, and also that the depression often remitted "spontaneously" once patients learned of their favorable prognosis but before vitamin-B_{12}-replacement therapy had begun.

While it would be unusual for a "pure" depressive syndrome to be the only finding in vitamin B_{12} deficiency, depression has been consistently reported in association with other mental changes. In an evaluation of 161 vitamin-B_{12}-deficient patients, Spatz et al. (quoted in Roos, 1978) found that "28% had mental changes consisting of apathy, difficulty of concentration, depression, lethargy, impaired memory and disorientation, while emotional lability and hallucinations were also found." Impaired intellectual function was the most consistent finding, an observation with which most authors are in agreement.

There is no constellation of mental findings that can be considered pathognomonic or even strongly suggestive of vitamin B_{12} deficiency. Early in the course of the illness, especially, complaints may be vague, subjective and nonspecific, thus suggesting a psychoneurotic problem. For example, one patient was referred for psychiatric evaluation after complaining of somnolence, fatigue, anorexia, weight loss, crying spells, and "numbness of his testicles." Further investigation, however, led to the diagnosis of pernicious anemia. Response to vitamin B_{12} was prompt, thus avoiding inappropriate treatment with psychotherapy or antidepressant drugs (Jefferson, 1977).

There is some evidence that the psychiatric manifestions of vitamin-B_{12} deficiency can occur in the presence of a normal blood picture and a normal neurological examination. Strachan and Henderson (1965) described three patients whose mental abnormalities occurred in the absence of hematological abnormalities or myelopathy and responded to treatment with vitamin B_{12}. Holmes (1956) reported 14 cases of vitamin B_{12} deficiency with cerebral manifestations, in whom spinal or peripheral nerve involvement was often slight and detectable only after careful examination. As will be described shortly, the presence of a normal serum vitamin B_{12} level is no absolute assurance that vitamin B_{12} deficiency does not exist.

Since vitamin B_{12} replacement is a specific and effective treatment if instituted early enough in the course of the disorder, it is especially tragic if diagnosis is delayed beyond the point of reversibility. Some authors have gone so far as to suggest that routine screening for vitamin B_{12} deficiency be mandatory in all mental patients even in the absence of hematological abnormalities. This issue is a thorny one, since mass-screening procedures are expensive, and even if laboratory tests are abnormal it may be difficult to establish a causal relationship to the clinical symptoms.

Screening studies of psychiatric patients for vitamin B_{12} deficiency have been reviewed by a number of authors (Shulman, 1967, 1972; Hällström, 1969; Lipton and Kane, 1972; Rose, 1976) without reaching consensus as to their merit. In general, for such screening to be productive, it would best be restricted to those patients at greater risk for vitamin B_{12} deficiency (e.g. the elderly, or postgastrectomy patient) or those showing clinical (organicity, peripheral neuropathy, or myelopathy) or laboratory (anemia) findings suggestive of the disorder.

Electroencephalogram. Electroencephalographic abnormalities are common in vitamin B_{12} deficiency (48–64% of patients), appear related to cerebral metabolic abnormalities rather than anemia, do not correlate well with the extent of neurological involvement, have no differential diagnostic value, and are likely to respond rapidly to treatment with vitamin B_{12} (Lipton and Kane, 1972; Roos and Willanger, 1977).

Neuropsychiatric Features—Folic Acid Toxicity

Hunter (1970) gave 5 mg of folic acid three times daily to 14 normal volunteers. The proposed three-month study was terminated after one month because of gastrointestinal and emotional symptoms which developed in 13 individuals. The emotional symptoms included irritability, excitability, overactivity, impaired judgment and concentration, and sleep disturbances with anxiety or vivid dreams.

Neuropsychiatric Features—Folic Acid Deficiency

For many years, folic acid deficiency was thought to be unrelated to nervous system dysfunction. In recent years, however, evidence to the contrary has accumulated, supporting an association between folate deficiency and disturbed mental function (Reynolds, 1976b; Thornton and Thornton, 1978).

Based on both his literature review and his own work, Reynolds (1976b) reached the following conclusions:

1. "The high incidence of folate deficiency in geriatric patients with mental symptoms and psychiatric patients is predominantly a secondary nutritional effect of the underlying mental state, although other causes such as drugs, malabsorption syndromes etc. must be considered. In epileptic patients, the cause is primarily anticonvulsant drug therapy." Low serum folate levels have been found in at least 10–20% of geriatric admissions (the percentage is higher if mental symptoms are present) and in 10–33% of psychiatric admissions.
2. "In many patients, probably most, a low serum folate level is of no neurological significance, but it does not follow that it will always remain so if untreated."
3. Available evidence supports the contention that in certain situations folic acid deficiency may cause neuropsychiatric complications. Although the clinical picture is variable, the most consistent finding is that of an organic brain syndrome. Reynolds feels that severe folate deficiency will gradually lead to "apathy, depression, social withdrawal and ultimately dementia," the specific presentation of which will be modified by biological and psychosocial factors.
4. When a neuropsychiatric disorder is present in association with a folic acid deficiency, there is no reliable way to determine if the deficiency is causing or aggravating the disorder, or if it is a secondary deficiency of no neuropsychiatric consequence. One must

assume that greater severity and duration of the deficiency will increase the likelihood of a causal relationship.

5. Folic acid deficiency should be viewed as having the potential for adversely affecting the nervous system and, consequently, should be corrected. The possibility of an associated vitamin B_{12} deficiency must always be considered. Caution should be exercised when treating anticonvulsant drug-induced folate deficiency, because of the chance of aggravating seizures.

In 1962, Herbert found that restricting his(?) dietary folic acid intake led to insomnia, irritability, and forgetfulness, which responded rapidly to replacement of the vitamin. Botez et al. (1967) described six patients with folate deficiency and neuropsychiatric conditions that responded to folic acid therapy. Three were "depressed and had permanent muscular and intellectual fatigue, mild symptoms of restless legs, depressed ankle jerks, diminution of vibration sensation in the legs, stocking-type hypoesthesia and long-lasting constipation" and all recovered after treatment. The other three patients had restless leg syndrome, diffuse muscle pain, and fatigability, which also responded to folic acid replacement.

A patient described by Freeman et al. (1975) had been previously diagnosed as schizophrenic by several psychiatrists, but was found to have homocystinuria secondary to a deficiency in methylenetetrahydrofolate reductase. Treatment with folic acid fully reversed the symptoms, which included withdrawal, hallucinations, and delusions, whereas discontinuation of treatment led to reemergence of psychotic behavior. Although this patient would be more properly diagnosed as having an organic brain syndrome with some "schizophreniform" features, psychiatric misdiagnosis resulted in a recommendation for admission to a state hospital, treatment with thioridazine, and delay of correct diagnosis and specific treatment.

Whether an abnormality in folate metabolism plays a role in schizophrenia is unknown and should be subjected to further investigation. In a retrospective study, Carney and Sheffield (1970) found that those patients with organic psychosis, endogenous depression, or schizophrenia who had been given folate replacement were discharged from the hospital earlier and were in better clinical condition at the time of discharge than were untreated patients.

Problems with establishing a causal relationship between folic acid deficiency and neuropsychiatric abnormalities are many. Surveys of psychiatric, geriatric, and epileptic populations are subject to numerous variables, and include complicating factors such as associated illnesses, drugs, and nutritional deficiencies. Case reports, while often dramatic, are usually uncontrolled, subject to spontaneous remission and observer bias and, hence, open to criticism. Results of therapeutic trials with folic acid may be difficult to evaluate, not only because of design faults, but also because the neuropsychiatric abnormalities may have passed the point of reversibility prior to initiation of treatment. Despite these difficulties, folic acid deficiency must be considered a potential cause of neuropsychiatric illness which, with timely recognition, can be specifically and successfully treated.

Neuropathology

The neuropathology of vitamin B_{12} deficiency has been thoroughly reviewed and summarized by Roos (1978) as follows:

> The main neuropathological lesions in vitamin B_{12} deficiency thus affect the thickly myelinated axons, both in the spinal cord and in the brain and peripheral nerves. The demyelination is pronounced, but perhaps secondary to axonal degeneration.

Diagnosis

Vitamin B_{12} Deficiency

The microbiologic assays for serum vitamin B_{12}, utilizing *Euglena gracilis* or *Lactobacillus leichmannii* have been largely replaced by radioisotope dilution assays. The former tests, which correlated well with clinical evidence of deficiency, were technically difficult, time consuming, and invalidated by the presence of certain drugs.

The reliability of the currently employed radioisotope-dilution techniques has been questioned, and it has been suggested that as high as 20% of patients with vitamin B_{12} deficiency are not diagnosed because of false normal serum vitamin B_{12} levels (Kolhouse et al., 1978). Whitehead and Cooper (1977) found that, of 42 patients with clinical evidence of vitamin B_{12} deficiency and low serum vitamin B_{12} levels by microbiologic assay, six had normal and nine had intermediate levels when measured by radioisotope dilution.

Apparently, the vitamin B_{12} binding protein used in most commercially available radioisotope dilution assay kits reacts with biologically inactive analogues of vitamin B_{12} present in the serum to give falsely elevated levels. To overcome this problem, pure intrinsic factor would have to be used as the binding protein (Cooper and Whitehead, 1978).

In 1975, Geagea and Ananth described a patient with a normal blood and neurological examination who developed psychiatric symptoms that included apathy, confusion, and paranoia, 7–9 years after a total gastrectomy. Treatment with antipsychotic drugs and electroconvulsive therapy was unsuccessful, but the patient responded dramatically to intramuscular vitamin B_{12}. Although the serum vitamin B_{12} level was normal, one suspects that this was a false normal value obtained by radioisotope-dilution assay.

Kolhouse et al. (1978) describe a tragic situation in which the false sense of security instilled by a "normal" serum vitamin B_{12} level by radioisotope-dilution assay resulted in a nine-month delay in diagnosis and treatment of a patient with neurological evidence of a peripheral neuropathy and macrocytic red blood cells. Over the ensuing months, she became unable to walk, was incontinent of urine and feces, and developed an organic brain syndrome and anemia. When repeated, the vitamin B_{12} level was again normal, but vitamin B_{12} absorption without and with intrinsic factor (Schilling test) established the diagnosis of pernicious anemia, which was further confirmed by a hematologic response to intramuscular vitamin B_{12}. When a sample of serum obtained prior to treatment was measured by microbiologic assay and by radioisotope dilution assay using intrinsic factor as the binding protein, strikingly low levels of serum vitamin B_{12} were discovered. Unfortunately, at followup four months after the start of treatment, marked neurological abnormalities were still present.

It cannot be overstressed that to rely on a single diagnostic test, especially in the face of clinical evidence to the contrary, is fraught with danger. As Donaldson (1978) aptly states: "Patients benefit most from physicians who are able to keep the whole patient in perspective when confronted with the vast array of data that modern diagnostic technology can generate."

Prior to accepting a normal serum vitamin B_{12} level as excluding a deficiency state (even when the correct assay is used), it is important to be sure that the patient has not recently received parenteral or even large oral doses of vitamin B_{12}.

Folic Acid Deficiency

For many years, serum folate levels were determined by a microbiologic assay utilizing *Lactobacillus casei*. New techniques involving radioisotope competitive binding which are faster and more reliable are currently being used. Hopefully, problems similar to those discovered with the vitamin B_{12} assays will not arise.

Therapeutic Trials

At times, diagnostic tests may give equivocal results, and a therapeutic trial will be embarked upon to help establish a diagnosis. When administering vitamin B_{12} or folic acid, it is important to give minimally effective doses to avoid the nonspecific response that higher doses may evoke. For example, the anemia of vitamin B_{12} deficiency may respond to large doses of folic acid while the neurological condition continues to deteriorate.

Treatment

Vitamin B_{12} Deficiency

Treatment is rather simple—adequate amounts of vitamin B_{12} must be given to induce a remission of the illness and replenish depleted body stores. Although sufficient vitamin can be asborbed if large oral doses are given, the preferred route of administration is intramuscular. Once remission has occurred, maintenance therapy consisting of monthly vitamin B_{12} injections must be continued indefinitely unless the underlying deficit can be corrected.

Response to treatment can be quite rapid, with normalization of the bone marrow beginning within hours, reticulocytosis peaking in 5–8 days, and improvement of electroencephalographic abnormalities after a week. Subjective improvement consisting of an increasing sense of well-being, mental alertness, and improved appetite may be apparent during the first few days. Hematologic normalization usually occurs within 6–8 weeks, while neurological abnormalities may take many months to stabilize. If treatment is unduly delayed, neurological damage will not be reversible.

Folic Acid Deficiency

Replacement of folic acid by the oral route in doses of 1–5 mg/day is generally sufficient to correct the deficiency, even in the presence of impaired absorption. According to Botez (1976), however, doses as high as 30–40 mg/day may be necessary to correct certain conditions. In cases of deficiencies produced by folic acid antagonists, folinic acid (citrovorum factor) is used (Bunn et al., 1977).

ASCORBIC ACID (VITAMIN C) DEFICIENCY

General Considerations

Ascorbic acid (vitamin C) is a water-soluble vitamin found in high concentrations in citrus fruits, tomatoes, potatoes, leafy vegetables, green peppers, and most grasses. The recommended daily dietary allowance ranges from 35 mg in infants to 80 mg in lactating women. Under experimental conditions, a daily dose as low as 10 mg for well over a year prevented the development of scurvy (Hodges et al., 1971).

In normally nourished adults, the body pool of ascorbic acid is about 1500 mg, and, depending on the extent of deficiency and the body requirements, clinical manifestations appear after two or more months of deficiency. Historically, scurvy was a major cause of disability and death during long ocean voyages until the therapeutic value of citrus fruits was recognized.

Deficiencies in ascorbic acid are usually caused by inadequate dietary intake due to lack of supplementary vitamin in infants or unbalanced or idiosyncratic diets in adults. The term "bachelor" scurvy has been applied to the illness developing in men living alone (Follis and Van Itallie, 1974). In the presence of pregnancy, lactation, inflammatory disease, surgical procedures, and burns, the requirement for vitamin C is substantially increased. Scurvy may have an iatrogenic cause if physicians recommend inappropriate diets for the treatment of various medical problems, especially if patient adherence is overzealous (Shafar, 1965).

Most mammals (but not man) are able to synthesize vitamin C, so, in a sense, scurvy is a genetic disease, since it occurs in those species lacking the enzyme necessary for synthesis. The vitamin is required for the synthesis of collagen, osteoid, and dentine, and for blood vessel integrity, tissue respiration, and wound healing. It also plays a role in folic acid metabolism.

Clinical Features

Scurvy occurs in scattered areas throughout the world, and occasional cases are still found in the United States. It can also be produced under experimental conditions by removing ascorbic acid from the diet. The naturally occurring illness tends to be more severe, perhaps because of associated nutritional deficiencies or additional illnesses.

General Features

Infantile scurvy usually occurs between 6–12 months of age and is characterized by irritability, anorexia, failure to thrive, and lower extremity swelling and tenderness associated with subperiosteal hemorrhage. Swelling and hemorrhage of the gums occurs in association with the eruption of teeth. Hemorrhages elsewhere in the body also occur (nose bleeds, hematuria, subdural bleeding).

Findings in adults include swollen, spongy, bleeding gums; perifollicular hemorrhage; poor wound healing; easy bruisability; spontaneous hemorrhages in almost any part of the body; arthralgias and arthritis; and anemia. The most characteristic finding is follicular hyperkeratosis with perifollicular hemorrhage.

Neuropsychiatric Features

Nonspecific symptoms such as fatigue, lassitude, weakness, anorexia, and depression have been reported as manifestations of naturally occurring scurvy (Cutforth, 1958; Shafar, 1965; Walker, 1968; Follis and Van Itallie, 1974). Cutforth (1958),for example, noted that over half of his 11 patients were lethargic, anorexic, depressed, resentful, and uncooperative, but that these symptoms resolved after a few days of ascorbic acid treatment. Walker (1968) mentioned that all seven of her patients were severely depressed at the time of admission, with mood elevations occurring after several days of treatment. Unfortunately, only one of the seven case reports described depression as a symptom. It was unclear if this depression was the cause of anorexia and subsequent dietary deficiency of vitamin C, if the depression was a primary manifestation of vitamin C deficiency, or if it was secondary to the other debilitating and painful aspects of scurvy.

In addition, in naturally occurring deficiency states it is often difficult to determine if behavioral manifestations are due to a specific vitamin lack or to multiple deficiencies, or whether associated but unrelated illnesses are responsible. This issue can be partially resolved by producing isolated ascorbic acid deficiency under experimental conditions in otherwise healthy subjects. Farmer (1944) described loss of interest and motivation and exaggeration of aggressive and submissive characteristics developing during experimental depletion.

A most intriguing report of the behavioral effects of experimentally induced ascorbic acid deficiency involved five healthy prison volunteers who were subjected to tests of mental function, psychomotor performance, physical fitness, and personality (Kinsman and Hood, 1971). Personality changes, as measured by the MMPI, occurred prior to the characteristic clinical manifestations of scurvy and prior to psychomotor changes. While the MMPI was normal at the start of the study and returned to normal following vitamin C replacement, depletion was associated with elevation of the Hypochondriasis, Depression, and Hysteria scales—the classic "neurotic triad." The changes were accompanied by findings of reduced arousal, decreased motivation, fatigue, and lassitude. Decreased performance on psychomotor tests (Digit Symbol Substitution Test and measures of hand–arm dexterity) developed later and were attributed to reduced arousal level.

The fact that the early phase of ascorbic acid deficiency can present with psychoneurotic symptoms in the absence of more suggestive signs of scurvy, emphasizes the need to obtain a thorough dietary history from patients to avoid the misdiagnosis of functional illness and to allow timely treatment that will avert more serious consequences.

Diagnosis

Once scurvy is fully developed, the constellation of clinical findings is characteristic. Support for the diagnosis is, of course, provided by a history compatible with a vitamin-C-deficient diet. Although x-rays in the adult are not particularly useful, certain characteristic radiographic findings may be present in infants.

Ascorbic-acid levels can be measured in the blood, with buffy coat concentrations most closely correlating with body stores. Whole blood, serum, and plasma levels are more easily measured, and concentrations below 0.2–0.3 mg/100 ml usually correlate with clinical scurvy. In the presence of depleted body stores, urinary output of ascorbic acid is markedly reduced even after a test dose of the vitamin.

Treatment

A diet rich in ascorbic acid (with supplemental vitamin C added if indicated) is effective treatment for both infantile and adult scurvy. Parenteral administration is usually not necessary. There is some evidence that the rate of recovery is proportional to the repletion dose of vitamin C (Hodges et al., 1971). Subjective improvement occurs within the first few days of treatment, while bruises and other hemorrhagic manifestations resolve more slowly. In chronic adult scurvy, 300–500 mg/day of ascorbic acid may be necessary for several months to insure a complete response.

REFERENCES

Adams PW, Wynn V, Seed M et al: Vitamin B_6, depression, and oral contraception. Lancet 2:516–517, 1974.

Anonymous: Folic acid and the nervous system. Lancet 2:836, 1976.

Anonymous: Wernicke's preventable encephalopathy. Lancet 1:1122–1123, 1979.

Baumblatt MJ, Winston F: Pyridoxine and the pill. Lancet 1:832–833, 1970.

Botez MI: Folate deficiency and neurological disorders in adults. Med Hypotheses 2:135–140, 1976.

Botez MI, Cadotte M, Beaulieu R, et al: Neurologic disorders responsive to folic acid therapy. Can Med Assoc J 115:217–222, 1976.

Brown RR, Rose DP, Leklem JE, et al: Effects of oral contraceptives on tryptophan metabolism and vitamin B_6 requirements in women. Acta Vitaminol Enzymol 29:151–157, 1975.

Brozek J: Psychological effects of thiamine restriction and deprivation in normal young men. Am J Clin Nutr 5:109–120, 1957.

Bunn HF, Lee GR, Wintrobe MM: Pernicious anemia and other megaloblastic anemias, in Thorn GW, Adams RD, Braunwalde, et al (eds): Harrison's Principles of Internal Medicine, ed 8. New York, McGraw–Hill, 1977, pp 1656–1664.

Carney MWP, Sheffield BF: Associations of subnormal serum folate and vitamin B_{12} values and effects of replacement therapy. J Nerv Ment Dis 150:404–412, 1970.

Cooper BA, Whitehead VM: Evidence that some patients with pernicious anemia are not recognized by radiodilution assay for cobalamin. N Eng J Med 299:816–818, 1978.

Cutforth RH: Adult scurvy. Lancet 1:454–456, 1958.

DiBenedetto RJ: Chronic hypervitaminosis A in an adult. JAMA 201:700–702, 1967.

Driskell JA, Geders JM, Urban MC: Vitamin B_6 status of young men, women, and women using oral contraceptives J Lab Clin Med 87:813–821, 1976.

Donaldson RM: "Serum B_{12}" and the diagnosis of cobalamin deficiency. N Engl J Med 299:827–828, 1978.

Farmer CJ: Some aspects of vitamin C metabolism. Fed Proc 3:179–188, 1944.

Feldman MH, Schlezinger NS: Benign intracranial hypertension associated with hypervitaminosis A. Arch Neurol 22: 1–7, 1970.

Follis RH, Van Itallie TB: Pellagra, in Wintrobe MM, Thorn GW, Adams RD, et al (eds): Harrison's Principles of Internal Medicine, ed 7. New York, McGraw–Hill, 1974a, pp 427–430.

Follis RH, Van Itallie TB: Scurvy, in Wintrobe MM, Thorn GW, Adams RD, et al (eds): Harrison's Principles of Internal Medicine, ed 7. New York, McGraw–Hill, 1974b, pp 434–436.

Freeman JM, Finkelstein JD, Mudd SH: Folate-responsive homocystinuria and "schizophrenia." N Eng J Med 292:491–496, 1975.

Frostig JP, Spies TD: The initial nervous syndrome of pellagra and associated deficiency diseases. Am J Med Sci 199:268–274, 1940.

Geagea K, Ananth J: Response of a psychiatric patient to vitamin B_{12} therapy. Dis Nerv Syst 36:343–344, 1975.

Hällström T: Serum B_{12} and folate concentrations in mental patients. Acta Psychiatr Scand 45:19–35, 1969.

Hart RJ, McCurdy PR: Psychosis in vitamin B_{12} deficiency. Arch Intern Med 128:596–597, 1971.

Herbert V: Experimental nutritional folate deficiency in man. Trans Assoc Physicians 75:307–320, 1962.

Hodges RE, Hood J, Canham JE: Clinical manifestations of ascorbic acid deficiency in man. *Am J Clin Nutr* 24:432–443, 1971.

Holmes JM: Cerebral manifestations of vitamin-B$_{12}$ deficiency. *Br Med J* 4:1394–1398, 1956.

Hunter R, Barnes J, Oakeley HF, et al: Toxicity of folic acid given in pharmacological doses to healthy volunteers. *Lancet* 1:61–63, 1970.

Jefferson JW: The case of the numb testicles. *Dis Nerv Syst* 38:749–751, 1977.

Kinsman RA, Hood J: Some behavioral effects of ascorbic acid deficiency. *Am J Clin Nutr* 24:455–464, 1971.

Kolhouse JF, Kondo H, Allen NC, et al: Cobalamin analogues are present in human plasma and can mask cobalamin deficiency because current radioisotope dilution assays are not specific for true cobalamin. *N Eng J Med* 299:785–792, 1978.

Le Boeuf A, Lodge J, Eames PG: Vasopressin and memory in Korsakoff syndrome. *Lancet* 2:1370, 1978.

Lipton MA, Kane FJ: The use of vitamins as therapeutic agents in psychiatry, in Shader RI (ed): *Psychiatric Complications of Medical Drugs*. New York, Raven Press, 1972, pp 333–368.

Malek-Ahmadi P, Behrmann PJ: Depressive syndrome induced by oral contraceptives. *Dis Nerv Syst* 37:406–408, 1976.

Mesulam M-M, Van Hoesen GW, Butters N: Clinical manifestations of chronic thiamine deficiency in the rhesus monkey. *Neurology* 27:239–245, 1977.

Mikkelsen B, Ehlers N, Thomsen HG: Vitamin A intoxication causing papilledema and simulating acute encephalitis. *Acta Neurol Scand* 50:642–650, 1974.

Muenter MD, Perry HO, Ludwig J: Chronic vitamin A intoxication in adults. *Am J Med* 50:129–136, 1971.

Nobbs BT: Pyridoxal phosphate status in clinical depression. *Lancet* 1:405–406, 1974.

Reynolds EH: The neurology of vitamin B$_{12}$ deficiency. *Lancet* 2:832–833, 1976a.

Reynolds EH: Neurological aspects of folate and vitamin B$_{12}$ metabolism. *Clin Haematol* 5:661–696, 1976b.

Roos D: Neurological complications in patients with impaired vitamin B$_{12}$ absorption following partial gastrectomy. *Acta Neurol Scand* 59(suppl 69): 1–7, 1978.

Roos D, Willanger R: Various degrees of dementia in a selected group of gastrectomized patients with low serum B$_{12}$. *Acta Neurol Scand* 55:363–376, 1977.

Rose DP, Strong R, Adams PW, et al: Experimental vitamin B$_6$ deficiency and the effect of oestrogen-containing oral contraceptives on tryptophan metabolism and vitamin B$_6$ requirements. *Clin Sci* 42:465–477, 1972.

Rose M: Why assess vitamin-B$_{12}$ status in patients with known neuropsychiatric disorder? *Lancet* 2:1191, 1976.

Shafar J: Iatrogenic scurvy. *Practitioner* 194:374–377, 1965.

Sheehan DV, Sheehan KH: Psychiatric aspects of oral contraceptive use. *Psychiatr Ann* 6:501–509, 1976.

Shulman R: Psychiatric aspects of pernicious anemia: A prospective controlled investigation. *Br Med J* 3:266–270, 1967.

Shulman R: The present status of vitamin B$_{12}$ and folic acid deficiency in psychiatric illness. *Can Psychiatr J* 17:205–216, 1972.

Spies TD, Aring CD, Gelperin J, et al:The mental symptoms of pellagra. Their relief with nicotinic acid. *Am J Med Sci* 196:461–475, 1938.

Spillane JD: *Nutritional Disorders of the Nervous System*. Baltimore, Williams & Wilkins, 1947a, pp 12–15.

Spillane JD: *Nutritional Disorders of the Nervous System*. Baltimore, Williams & Wilkins, 1947b, pp 29–47.

Spivak JL, Jackson DL: Pellagra: An analysis of 18 patients and a review of the literature. *Johns Hopkins Med J* 140:295–309, 1977.

Stokes J, Mendels J: Pyridoxine and premenstrual tension. *Lancet* 1:1117–1178, 1972.

Strachan RW, Henderson JG: Psychiatric syndromes due to a vitaminosis B$_{12}$ with normal blood and marrow. *Quart J Med* 34:303–317, 1965.

Sydenstricker VP: The history of pellagra, its recognition as a disorder of nutrition and its conquest. *Am J Clin Nutr* 6:409–414, 1958.

Thornton WE, Thornton BP: Folic acid, mental function, and dietary habits. *J Clin Psychiatry* 39:315–322, 1978.

Van Itallie TB: Thiamine deficiency, ariboflavinosis, and vitamin B_6 deficiency, in Thorn GW, Adams RD, Braunwald E, et al(eds): *Harrison's Principles of Internal Medicine*, ed 8. New York, McGraw–Hill, 1977, pp 455–459.

Van Itallie TB, Follis RH: Thiamine deficiency, ariboflavinosis, and vitamin B6 deficiency, in Wintrobe MM, Thorn GW, Adams RD et al (eds): *Harrison's Principles of Internal Medicine*, ed 7. New York, McGraw–Hill, 1974a, pp 430–432.

Van Itallie TB, Follis RH: Defciencies of vitamins A, E, and K. Hypervitaminosis A, in Wintrobe MM, Thorn GW, Adams RD, et al (eds): *Harrison's Principles of Internal Medicine*, ed 7. New York, McGraw–Hill, 1974b, pp 436–441.

Victor M, Adams RD, Collins GH: *The Wernicke–Korsakoff Syndrome*. Philadelphia, FA Davis, 1971.

Vollbracht R, Gilroy J: Vitamin A induced benign intracranial hypertension. *Can J Neurol Sci* 3:59–61, 1976.

Walker A: Chronic scurvy. *Br J Dermatol* 80:625–630, 1968.

Waxman S, Corcing JJ, Herbert V: Drugs, toxins and dietary amino acids affecting vitamin B_{12} or folic acid absorption or utilization. *Am J Med* 48:599–608, 1970.

Whitehead VM, Cooper BA: Failure of radiodilution assay for vitamin B_{12} to detect deficiency in some patients. *Blood* 50(suppl 1):99, 1977.

Winston F: Oral contraceptives, pyridoxine, and depression. *Am J Psychiatry* 130:1217–1221, 1973.

Wynn V: Vitamins and oral contraceptive use. *Lancet* 1:561–564, 1975.

Infectious Disorders

The number of organisms that can affect the central nervous system to produce mental or behavioral changes is legion. Virtually any infection may alter brain functioning, either by direct invasion, secondary systemic effects, or postinfection allergic responses. The result may be vague neuropsychiatric disturbances, or the most commonly diagnosed psychiatric disorder associated with infection, delirium. In general, mental status changes produced by infection are nonspecific and have no direct relationship to the specific organism involved. Neuropsychiatric changes may be noted in response to a wide variety of bacterial, viral, mycotic, spirochetal, rickettsial, and protozoal infections. Although syphilis, malaria, and tuberculosis were once prominent offenders, viral infections are probably most common at the present time. Certain infectious diseases that merit special attention because psychiatric features may be marked are discussed below. (See Hepatic section for infectious hepatitis.)

VIRAL ENCEPHALITIS

There are more than 40 known viruses capable of infecting and causing injury to the central nervous system. For some, the neurologic manifestations are part of a generalized disease that has its own peculiarities and is easy to identify, such as mumps or chicken pox. For others, evidence of the infection may be limited to the nervous system, and the resulting syndrome may be highly varied. Occasionally, seasonal or geographic associations, knowledge of recognized current epidemics, or associated systemic illnesses may provide clues to etiology. In many of these conditions, one must rely upon complicated laboratory procedures for specific identification of the causative agent, or presume an etiology based on features of the illness. In 30–50% of cases, the disease remains undiagnosed while the patient is living (Kakulas and Adams, 1977). In some cases of known viral infection, it is uncertain whether the virus actually has gained access to the central nervous system or whether the signs and symptoms represent an autoimmune hypersensitivity reaction to the presence of viral infection elsewhere in the body.

Clinical Features

The central encephalitic syndrome is that of a febrile illness of acute onset proceeding directly to more severe neurologic manifestations. Though this is the common course, occasionally signs of central nervous system involvement may be preceded by nonspecific illness one to three weeks earlier. The history is usually that of a brief upper respiratory illness with fever, malaise, coryza, and occasional mild headache.

Though the syndromes of aseptic meningitis and encephalitis are usually discussed separately, in fact the symptoms are often mixed (meningoencephalitis), and delineation of one illness from another is quite difficult. Symptoms may include headache, stiffness of the neck or spine upon bending forward, disturbance of consciousness ranging from mild somnolence to coma, disorientation, photophobia, nystagmus, hallucinations, ataxia and/ or myoclonic jerks, various kinds of seizures, ocular palsies, facial weakness, and occasional incontinence of urine or stool. With progression of the illness, stupor, coma, and eventually death may occur. At present, there is an estimated 5–20% mortality of patients with viral encephalitis.

Both meningitis and encephalitis are associated with personality or mental status changes; in some instances definitive neurologic symptoms never develop, and these changes are the only symptoms. Different groups of these syndromes will predominate in different types of encephalitis or during different stages of illness in the same individual, but the basic diagnosis rests upon the demonstration of derangement of function of the cerebrum, brain stem, or cerebellum. Because the single most common cause of nonepidemic viral encephalitis is herpes simplex virus, a history of recurrent lip lesions may be useful.

Residual effects vary widely, depending upon the agent, the severity of the illness, the age of the patient, and the timing and effectiveness of the treatment modalities used. The common chronic sequelae are change of personality, mental deficits, and parkinsonian symptomatology. Infants and children tend to develop mental deficits and personality disturbances, while adults tend more toward parkinsonism. Amnesic deficits, personality changes, and other signs of mental deterioration may be seen in approximately 20% of patients (Thorn, 1977). (See following sections.) Headache, irritability, and sleep disturbances are often persistent symptoms. Postencephalitic parkinsonism, the most common neurologic sequela, develops insidiously, with initial weakness and slowing of movements and then gradual development of a stiff and unnatural posture. The ensuing picture resembles other forms of parkinsonism, with masklike facies, stooping posture, festinate gait, and excessive salivation. Tremor is commonly seen. Occasionally, repetitive motor phenomena such as tics, torticollis, sighing and yawning spells, or complex respiratory spasms may be present. Sacks (1973) has provided a striking account of motor and behavioral abnormalities encountered in a group of very long-term institutionalized survivors.

Laboratory Findings

Laboratory studies in the diagnosis of these disorders are often of minimal value. Changes sometimes found in the cerebrospinal fluid consist mainly of pleocytosis (mainly mononuclear cells, except in the initial stages), small and variable increases in protein level, and the absence of other demonstrable microorganisms by smear or culture. Normal concentrations of glucose are found (low glucose concentrations indicate the possibility of other infectious diseases, such as tuberculosis or mycotic meningitis). Spinal fluid findings, however, may remain normal for prolonged periods of time. The postinfectious encephalopathies (believed to be allergic phenomena) commonly manifest little or no cellular reaction in the spinal fluid. Presumptive diagnosis rests upon finding serological evidence, i.e., increased antibody titers, particular viruses, or positive cultures from other areas of the body. Postmortem examination involving isolation of these viruses from the brain results in a definite diagnosis.

Neuropsychiatric Features

Viral encephalitis may present with personality changes or other psychiatric symptoms, occurring considerably in advance of neurologic signs, as the only signs of infection, thus causing difficult and often mistaken diagnoses. In one series, seven of eight patients had originally been misdiagnosed as having functional psychiatric disorders (Himmelhoch, 1970). Many of these patients present initially to other physicians, and are referred to the psychiatrist, who may be falsely reassured that organic etiologies have been "ruled out" by the referring physician.

A major diagnostic dilemma is that the early encephalitic picture occurring without an acute febrile illness is difficult to distinguish from other psychiatric disorders. In this form, subacute changes in the mental status and/or behavior of an adolescent or young adult may evolve over a time period of one to three weeks. These early changes are quite variable, but usually involve distinct alterations from the normal personality of the individual. Behaviors are often described by the family as "odd." They include restlessness, agitation, irritability, negativism, and, occasionally, overt anger and uncharacteristic violent outbursts. Conversely, some patients initially present with lethargy, withdrawal, and depressive appearing affects (Sorbin and Ozer, 1966; Misra and Hay, 1971). Careful psychiatric histories will usually reveal an absence of prior psychiatric problems and of recent events that would contribute to psychological stress.

With progression of the clinical picture in the absence of fever or neurologic signs, the syndrome begins to closely resemble that of schizophrenia or other "nonorganic" psychoses. Bizarre behaviors, rambling speech, inappropriate laughter and giggling, paranoia, grandiosity, delusions, and auditory hallucinations are common (Weinstein et al., 1955; Glaser and Pincus, 1969). These characteristically schizophrenic symptoms occur in many patients in the presence of clear consciousness. Steinberg et al. (1972) presented a case of viral encephalitis in which a diagnosis of manic–depressive psychosis was based upon pressure of speech, flight of ideas, distractibility, grandiosity, and overresponsiveness to environmental cues.

It is important to note the high frequency of reported cases in which patients appear to be catatonic (Hollander et al., 1965; Wilson, 1976; Misra and Hay, 1971). Rasken (1974) described a woman who was diagnosed as having herpes simplex encephalitis who became akinetic, mute, and eventually lapsed into a coma. All of Wilson's (1976) reported cases showed catatonic features, including mutism (a very commonly reported symptom), staring, exaggerated poses, immobility, posturing for prolonged periods, and waxy flexibility. Penn et al. (1972), in addressing the syndrome of fatal catatonia, noted that in 1832, Calmeil, a student of Esquirol, had described agitated, hyperactive patients with auditory hallucinations who precipitously became stuporous and died, with hyperthermia as high as 43.3°C. Since that time, there has been much puzzlement and debate over the group of disorders variously called fatal catatonia, lethal catatonia, mortal catatonia, catatonic delirious state, hypertoxic schizophrenia, confusocatatonia, delirium acutum, delire aigu, exhaustion syndrome, and pernicious catatonia, all of which present with remarkably similar onset, course, and prognosis. Penn et al. presented a case in which a patient who appeared to have schizophrenia later developed catatonic features, became hyperthermic, and died. They suggested that viral infections may be the underlying etiologic agent in some cases of fatal catatonia. Other authors have also emphasized that catatonia is by no means synonymous with schizophrenia (Joyston-Bechal, 1966; Rasken, 1974).

Diagnosis

In most cases of viral encephalitis in which the mistaken diagnosis of schizophrenia or other psychiatric disorders has been made, the etiology becomes clear with the onset of recognizable signs of organic dysfunction. Caution must be taken that an initial diagnosis of psychiatric disorder not lead to a bias that may impede careful observation or result in minimizing of observations that would ordinarily indicate an organic process. Some of the earliest signs that are not typical of functional psychoses are a clouded sensorium, diminished recall, and disorientation. Careful formal mental status examination plays a critical role as the major test aiding in prompt diagnosis of these patients. Any evidence of disorientation or other "minor" disturbances of sensorium, no matter how well explained by presumed severe psychopathology, should raise suspicions. Since fluctuations in mental status are characteristic of the encephalitides, repeated and documented examinations are most helpful.

The onset of other atypical symptoms further confirms a diagnosis of organic illness. These include olfactory, gustatory, tactile, and visual hallucinations, dysarthria, and pronounced muscle weakness. Feelings of strangeness or impending doom are features consistent with pathological changes in the temporal and frontal lobes. Stewart and Baldessarini (1976) noted a "remarkable disinhibition of behavior, with acute loss of verbal, social, and sexual continence (and later urinary and fecal continence); and profound regression more typical of chronic schizophrenia." In addition to primitive behaviors such as open masturbation and smearing of feces, hebephrenic features were noted.

The presence of a fever is helpful in indicating the correct nature of the underlying process, but often, in subacute courses, the temperature elevation is minimal, intermittent, or easily ascribed to other phenomena (occasionally to phenothiazines). Headache and nausea and vomiting, of course, are not typically present in most psychiatric illnesses.

In his discussion of herpes encephalitis presenting with catatonic stupor, Rasken (1974) notes that the following features of a brief neurologic examination are helpful in a differential diagnosis of catatonic stupor. (1) Examination of the pupils and eyelids: In depression, schizophrenia, or neurosis, pupillary responses are intact. If the eyelids are closed, the patient will resist the examiners opening them; once the lids are released, they do not drift back slowly into the closed position as in organic stupor. (2) Eye movements: In schizophrenia, depression, and neurosis there are no roving eye movements. (3) Respiration should be normal in these disorders. (4) Motor movements should not include seizures, asterixis, myoclonic movements, decerebrate rigidity, or decorticate posture.

Rasken (1974) and others have used an amytal interview as an aid in differentiating certain psychotic disorders from neurologic diseases (Weinstein et al., 1955; Wilson, 1976). In catatonia unrelated to organic disease, the amytal will usually allow the patient to communicate, revealing psychotic or depressive content. With encephalitis or other organic impairment, the usual pattern is a deterioration in communication abilities, with increased disorientation and occasional anosognosia.

An EEG may be helpful. Though early readings may be normal in encephalitis, with progression of symptoms there are often demonstrable abnormalities. Strauss et al. (1952) found abnormal records in 37 of 55 patients diagnosed as having encephalitis. Most commonly, a diffusely abnormal pattern with slow delta or theta waves is reported. Occasional slow foci in the frontal temporal region have been seen (Rasken, 1974). The EEG in schizophrenia is, of course, usually normal. Brain scans, skull films, angiography, and computer-augmented tomographic radiography are generally noncontributory.

Postencephalitic Changes

A variety of mental status changes during both the immediate recovery period following encephalitis and upon subsequent long-term followup has been reported. In some reported cases, viral infection of the central nervous system was probably still present or recurrent. Shearer and Finch (1964) reported a case in which 17 episodes of an organic psychosis associated with recurrent herpes-simplex labialis occurred in a 9-year-old boy. In other reported cases of psychosis found during this stage, it is likely that the pathology is created by a postinfectious allergic response rather than direct viral invasion of the brain. These postinfectious encephalopathies may closely resemble functional psychoses, with relatively clear sensorium (Misra and Hay, 1971; Spittle et al., 1977). Nikolovski and Fernandes (1978) reported a case of Capgras syndrome as an aftermath of varicella encephalitis. They may also have classic organic features, and in Still's (1958) series of 19 cases of postinfluenzal psychosis, a number were confusional and seven had unusual olfactory hallucinations. The relationship to the infection was not clear, and cerebrospinal fluid in these cases usually showed little change. In general, it is felt that the prognosis is better than in encephalitis secondary to a direct viral invasion, although recurrences of postinfectious encephalopathy are common.

The evidence of long-term personality changes is highly equivocal. Chronic sequelae of encephalitis are less frequently reported in adults than in children (Klein, 1951). Depression, anxiety, and heightened emotionality appear to be common psychiatric symptoms occurring after infection by neurotropic viruses (Warm and Alluisi, 1967). Other personality changes reported in adults include impulsiveness, aggressiveness, marked dependency, hypochondriasis, and chronic fatigue (Wallin, 1949; Brill, 1959; Spittle et al., 1977).

A number of uncontrolled studies suggest a long-term relationship of encephalitis to more serious psychiatric disease. Meninger (1926) described a series of 200 postinfluenzal psychoses following the 1918 epidemic, and claimed that one third of these resembled dementia praecox. However, the time between the influenza and psychosis was highly variable, and many of these patients would not be diagnosed as schizophrenic by modern criteria. Fairweather (1947) noted that 25% of men and 12% of women after encephalitis lethargica had delusions with paranoid features and showed a "schizoid emotional imbalance." Davison and Bagley (1969) reviewed the evidence concerning schizophrenia and its relationship to encephalitic illness. They estimated that paranoid–hallucinatory psychoses occurred in 15–30% of postencephalitics, and found psychoses indistinguishable from dementia praecox in 10% of those admitted to mental hospitals.

Slow Viruses and Other Syndromes

There is speculation that some patients treated for behavioral syndromes are really suffering from undiagnosed mild and/or chronic forms of subacute encephalitis, which may be more common than is currently realized. Whether viruses contribute significantly to diseases, such as the functional psychoses, whose etiology at present is obscure, is an area of speculation. Recent interest stems from the discovery of a transmissible agent in Creuz-feldt–Jakob Disease, and the recognition that the nature of the infection in this illness has unusual features, such as the lack of an antibody response. Other slow-virus infections of the nervous system have been identified, such as subacute sclerosing panencephalitis and progressive multifocal leucoen-cephalopathy. These are known as chronic, latent, or slow viruses.

Rimon and Halonen (1969) found, in a survey of psychiatric patients, that levels of type I herpes antibodies were higher in patients with psychotic depression than in other psychiatric patients and healthy control subjects (Halonen et al., 1974). Lycke et al. (1974) reported an increase in comple-ment-fixing antibodies to herpes virus in patients with depression and to herpes virus and cytomegalovirus in patients with dementia. Cleobury et al. (1971) found that aggressive psychopathic patients had higher levels of serum antibodies to herpes virus I than patients with other psychiatric dis-orders or controls. These findings were not confirmed by Pokorny et al. (1972). The recognition of these slow viruses, which cause diseases char-acterized by long asymptomatic periods, often on the order of months or years, between the introduction of the infectious agent and the appearance of clinical illness, has far-reaching theoretical importance for future behav-ioral neurology and psychiatry.

Treatment

Attempts at treatment of the supposed psychiatric condition have had variable results. Occasionally, there is brief improvement following anti-psychotic medication or treatment with ECT (usually given for extreme agi-tated behavior). Schreier (1979) reported a case of an organic psychosis secondary to viral encephalitis that responded successfully to propranolol; the rationale for using this drug is its reported success in controlling bel-ligerent behavior following acute brain damage (Elliott, 1977). In some cases, parkinsonian features seen during the treatment period are mistakenly at-tributed to drugs. Most often, any improvement is brief, and behavioral deterioration continues. An overall poor response to pharmacologic interventions is characteristic of the encephalitic syndromes and should be seen as a further clue to diagnosis.

Early recognition of viral encephalitis can be critical, for many of the viral diseases are associated with high mortality. Treatment with various agents, though not of certain effectiveness, seems beneficial in some cases. The availability and quality of symptomatic treatment is also important. Three of Wilson's (1976) patients developed aspiration pneumonitis and two required tracheostomies, which earlier intensive nursing care, usually unavailable on a psychiatry ward, might have prevented. Intensive medical management of associated phenomena (e.g., cerebral edema) may prevent some of the morbidity of the illness. Unfortunately, the quality of treatment of residual defects may also vary depending on whether the basic illness is seen as psychiatric or "medical."

INFECTIOUS MONONUCLEOSIS

Infectious mononucleosis has received special attention owing to occasional associated neuropsychiatric symptomatology. It has a yearly incidence of 38 cases per 100,000 population and commonly occurs among adolescents or young adults. Characteristic presenting symptoms are fever, sore throat, swollen lymph nodes, enlargement of the spleen and liver, malaise, and myriad other complaints (Penman, 1970). Inflammation of the pharyngeal tissue with a grayish-white exudative tonsillitis is found in one half of the cases, and petechiae may be found on the palate in about one third of patients. Typical laboratory findings include an increase in peripheral lymphocytes, with a high proportion of atypical cells, and the development of heterophile and persistent Epstein–Barr virus antibody responses. Usually the clinical course is benign, with approximately 85% of patients resuming relatively good health within a few months. Ultimate prognosis is also good, with the fatality rate estimated at 1 per 3000 (Penman, 1970).

Neuropsychiatric Features

It is considered rare for neurologic manifestations to herald the onset of infectious mononucleosis, although Silverstein et al. (1972) reported neurologic complications as the presenting signs in 6 of 15 patients. Schnell et al. (1966) found no instances of this occurrence among 1285 patients. They did, however, report one case in which an acute psychosis developed after a very brief prodromal illness and remained the predominant feature of the illness.

The incidence of neuropsychiatric complications during the acute illness is estimated to be approximately 1% (Schnell et al., 1966), though Hafstrom (1963) estimated that 50% of patients exhibit slight mental disturbances during the acute course of the illness. Manifestations may include altered states of consciousness, disorientation, memory loss, irrational behavior, inappropriate affect, and acute psychosis. Several authors have reported cases of psychoses in which the patient showed initial schizophrenic-like pictures rather than obvious delirium (Landes et al., 1941; Raymond and Williams, 1948). More recently, Rubin (1978) described an adolescent with an acute catatonic schizophrenic-like illness associated with mononucleosis.

Reported neurologic signs secondary to meningoencephalitis are evidence of meningeal irritation, aphasia, dysarthric speech, transient hemiparesis, generalized and focal seizures, scotoma, involvement of any of the cranial nerves, cerebellar signs, and peripheral nerve involvement of the Guillain–Barré type. Nonspecific EEG findings, consisting of either focal or general slow activity in the theta or delta frequency ranges, are commonly reported in these cases.

Chronic Sequelae

It is a common clinical observation that some patients seem to recover especially slowly from infectious mononucleosis, and patients themselves often attribute psychological malaise to the illness. Several workers have suggested that psychological variables determine the length of recovery from infectious mononucleosis (Imboden, 1972; Lipowski, 1975). Greenfield et al. (1959) noted that slow recovery was associated with low scores of ego strength. Peszke and Mason (1969), however, found that elevated heterophile antibody titers of 1/96 or more correlated positively with seeking psychiatric help, whereas low ego-strength scores did not; they suggested that the severity of the illness and possible residual changes were the critical factors.

Cadie et al. (1976), in observing 36 patients who had had infectious mononucleosis, found that 13 of 20 women suffered depression and anxiety felt to be related to the disease more than one year later. The possibility of residual changes should not be surprising, for pathological changes may be found in the blood and spinal fluid up to one and one half years after the acute stage of the disease. Thus, a history of infectious mononucleosis may be important in evaluating these complaints.

Hendler and Leahy (1978) reported two cases of neuropsychological sequelae presenting to a psychiatric clinic. In the first, a 14-year-old male reported an inability to concentrate, loss of athletic ability, feelings of depression, irritability, and suicidal ideation for five months after an episode of documented infectious mononucleosis. Despite a negative mental status examination and neurologic examination, an EEG revealed diffuse slow wave activities (2–7 CPS) and diffuse low voltage fast activity (15–25 CPS). Testing revealed a verbal IQ of 145 and a performance IQ of 122. Following an ineffective trial of imipramine, the patient was placed on tranylcypromine, 20 mg b.i.d., and the depression lifted. Repeat psychological testing nine months after the initial visit resulted in a verbal IQ of 147 and a performance IQ of 131. School performance, athletic ability, and social functioning were marked by a return to premorbid levels.

In the second case, a 16-year-old student presented to an inpatient unit with a suicide attempt. History revealed a psychiatric disturbance that had begun following infectious mononucleosis (documented by heterophile titer) at age nine. Subsequently, reduced concentration, an inability to calculate, impairment of fine motor coordination, and general difficulty with school-work ensured. The history prior to the illness revealed good school performance and normal adaptation.

This patient's EEG showed diffuse low-voltage activity. Echo results were suggestive of an enlarged right ventricle, and the cerebral mantle thickness appeared abnormal. Therapy centered around adjustment of parental expectations (the patient had verbal and performance IQs of 104).

These two cases illustrate persistent neurologic dysfunction as sequelae of infectious mononucleosis. Although postinfective reactive depressions are commonly reported, one must be alert to organically caused components and not dismiss intellectual, affective, or motor abnormalities as "purely psychological." The authors further suggest that the success of the mono-amine-oxidase inhibitor, tranylcypromine, may be related to its amphetamine-like structure. Central nervous system involvement after infectious mononucleosis may be similar to minimal brain dysfunction in that both respond to amphetamine-like substances.

NEUROPSYCHIATRIC EFFECTS OF INFECTIOUS DISEASE DRUGS

Amantadine

Amantadine HCl (Symmetrel), a drug initially introduced to prevent A_2 influenza and now being used for other purposes (parkinsonism), has also been reported to cause confusion, hallucinations, and full-blown toxic psychoses (Schwab et al., 1969; Fahn et al., 1971). Of particular note is that these symptoms have been found among patients taking both amantadine and near-maximum doses of trihexyphenidyl (Artane) and benztropine (Cogentin). Amantadine is felt to potentiate the anticholinergic side effects of these agents, and this may be the etiology of the psychosis (Hansten, 1976). Amantadine has also been shown to have psychotogenic properties when used in elderly patients with renal disease (Postma and Van Tilburg, 1975; Borison, 1979).

Antibiotics

The psychiatric side effects caused by this group of drugs may easily be overlooked, since the primary infection and associated medical conditions, especially fever, can seem to be plausible explanations of any adverse reactions. It appears that most antibiotics have the potential for adverse neuropsychiatric reactions. Toxic psychoses have been specifically reported for drugs commonly used for urinary infection, such as nitrofurantoin nalidixic acid, and gentamicin (Johnson, 1972; Wadlington et al., 1972; Kane and Byrd, 1975). Chloramphenicol, isomiazid, rifampin, and cephalexin have also been associated with toxic encephalopathies (Levine, 1970; Saker, 1973; Pratt, 1979; Reilly, 1979). The sulfonamides commonly produce minor symptoms such as headache, dizziness, drowsiness, and mood changes. Acute toxic states have also been observed (Johnson, 1972). They are of particular interest because of their propensity to precipitate porphyric attacks.

Penicillin

It has been estimated that 1–5% of all patients receiving penicillin exhibit some untoward manifestations. Among these reactions are occasional acute psychotic episodes associated with the administration of procaine penicillin (Tompsett, 1967). These reactions seem to be of two different types. In the first, the psychotic symptoms are concurrent or associated with an allergic response. Apprehension, restlessness, confusion, and disorientation are found, along with varying degrees of allergic phenomena such as urticaria, wheezing, edema, and arthralgias. Cardiovascular findings may be those of anaphylactic shock, with decreased blood pressure and increased pulse rate. It is believed that the associated neuropsychiatric symptoms are secondary to cerebral edema of allergic origin. Antihistamines seem to be the treatment of choice for both the allergic and secondary psychotic symptoms.

The second category of psychotic reaction was first described in 1951 (Batchelor et al., 1951). Administration of intramuscular aqueous procaine penicillin G is closely followed by symptoms such as sensations of imminent death, anxiety, sensory phenomena such as visual, auditory, and tactile hallucinations, and increased psychomotor activity (Bjornberg and Selstam, 1960; Bradberry and Ownes, 1975). The reaction seems to be immediate and directly related to the injection of the penicillin. There are no findings of allergic phenomena and, in contrast to an anaphylactic reaction, the blood pressure is usually elevated, as is the pulse rate. In several of the reported cases, without treatment, the episode ended abruptly within 15 min and all vital signs returned to normal. In others, a chronic sense of apprehension and anxiety remained for several months. This type of reaction has been called "pseudoanaphylactic," since the definitive signs of an anaphylactic reaction such as hypotension are conspicuously absent from all reported cases.

The exact cause of the psychotic reaction is not known. There are several theories, all of which rest on the assumption that the injection consists of an inadvertent intravenous administration of the drug. It has been suggested that the aqueous combination of procaine and penicillin G existing in the form of insoluble particles may act directly on certain areas of the brain as temporary microemboli (Utley et al., 1966). Tompsett (1967), also implicating particles in the insoluble suspension, pointed out the similarities of the symptoms to those of fat emboli. Bell (1954) indicated that a chemical rather than a physical explanation was more likely, the cerebral tissues having an affinity for this compound. Downham and Ramos (1973) noted that the penicillin itself is unlikely to produce such psychotic symptoms, but that the high local concentration of free procaine might do so. They postulate that there may be enough free procaine to produce cortical stimulation and that the reaction is short lived due to the hydrolysis of the procaine by plasma procaine esterase.

Downham and Ramos (1973) also reported that the treatment of choice consists of phenobarbital i.m., which yielded improvement in every case. Diphenhydramine hydrochloride (Benedryl) was also successfully used. Physical restraint and reassurance may be necessary in order to protect the patient during this initial period. When particular precautions have been taken to avoid injection within a vessel, the reaction has not been described.

REFERENCES

Batchelor RB, Horne GO, Rodgerson HL: An unusual reaction to procaine penicillin in aqueous suspension. *Lancet* 2:195–198, 1951.
Bell RC: Sudden death following injection of procaine penicillin. *Lancet* 1:13–17, 1954.
Bjornberg A, Selstam J: Acute psychotic reaction after injection of procaine penicillin—a report of 33 cases. *Acta Psychiatr Scand* 35 (suppl):129–139, 1960.
Borison RL: Amantadine-induced psychosis in a geriatric patient with renal disease. *Am J Psychiatry* 136:111–112, 1979.
Bradberry JC, Owens J: Acute psychotic reactions to procaine penicillin. *Am J Hosp Pharm* 32:411–413, 1975.
Brill H: Post-encephalitic psychiatric conditions, in Arieti S (ed): *American Handbook of Psychiatry.* New York, Basic Books, pp 1163–1174, 1959.
Cadie M, Nye FJ, Storey T: Anxiety and depression after infectious mononucleosis. *Br J Psychiatry* 128:559–561, 1976.
Cleobury JF, Skinner GRB, Thouless ME: Association between psychopathic disorder and serum antibody to herpes simplex virus (Type I). *Br Med J* 1:438–439, 1971.
Davison K, Bagley CR: Schizophrenia-like psychoses associated with organic disorders of the central nervous system: A review of the literature, in Harrington RN (ed): *Current Problems in Neuropsychiatry.* Brit J Psychiat Special Publication No. 4, Ashford Kent, Headley Brothers, 1969.
Downham TF II, Ramos DP: Non-allergic adverse reactions to aqueous procaine penicillin G. *Mich Med* 72:223–227, 1973.

Elliott FA: Propanolol for the control of belligerent behavior following acute brain damage. *Ann Neurol* 1:489–491, 1977.

Fahn S, Craddock G, Kumin G: Acute toxic psychosis from suicidal overdosage of amantadine. *Arch Neurol* 25:45–48, 1971.

Fairweather, DS: Psychiatric aspects of the post-encephalitic syndrome. *J Med Sci* 93:201–254, 1947.

Glaser GH, Pincus JH: Limbic encephalitis. *J Nerv Ment Dis* 149:59–67, 1969.

Greenfield NS, Roessler R, Crosley AP: Ego strength and length of recovery from infectious mononucleosis. *J Nerv Ment Dis* 128:125–128, 1959.

Hafstrom N: Neurologic complications of mononucleosis. *Acta Neurol Scand* 39:69–81, 1963.

Halonen PE, Arohonka K, Jantti V, et al: Antibody levels of herpes simplex type I, measles and rubella viruses in psychiatric patients. *Br J Psychiatry* 125:461–463, 1974.

Hansten PD (ed): *Drug Interactions*, ed 3. Philadelphia, Lea & Febiger, 1976.

Hendler N, Leahy W: Psychiatric and neurologic sequelae of infectious mononucleosis. *Am J Psychiatry* 135:842–844, 1978.

Himmelhoch J, Pincus J, Tucker G, et al: Sub-acute encephalitis: Behavioral and neurologic aspects. *Br J Psychiatry* 116:531–538, 1970.

Hollander MC, Duffy TE, Feldman HA, et al: Encephalitis or schizophrenia? *Int Psychiatry Clin* 2:691–709, 1965.

Imboden J: Psychosocial determinants of recovery. *Adv Psychosom Med* 8:128–137, 1972.

Johnson DW: The psychiatric side effects of drugs. *Practitioner* 209:320–326, 1972.

Joyston-Bechal MP: The clinical features and outcome of stupor. *Br J Psychiatry* 112:967–981, 1966.

Kakulas B, Adams RD: Viral Infections of the nervous system: Aseptic meningitis and encephalitis, in Thorn GW, Adams RD, Braunwald E (eds): *Harrison's Principles of Internal Medicine*. New York, McGraw-Hill, 1977, pp 1895–1899.

Kane, FJ Jr., Byrd G: Acute toxic psychosis associated with gentamicin therapy. *South Med J* 68:1283–1285, 1975.

Klein DB: *Abnormal Psychology*. New York, Holt, 1951.

Landes R, Reich JP, Perlow S: Central nervous system manifestations of infectious mononucleosis. *JAMA* 116:2482–2484, 1941.

Levine PH, Regelson W, Holland JS: Chloramphenicol-associated encephalopathy. *Clin Pharm Ther* 11:194–199, 1970.

Lipowski ZJ: Physical illness, the patient and its environment: Psychosocial foundations of medicine, in organic disorders and psychosomatic medicine, in Reiser MF, Arieti S (eds): *American Handbook of Psychiatry*, ed 2. New York, Basic Books, vol 4, 1975.

Lycke E, Norrby R, Roos BE: A serological study on mentally-ill patients. *Br J Psychiatry* 124:277, 1974.

Meninger KA: Influenza and schizophrenia. An analysis of post-influenzal "dementia praecox" as of 1918 and five years later. *Am J Psychiatry* 5:469–474, 1926.

Misra PC, Hay GG: Encephalitis presenting as acute schizophrenia. *Br Med J* 1:532–533, 1971.

Nikolovski OT, Fernandes JV: Capgras Syndrome as an aftermath of chicken pox encephalitis. *Psych Opinion* 15:39–43, 1978.

Penman HG: Fatal infectious mononucleosis: A critical review. *J Clin Pathol* 23:765–769, 1970.

Penn H, Racy J, Lapham L, et al: Catatonic behavior, viral encephalopathy, and death: The problem of fatal catatonia. *Arch Gen Psychiatry* 27:758–761, 1972.

Peszke MA, Mason WM: Infectious mononucleosis and its relationship to psychological malaise. *Conn Med* 1:260–262, 1969.

Pokorny Ed, Rawls WE, Adam E, et al: Depression, psychopathology and herpes virus type I antibodies. *Arch Gen Psychiatry* 29:820–824, 1972.

Postma JU, Van Tilburg W: Visual hallucinations and delirium during treatment with amantadine (Symmetrel). *J Am Geriatr Soc* 23:212–215, 1975.

Pratt TH: Rifampin-induced organic brain syndrome. *JAMA* 241:2421–2422, 1979.

Rasken DE: Herpes encephalitis with catatonic stupor. *Arch Gen Psychiatry* 31:544–546, 1974.

Raymond RW, Williams RL: Infectious mononucleosis with psychosis: Report of a case. *N Engl J Med* 239:542–544, 1948.

Reilly DK: Isomiazid-related CNS toxicity. *Drug Ther* 9:187–188, 1979.

Rimon R, Halonen P: Herpes simplex virus infection and depressive illness. *Dis. Nerv Syst* 30:338–340, 1969.

Rubin RL: Case reports: Adolescent infectious mononucleosis with psychosis. *J Clin Psychiatry* 39:63–65, 1978.

Sacks O: *Awakenings.* London, Duckworth, 1973.

Saker BM, Musk AW, Hayward EF, et al: Reversible toxic psychosis after cephalexin. *Med J Aust* 1:497–498, 1973.

Schnell RG, Dyck TJ, Bowie EW, et al: Infectious mononucleosis: Neurologic and EEG findings. *Medicine* 45:51–63, 1966.

Schreier HR: Use of propranolol in the treatment of post-encephalitic psychoses. *Am J Psychiatry* 136:840–841, 1979.

Schwab JJ: Psychiatric illnesses produced by infections. *Hosp Med* 5:98–108, 1969.

Schwab RS, England AC Jr., Poskanzer DC: Amantadine in the treatment of Parkinson's disease. *JAMA* 208:1168–1170, 1969.

Shearer ML, Finch SM: Periodic organic psychosis associated with recurrent herpes simplex. *N Eng J Med* 271:494–497, 1964.

Silverstein A, Steinberg G, Nathanson M: Nervous system involvement in infectious mononucleosis. *Arch Neurol* 26:353–359, 1972.

Sorbin A, Ozer MN: Mental disorders in acute encephalitis. *J Mt Sinai Hosp* 33:73–75, 1966.

Spittle BJ, Fliegnar J, Faed JA, et al: Post-infectious encephalopathy simulating functional psychosis. *New Eng Med J* 85:180–181, 1977.

Steinberg D, Hirsch SR, Marston SD, et al: Influenza infection causing manic psychosis. *Br J Psychiatry* 120:531–535, 1972.

Stewart RM, Baldessarini RJ: Viral encephalopathy and psychosis. *Am J Psychiatry* 133:717, 1976.

Still RML: Psychosis following Asian influenza in Barbados. *Lancet* 2:20–21, 1958.

Strauss H, Ostow M, Greenstein L: *Diagnostic Electroencephalography.* New York, Grune & Stratton, 1952.

Thorn GW, Adams RD, Braunwald E, et al (eds): *Harrison's Principles of Internal Medicine,* ed 8. New York, McGraw-Hill, 1977.

Tompsett TR: Pseudoanaphylactic reactions to procaine penicillin G. *Arch Intern Med* 120:565–567, 1967.

Utley PM, Lucas JB, Billings GE: Acute psychotic reactions to aqueous procaine penicillin. *South Med J* 59:1271–1274, 1966.

Wadlington WB, Hatcher H, Turner DJ: Osteomyelitis of the patella—gentamicin therapy associated with encephalopathy. *Clin Pediatr* 10:577–580, 1972.

Wallin JW: *Children with Mental and Physical Handicaps.* New York, Prentice–Hall, 1949.

Warm JS, Alluisi EA: Behavioral reactions to infection: Review of the psychological literature. *Precept Skills* 24:755–761, 1967.

Weinstein EA, Linn L, Kahn RL: Encephalitis with a clinical picture of schizophrenia. *J Mt Sinai Hosp* 21:341–354, 1955.

Wilson LG: Viral encephalopathy mimicking functional psychosis. *Am J Psychiatry* 133:165–170, 1976.

13

Toxin Disorders

MERCURY

Neuropsychiatric manifestations may be seen following exposure to mercury. The signs and symptoms vary with the form and type of compound involved. Although elemental mercury is not absorbed, poisoning may occur from mercury vapors, organic compounds, and soluble and insoluble inorganic compounds. Acute mercury poisoning, usually the result of ingestion of soluble salts such as mercury chloride, either by accident or with suicidal intent, is an acute medical crisis. Symptoms occur quickly and are caused by severe local inflammation of the gastrointestinal tract and renal toxicity. Anuria and uremia are the usual causes of death.

Chronic poisonings, typically occurring secondary to medicinal use or industrial exposure, are of more relevance to the psychiatrist. Intoxication is almost always by way of dust or vapor inhalation, but occasionally may occur with heavy exposure to the skin. Several cases have been reported of intoxication caused by application of an organic mercury compound for skin fungus infections (Okinaka et al., 1964). Original reports of chronic mercurialism emanated from the hatters' fur-cutting industry (Freeman 1860). Opinions differ on whether this was the source of the expression "mad as a hatter." Mercury compounds are also employed as herbicides and fungicides, and may be found in water-based paints. Many industries use mercury processes for the extraction of metal from ores, the production of phosphate or cement, or the burning of fossil fuels. Mercury vapors are an occupational hazard in mining and in industries concerned with the extraction of mercury from cinnabar, in the production of chlorine, paper pulp, and electrical equipment, and in various laboratories, including those in hospitals.

Clinical Features

Systemic signs and symptoms characterizing chronic mercury poisoning are gingivitis, stomatitis, loosening of the teeth, excessive salivation, a metallic taste, colitis, loss of appetite, progressive renal damage, anemia, hypertension, and peripheral neuritis. A variety of neurologic signs and symptoms may be produced, including tremor, ataxia, dysarthria, and, in several cases, mental deterioration. Some observers have noted a characteristic concentric narrowing of the visual field (Study Group of Minamata Disease, 1968). Synder (1972) emphasized that the occurrence of otherwise unexplained involuntary movements could suggest the diagnosis of mercury poisoning. Ross et al. (1977) felt that typical signs of mercurialism are a fine intention tremor and a coarse jerking of some muscles (especially of the face or arms).

Neuropsychiatric Features

Documenting mercury poisoning in the fur-cutting industry, Neal and Jones (1938) noted that 37.2% of their patients suffered psychic disturbances. They described the following abnormalities: irascible temper, discouragement without cause, feelings of depression or despondency, excessive embarrassment in the presence of strangers, timidity, a desire for solitude, anxiety, excitability, an inability to take orders, or a strong feeling of self-consciousness. Hunter (1939), describing the same group of patients in the felt hat industry, confirmed the depresssion and timidity, and noted that patients seemed to lose control of themselves, "thus, if visitors stopped to watch him, he will sometimes throw down his tools and turn in anger towards the intruder."

Many of the subsequent reports are fascinating. Several case histories from London and Australia describe detectives who, for no readily explicable reason, became anxious, weak, and tremorous, and developed a strange clinical phenomenon called "erythism" wherein they ceased being able to function in front of their superiors (Agate and Buchnell, 1949; Blench and Brindle, 1951; Felton et al., 1972). Investigation demonstrated mercury toxicity acquired from the powder used in their law enforcement work to bring out latent fingerprints.

In 1953, a mysterious and infamous illness broke out in the Japanese fishing village of Minamata. The illness affected 111 persons, resulting in 41 fatalities. It was later discovered that the cause was the dumping of some 100 tons of methyl mercury into an adjacent bay. The report of that incident documented a vague set of objective and psychological symptoms, including irritability, insomnia, forgetfulness, inability to concentrate, and numbness, particularly of the extremities and around the mouth (Study Group of Minamata Disease, 1968).

Several other reports from industrial situations have confirmed similar symptoms. Miller et al. (1967) emphasized lassitude, headache, and clumsiness in 50% of their cases, and described attacks of tremulousness and crying and marked feelings of fatigue that would be brought on in some patients by only five to ten minutes of exertion. Benning (1958) described similar symptoms, and also noted lability of mood in 42% of her patients.

Although depression or discouragement had been mentioned in prior reports, Maghazaji (1974), who studied methyl mercury poisoning secondary to ingestion of homemade bread prepared from wheat contaminated with a fungicide, highlighted this feature. Depression, varying from mild to moderate in degree and consisting of a lack of interest, the wish to be left alone, and deficient concentration, occurred in 74.4% of the 43 patients he studied. Suicidal tendencies were not seen. The author compared depressive symptoms with average blood levels of total and inorganic mercury and found a considerable positive correlation. Interestingly, none of their patients exhibited delusions or evidence of a thought disorder. Most reports indicate that toxicity at mild to moderate levels causes relatively minimal defects in orientation, abstract thinking, and judgment. There is some disagreement over the effect on memory functions. Ross et al. (1977) specifically noted that they felt that memory difficulties were due to defects in registration resulting from distractability and lack of concentration rather than from failure of short-term retention per se. Perceptual abnormalities such as illusions and visual hallucinations are rarely reported, as are delusions. Hunter's (1939) report is an exception to this.

Because many behavioral disorders have been associated with mercury poisoning, Gowdy and Demers (1978) investigated the possibility that chronic mercury accumulation may be a hidden factor in the mental illnesses of hospitalized patients. They measured whole blood mercury levels of 91 patients at a Veterans Administration hospital. The mean level in the patient group was 7.82 parts per billion (ppb), which was slightly lower than the 8.1 ppb mean previously reported for an urban population (Gowdy et al., 1978). Values were higher in patients with organic brain syndromes, but only three subjects were at or above the theoretically normal limit of 20 ppb blood mercury content. One of these patients was depressed, and two others had been hospitalized for senile dementia.

The treatment of chronic poisoning is largely symptomatic, including immediate removal from all contact with mercury and efforts to improve the nutritional state of the patient. While penicillamine does promote excretion of mercury, patients often improve slowly and may remain in ill health for years.

LEAD

Lead poisoning continues to be common, even though many historically toxic sources have been eliminated. Although the disappearance of lead plumbing, the use of ceramic glazes with low lead content, the decline in the use of lead-base paints, and industrial hygienic measures have contributed to the reduced incidence of poisoning, cases are still reported among workers involved with battery production, printing, or spray painting. The most common victims of lead toxicity continue to be children who ingest the lead-containing paint that is still found in older homes. Other sources of exposure have also been described. High blood levels are found among parking lot attendants, traffic policemen, law enforcement personnel using indoor firing ranges, and tunnel employees, who absorb airborne lead (Needleman and Scanlon, 1973, Fischbein et al., 1979). Lead poisoning has also been reported among gasoline sniffers. There are many reports of lead intoxication from illicit whiskey ("moonshine"), much of which is distilled through auto radiators or other lead-containing apparatus (Morris et al., 1964; Crutcher, 1963; Morgan et al., 1971; Cheatham and Chobot, 1968). It is also possible to absorb toxic amounts of lead from foreign objects, such as bullets or buckshot, lodged in serous cavities within the body. Cases of lead poisoning have also been reported among artists working with leaded glass.

Absorption of lead is slow by any route, and only prolonged exposure results in the cumulative amounts necessary for poisoning. However, the rate of excretion is so limited that only a slight excess may result in a positive lead balance. Most absorbed lead is deposited in the bones and soft tissue, with blood, urine, and feces containing only small amounts.

Clinical Features

General systemic manifestations of poisoning are colic, anemia, peripheral neuritis, and encephalopathy. Abdominal symptoms usually begin with vague complaints, such as anorexia, muscle discomfort, and malaise. Constipation is usually an early sign; as severity increases nausea and vomiting are usually present. The most prominent feature is colic (painters' cramps), considered to be the result of intestinal spasm; it is paroxysmal and excruciating. Abdominal muscles become rigid and the pain is wandering and poorly localized. No fever or leukocytosis is present, morphine has little effect upon the pain, and the attacks of colic seem to be precipitated by alcoholic excesses.

Mild anemia, characterized by large numbers of erythrocytes with basophilic stippling is usually found. Although pallor may be present, it is thought to be due to spasm of small vessels in the skin rather than to anemia. A "lead line" of black lead sulfide may develop along the gingival margins, but is often absent in adults.

Neuromuscular findings, also known as lead palsy, are manifestations of advanced poisoning. Muscle weakness and easy fatigue occur in advance of actual paralysis and may be the only symptoms to develop. The muscle groups involved are usually those most actively used, resulting in wrist drop or, to a lesser extent, foot drop. Central nervous system signs and symptoms occur most often in children and are relatively rare in adults (see following section). The encephalopathy occurring in children has a significant mortality and causes severe permanent brain damage in 25% of survivors (Poskanzer, 1977).

Laboratory Findings

In addition to the characteristic stippling seen in erythrocytes, patients with lead poisoning excrete increased amounts of coproporphyrin III in the urine. Examination of a urine specimen for porphyrin is the best screening test in suspected cases. When encephalopathy is present, the cerebrospinal fluid is usually under increased pressure, with pleocytosis· and elevated proteins. Urinary lead determinations are of aid in confirming the diagnosis; a level of 0.15–0.2 mg/liter is considered significant, although interpretations vary. Concentrations in blood in excess of 0.07 mg/100 ml of whole blood are indicative of recent lead exposure, while those in excess of 0.10 mg/100 ml indicate severe toxicity.

Neuropsychiatric Features

Central nervous system findings of lead encephalopathy are the most serious manifestations of lead poisoning, with a mortality of greater than 25% (Segal et al., 1974). Encephalopathy resulting from lead intoxication occurs rarely in adults and is not distinguishable on a clinical basis from acute brain syndromes secondary to other etiologies. Onset is often acute; first signs may include clumsiness, vertigo, ataxia, headache, insomnia, and restlessness. Several studies have emphasized the irritability (Baloh et al., 1975; Repko and Corum, 1979). No evidence has been reported which attempts to determine whether it is related to sleep loss, general discomfort, or other factors. A recent study of workers in the battery manufacturing industry found evidence that the psychological impact of working in a leaded environment is one of increased hostility, depression, and general dysphasia (Repko and Corum, 1979).

These symptoms are usually followed by excitement and confusion, impairment of memory, and auditory or visual hallucinations. With progression of encephalopathy, convulsions of the grand mal type and signs of increased intracranial pressure, such as papilledema or projectile vomiting may occur. When the onset is slower, the chronic patient may show general mental dullness, poor memory, trembling, and, occasionally, deafness or seizures. Once encephalopathy occurs, approximately 40% of survivors will have neurologic sequelae such as mental retardation, seizures, or cerebral palsy (Pearlstein and Attala, 1966).

Since the clinical picture of encephalopathy does not differ significantly from that of chronic alcohol abuse and withdrawal, awareness of the possibility of lead poisoning from ingestion of illicit distilled whiskey must be maintained, particularly in the southeastern areas of the United States. In these situations, history is usually not helpful, although a relative may admit to the patient's ingestion of illicit alcohol. In most of the reported cases of lead encephalopathy from this source, clinical suspicions were raised by alcohol withdrawal states that were uncharacteristic, i.e., were unusually protracted and nonresponsive to customary interventions (Cheatham and Chobot, 1968). The finding of hypochromic anemia with basophilic stippling and an increase in reticulocytes was important in directing attention toward the diagnosis of lead intoxication. Ultimately, clinical differentiation was made possible only by the finding of elevated cerebrospinal fluid protein and abnormally high serum and urine lead levels.

Encephalopathy has also been reported secondary to organic lead poisoning. Symptoms are similar to those of inorganic lead poisoning, as the lead in the body is eventually converted to inorganic lead. The encephalopathy may be secondary to accidental or purposeful inhalation of vapors of commercially available gasoline containing tetraethyl or tetramethyl lead (Law and Nelson, 1968). If exposure is not intentional, intense, and methodical, it appears that a period of weeks to months is needed for lead absorbed from this source to reach hazardous levels. Early symptoms include insomnia and disturbing dreams; these are followed later by anorexia, nausea and vomiting, diarrhea, headache, muscular weakness, and emotional instability. Irritability, restlessness, and anxiety are also evident, and, with continued exposure, progress to a typical acute brain syndrome. It appears that chronic gasoline intoxication can produce its own symptoms, such as anorexia, weight loss, fatigue, nervousness, insomnia, memory loss, and tremor, but florid organic psychoses have not been reported in the absence of lead intoxication (Sanders, 1964; Cassells and Dodds, 1946; Law and Nelson, 1968). Early recognition of this syndrome is important, since treatment seems to be effective.

Treatment

The most important single feature of treatment is prevention of further lead absorption by the patient. This necessitates a definitive history of the exposure. It takes approximately twice as long to excrete a given burden of lead as it does to accumulate it. Treatment of encephalopathy is begun once urine flow is established, and a combination of British Anti-Lewisite (BAL) and calcium disodium versenate is commonly employed. Symptomatic treatment of increased intracranial pressure may also be needed. Oral penicillamine is often used when blood levels exceed 100 mg lead/100 g blood (Poskanzer, 1977).

BISMUTH

Bismuth toxicity was once almost entirely a complication of antisy-philitic therapy. At present, complications are secondary to bismuth salts taken orally for intestinal disorders or to bismuth used in skin powders or ointments. Harvey (1970) feels that there is little reason for use of bismuth in modern therapeutics, and no case reports of adverse reactions are to be found in the North American literature.

In 1974, Burns et al. (Australia) first described four patients with ster-eotyped recurrent and reversible neurologic syndromes consisting of con-fusion, tremulousness, clumsiness, myoclonic jerks, and difficulty walking. The patients, who had all undergone abdominoperineal resection, were tak-ing oral bismuth subgallate for colostomy regulation. Symptoms progressed until the bismuth was stopped. Eventually, a national committee tabulated 29 similar cases in Australia (Robertson, 1974a,b), and Buge et al. (1974) (France) added 20 other patients with a similar picture.

Krúger and Thomas (1976) reported two patients with an organic brain syndrome thought to be secondary to bismuth absorbed from a skin cream. The patients had been using the cream to lighten skin blemishes for 19 and 20 years, respectively. Both demonstrated intelluctual impairment with memory loss, and periods of confusion, tremulousness, clumsiness, diffi-culty in walking, and myoclonic jerks. Both patients were initially diagnosed as neurotic. Cerebral venous blood levels of bismuth were found to be 160 μg/ml and 100 μg/ml, respectively. No bismuth was detectable in the blood three weeks after use of the cream was discontinued.

In 1977, a French group studied 45 patients admitted with "myoclonic encephalopathy" due to ingestion of insoluble bismuth salts (subnitrate) for various colon disorders and constipation (Supino-Viterbo et al., 1977). The patients had been taking 5–20 g daily, over a period ranging from 4 weeks to 30 years. The physicians described two phases. A first, insidious period lasted from one week to several months, with gradual onset of nonspecific symptoms such as depression, anxiety, irritability, intermittent delusions or phobias, and occasional sleep disorders with prolonged insomnia. Fifteen of the patients complained of headache. The symptoms of toxicity often aggravated the primary intestinal problem, inducing patients to increase the dose of bismuth.

The second phase consisted of confirmed encephalopathy that began abruptly over a 24- to 48-h period. Four symptoms were constant and felt to be of considerable diagnostic value: (1) mental confusion, (2) pseudotre-mor accompanied by myoclonic jerks, (3) dysarthria, and (4) disturbances of walking and standing. The myoclonic jerks were always present if the patient was examined carefully, hence the designation of "myoclonic encephalopathy."

In 31 of the patients there was a distinctive EEG pattern, consisting of monomorphic waves at 3–5 Hz involving both temporal–rolandic and frontal areas, which were unaffected by eye opening. In most patients there was also a diffuse beta rhythm of low voltage. No spikes or other paroxysmal features were present. This observation confirmed findings of previous investigators (Gastaut et al., 1975).

Bismuth blood levels measured on the same day as the EEG ranged from 150 to 1600 μg/liter (normal is less than 20 μg/liter). EEG features did not correlate closely with bismuth blood levels, suggesting a poor correlation between blood levels and concentration in brain tissue.

Monseu et al. (1976) summarized the literature and noted that in all reported cases of bismuth encephalopathy the encephalopathy is reversible and parallels the symptoms. As noted, this new iatrogenic entity is not yet a problem within the United States, but more than 100 cases have now been reported in other countries.

ARSENIC

Arsenic, a popular poison in ancient times, was quite common as a source of toxicity in the United States before the second World War due to the use of medicinal arsenic, arsenic used with homicidal intent, and contamination from agricultural arsenical sprays. In current human therapeutics, arsenicals are important only for treatment of certain tropical diseases and amebiasis. Development of chemical methods of detecting minimal amounts of arsenic and alertness on the part of physicians to possible poisoning have reduced the incidence of criminal poisoning by this agent (Harvey, 1975). Control of arsenic in farm produce has been helpful in reducing accidental toxicity. Most poisonings now are the result of accidental or suicidal ingestion of insecticides or rodenticides containing copper acetoarsenate (Paris green) or calcium or lead arsenate. Some chronic poisoning may still be found among workers in the metal, paint, dye, cosmetic, or insecticide industries.

Clinical Features

Arsenic may be absorbed through all mucous membranes, the toxic dose varies considerably, depending on individual susceptibility. Symptoms of acute poisoning are nausea, vomiting, diarrhea, severe burning of the mouth and throat, and very severe abdominal pain. The vomitus often contains blood. Headache, delirium, convulsions, coma, and death may occur within a few hours.

Of more relevance to the psychiatrist are patients who may suffer from chronic intoxication. Systemic signs of poisoning usually include weakness, muscle aching, anorexia, dermatitis, and nervous system involvement. Cutaneous manifestations appear within several weeks and are characterized by a diffuse, dry, scaly appearance, with occasional hyperpigmentation over the trunk and extremities. After about five weeks of exposure to arsenic, a transverse white stria, 1–2 mm in width, appears above the lunula (white portion) of each fingernail; this is called the Mees line.

Laboratory Findings

No clinical or laboratory findings are specific for arsenic poisoning. General findings usually include moderate anemia and leukopenia of 2000–5000 white blood cells/mm^3. There is slight proteinuria and liver function tests may be mildly abnormal. The spinal fluid is normal. Diagnosis depends upon an accurate history of ingestion or laboratory confirmation of absorption. It may be detected in urine, hair, or nails, but because arsenic is found widely in nature, and hence in food and water, its presence may not be diagnostic of poisoning. Arsenic in the hair or nails may represent quantities taken several months or even years earlier. Measurement of urine arsenic levels is generally most helpful in diagnosis; patients with clear evidence of intoxication have been found to excrete more than 0.1 mg/ml. This level may be much higher after acute exposure. The treatment of arsenic poisoning consists of gastric lavage and treatment with BAL (see general medical text for specific instructions).

Neuropsychiatric Features

General central nervous system symptoms include headache, drowsiness, confusion, and convulsions. Frank (1976) described delayed personality changes and neuropathy in six patients following arsine poisoning. Their symptoms included malaise, emotional lability, insomnia, and depression, all of which abated without specific therapy within two years. Harvey (1975) noted an "apathetic, idiotic condition" that results from long and severe exposure. Schenk and Stolk (1967) described a 56-year-old woman in whom arsenic poisoning was followed by a permanent organic psychosis characterized by agitation, paranoid-delusional thinking, and progressive disturbance of judgment and self-care function.

Differentiating neuropathy and encephalopathy that may be associated with relatively acute arsenic toxicity from that occurring with ethanol abuse constitutes a major clinical difficulty. Freeman and Couch (1978) report a case of prolonged encephalopathy with features of Korsakoff psychosis occurring with severe peripheral neuropathy. The clinical picture was that of a rather typical organic brain syndrome, including symptoms of disorientation, confusion, intermittent agitation, and visual hallucinations. Arsenic encephalopathy was suspected when there was no improvement after five

weeks of thiamine therapy for Wernicke–Korsakoff syndrome. Most patients
with the global confusion of Wernicke encephalopathy improve within two
weeks after treatment is initiated (Victor et al., 1971). Once treated with
BAL, the arsenic encephalopathy cleared, and the patient did not demonstrate the long-term disorder of memory and learning characterized by the
Korsakoff psychosis.

It is often difficult to trace the origin of arsenic exposure. Jenkins (1966)
suspected "moonshine whiskey" in some of his patients. There are also
several reports of arsenical encephalopathy due to the use of the medication
glycobiarsol (Milibis) (Cole et al., 1966; Browne et al., 1950). The patients
described in both of these reports had been treated for amebiasis; this suggests that a heightened suspicion is necessary when patients have a history
of international travel.

Encephalopathies are relatively rare, the most typical neurologic symptom seen among patients with chronic arsenic intoxication being that of
peripheral neuropathy. Symptoms include numbness with tingling paresthesias in the extremities, a burning sensation in the hands and particularly
in the soles of the feet, and complaints of muscular weakness. There may
also be a decrease in touch, pain, and temperature sensation in the extremities, which often has a symmetrical "stocking–glove" distribution. Diminished or absent tendon reflexes are early signs; continued exposure results
in distal weakness with an inability to stand or walk. The peripheral neuropathy associated with arsenical ingestion, while similar to that of alcoholism, is more rapid in onset and differs somewhat in that the early impairment of the motor system leads to severe crippling (Jenkins, 1966). The
prognosis for recovery from neuropathy depends upon its severity, with
recovery occurring in early sensory and mild sensory–motor cases, while
permanent changes are found in more severe cases.

BROMIDES

Bromides were widely used as sedatives and antiepileptics in the late
19th and early 20th centuries. In the late 1800's, up to 2 ½ tons of bromides
were dispensed annually by one London hospital (Ewing and Grant, 1965).
In 1927, Wuth (1927) reported that of 238 admissions over a 6-month period
to the psychiatric division of Johns Hopkins Hospital, 21% had elevated-
bromide levels and 8.4% showed signs of intoxication. Although the use of
bromides has decreased markedly since then, bromism has continued to be
a health hazard. In the mid-1960's, a survey of psychiatric admissions to
four North Carolina hospitals found toxic serum bromide levels (greater than
65 mg%) in 1% of 2580 patients (Ewing and Grant, 1965). Since then, there
has been a further decrease in availability of both prescription and proprie-
tary bromide preparations, yet cases of bromism continue to be reported
(Muller, 1968; Carney, 1971; Reick, 1971; Serpe, 1972; McDanal et al., 1974;
Pleasure and Blackburn, 1975; Raskind et al., 1978).

Pharmacology and Pathophysiology

Bromide is readily absorbed from the gastrointestinal tract and distributed throughout the body much the same as chloride. Although its distribution is mostly extracellular, a substantial intracellular concentration occurs, especially in red blood cells and nerve cells. The bromide level in brain and cerebrospinal fluid is about ⅓ that found in blood. While it is not fully known how bromide exerts its effects on the central nervous system, it may work through ion substitution with chloride. Bromide is excreted from the body by the kidneys, but because it is selectively reabsorbed in preference to chloride, it disappears slowly. Its serum half-life is *12 days*, a factor which accounts for its accumulation and persistence over time and the ease with which chronic intoxication can occur (Sharpless, 1970). Acute bromide intoxication, on the other hand, is quite rare, since gastric irritation usually results in vomiting and failure to absorb a toxic quantity.

Bromide-Containing Preparations

In 1938 it was estimated that more than 200 bromide-containing preparations were available in this country. Today, bromides are far less in evidence, yet continue to be manufactured for both over-the-counter and prescription use. The following are preparations which were available in 1978 and contained enough bromide to cause chronic intoxication:

Alva Tranquil	Fello-sed
Lanabrom Elixir	Broniacin
Neurosine	Neo-Sedaphen
Peacock's Bromides	Triple Bromides
Carbrital	Elixsed
Bromural	

This list should be considered representative rather than complete. For more comprehensive and up-to-date information, a regional drug information center should be consulted.

The bromide was removed from Bromo-Seltzer in 1973 and from Miles Nervine in 1977, and although many of the over-the-counter sleeping aids do contain scopolamine HBr, the bromide concentration in them is quite low (less than 1 mg per capsule). Although one case of bromism has been attributed to Sleepeze (Serpe, 1972), it is generally felt that these preparations are unlikely to cause bromide toxicity (the risk of an anticholinergic delirium is much greater).

Clinical Features

The predominant manifestations of chronic bromide intoxication are neuropsychiatric in nature. Skin lesions do occur in 20–30% of patients, and are usually acne-like, but may also be erythema multiforme-like, pustular, ulcerative, pemphigus-like, or nodular (proliferative nodular lesions known as *nodose bromoderma* may be mistaken for tertiary syphilis). Other non-neuropsychiatric findings include foul breath, furry tongue, gastric distress, anorexia, constipation, and mild conjunctivitis.

Although Levin (1948) described four varieties of bromide psychoses ("simple bromide intoxication," "delirium," "transitory schizophrenia with paranoia," and "bromide hallucinosis"), it is generally agreed that bromide intoxication has no specific identifying characteristics. Presenting features will be determined by factors such as magnitude of intoxication, underlying illnesses, and premorbid personality. The incidence of bromism in alcoholics is higher than in the general population, and this combination of conditions may present special diagnostic problems (Rollins and Cefalu, 1968; Wilkinson et al., 1969; McDanal et al., 1974).

Symptoms of mild bromism are nonspecific and include fatigue, drowsiness, weakness, emotional lability, depression, impaired memory and concentration, self-neglect, disturbed sleep, and confusion. More advanced intoxication may exaggerate these findings as well as cause delirium, disorientation, stupor, coma, excitement, delusions, hallucinations, paranoia, slurred speech, ataxia, and seizures (Rollins and Cefalu, 1968; Trump and Hochberg, 1976; Raskind et al., 1978).

In Perkins' (1950) series of 27 well-documented cases of bromism, the commonest presenting problems were drowsiness (ranging from mild to coma) and weakness. The overall frequency of symptoms were as follows:

Weakness	78%
Aches and pains	41%
Depression	37%
Sleepiness	30%
Coma	22%
Irritability	15%
Stupor	11%

When the patients were evaluated for "psychiatric" changes, Perkins found the following:

Excitement	78%
Confusion	63%
Disorientation	56%
Lack of cooperation	48%
Hallucinations	44%
Memory defects	37%
Delusions	30%
Confabulation	15%

Findings on neurological examination included slurred speech and abnormal reflexes in 74%, ataxia in 37%, and tremor in 30%. Patients were frequently described as appearing intoxicated with alcohol.

Misdiagnosis

Given the varied clinical manifestations of bromism, the often surreptitious use of bromides, and the relatively uncommon nature of the problem, the possibility of misdiagnosis is high.

Bromism in an alcoholic is likely to be overlooked, since both conditions may present as acute organic brain syndromes, and the likelihood of obtaining a reliable history is low. Localized neurological findings suggesting a space-occupying lesion may occur but will resolve with discontinuation of the drug (Perkins, 1950). Especially in the elderly, the early symptoms of bromism can be mistaken for senility. Among the cases presented by Raskind et al. (1978) was a 67-year-old woman misdiagnosed as "senile" and referred for nursing home placement and her daughter who had been hospitalized for "schizophrenia." Both were found to be bromide-toxic secondary to Miles Nervine ingestion. Unless maternal bromism is recognized, central nervous system depression in the newborn may not be diagnosed as bromide intoxication (Pleasure and Blackburn, 1975).

Carney (1973) refers to patients initially diagnosed as having Huntington chorea, paraplegia, dementia, temporal lobe epilepsy, delirium tremens, and one patient who was "successively investigated for coronary thrombosis (chest pain), Addison disease (pigmentation and weakness), dementia (confusion), and acute psychosis (hallucinations of strange women in her room), all with negative results before the correct diagnosis was made."

Other common misdiagnoses include toxic encephalopathy in which bromism was not suspected, depression, schizophrenia, and psychoneurosis. Hanes and Yates (1938) stressed that the early manifestations of bromide intoxication were those of a "mild neurosis" which, if unrecognized, was often inadvertently treated with bromide sedation. They further stated that "although experience may sharpen one's suspicions, the clinical manifestations of bromide intoxication are so varied and withal so subtle, simulating every neuropsychiatric condition, that only the positive evidence of bromide in the blood can substantiate the tentative diagnosis." And that was at a time when bromides were extensively used!

A further problem with bromide is that currently available over-the-counter preparations are recommended for symptoms similar to those produced by bromide intoxication. Thus, a patient with worsening of insomnia, tension, irritability, restlessness, and headache who increases the bromide dose hoping to alleviate the symptoms will actually aggravate the intoxication.

Diagnosis

Bromism should always be considered when confronted by a patient with vague, ill-defined, unexplained psychiatric or neurological symptoms. The determination of serum-bromide level is central to the diagnosis. Given the long half-life of bromide, a blood level even several days after hospitalization can be of value. According to Sharpless (1970), a level of 150 mg% (19 mEg/liter) or above is almost always associated with clinical manifestations, while a level of 72 mg% (9 mEq/liter) or greater in a patient with unexplained symptoms is highly suspect. The relationship of serum levels below 72 mg% (9 mEq/liter) to symptoms is less clear, but it seems reasonable that predisposing factors such as age and associated illness may lower the threshold of susceptibility. Also, a blood sample drawn days after bromide discontinuation may give a deceptively low value. Even though separating cause from coincidence may be difficult, observation of the patient after removing all bromide sources may be of diagnostic and therapeutic value.

Extracellular electrolyte balance is regulated in such a way that halide concentration remains relatively constant. Thus, when bromide is added, an equal amount of chloride is displaced, decreasing extracellular fluid chloride. Because clinical laboratory techniques used to measure chloride concentration are not specific, total halide concentration is reported as chloride, and the lowered chloride concentration is not recognized. In fact, since the reagents in the commonly used AutoAnalyzer method have a greater affinity for bromide, serum "chloride" levels will actually appear elevated. This apparent elevation in serum chloride may be the first clue to a diagnosis of bromide intoxication. Because the reagents used in the Cotlove coulimetric chloride titrator have similar affinities for chloride and bromide, serum "chloride" levels determined by this method tend to be normal (Blume et al., 1968; Palatucci, 1978).

Treatment

Bromide is eliminated from the body almost entirely by the kidneys, and most treatment approaches are directed at increasing the rate of excretion. The administration of chloride salts (sodium chloride, ammonium chloride) can decrease the serum half-life of bromide from 12 days to 3 days. The use of various diuretics can further reduce the serum half-life to as low as 1.65 hours. This latter figure, obtained in a single case with the use of ethacrynic acid and osmotic diuresis compares favorably to half-lives obtained by hemodialysis (Adamson et al., 1966).

Because a portion of bromide is distributed intracellularly, rapid removal of the ion from the blood by diuresis or dialysis can be followed by a rebound increase in serum level. Whether clinical relapse can be associated with this rebound is not clear. Even when treatment consisted only of chloride loading, a patient's clinical course was often one of "pronounced, sudden and unpredictable ups and downs" (Perkins, 1950). Clinical improvement characteristically lags behind the fall in serum bromide level, and even with active treatment full recovery may take 4–10 days. With timely treatment, the prognosis for restoration of premorbid function is good.

ORGANOPHOSPHATE

Organic phosphates are a group of compounds with a variety of uses, including treatment of glaucoma and myasthenia gravis, and as "nerve gases." They are most commonly used as insecticides (e.g., Parathion, Malathion, Systox, Diazinon, DFP, TEPP, HEPP, OMPA). The toxicity of these compounds depends on the preparation; they are often diluted with powders, organic solvents, or water, and may consist of from 1% to 95% active ingredients. Poisoning occurs by ingestion, inhalation, or, particularly important, by rapid absorption through intact skin. Thus, those at highest risk are farm workers, crop dusters, persons in particular industries, or people, particularly children, who may accidentally come into contact with the compounds (often from discarded containers).

The pharmacologic and toxicological effects of organophosphates are primarily due to the inhibition of acetylcholinesterase of the nervous system, resulting in accumulation of acetylcholine at the synapses. The overabundance of acetylcholine initially stimulates, but then blocks, transmission at cholinergic synapses in the central nervous system and somatic nerves, at ganglionic synapses of autonomic nerves, at parasympathetic nerve endings, and at some sympathetic nerve endings, such as sweat glands.

Clinical Features

The route and degree of exposure determines the time interval between exposure and onset of symptoms. This interval may be as little as 5 min with massive ingestion, is usually less than 12 hr, and is always less than 24 hr. Therefore, symptoms beginning more than 24 hr after exposure cannot be attributed directly to acute organophosphate poisoning. Systemic symptoms include signs of respiratory depression, such as tightness in the chest, wheezing, dyspnea, increased bronchial secretion, and, ultimately, pulmonary edema and cyanosis. Gastrointestinal symptoms include nausea, vomiting, abdominal cramps, diarrhea, and fecal incontinence. Sweating, salivation, lacrimation, and blurring of vision are common. Either bradycardia with hypotension or tachycardia with hypertension may be seen, depending on whether muscarinic (parasympathetic) or nicotinic (sympathetic and motor) innervation is predominantly stimulated. Miosis (pupillary constriction) is one of the most characteristic signs and is found in almost all patients with moderately severe or severe poisoning (10% of patients fail to have miosis.) Persistence of acetylcholine at the neuromuscular junctions also results in muscular tremors, cramps, fasciculations (a very common finding), and, ultimately, muscle weakness and flaccid paralysis. (See below for central nervous system manifestations.)

Laboratory Findings

The most specific test for systemic absorption is evidence of the inhibition of cholinesterase activity of the blood. Although estimation of erythrocyte cholinesterase is theoretically preferable, since it reflects the degree of inhibition of synaptic cholinesterase, plasma cholinesterase levels are often done instead because the measurement is simpler and more accurate. In acute poisoning, manifestations occur only after more than 50% of serum cholinesterase is inhibited, and the severity of manifestations parallels the degree of remaining serum cholinesterase activity: 20–50% of normal in mild poisoning, 10–20% of normal in moderately severe poisoning, and less than 10% in severe poisoning. This is pertinent only for cases of acute poisoning, since inhibition of serum cholinesterase activity remains even after clinical signs of the illness have disappeared. This lag period may be up to four weeks in duration.

Neuropsychiatric Features

In 1961, Gershon and Shaw reported on 16 patients with psychiatric sequelae subsequent to prolonged exposure to organophosphate insecticides. These patients displayed a variety of minor signs and symptoms, such as insomnia, anxiety, restlessness, irritability, and lethargy; they also displayed symptoms of disorientation, hallucinations, and delusions. Seven of the patients were diagnosed as depressed and five as schizophrenic, even though a predominant finding in all of them was impaired recent memory and ability to concentrate. Eleven of the group had classical systemic signs and symptoms of acute poisoning.

This report stimulated much interest and controversy over the theoretical and practical ramifications of organophosphate use. Gershon and Shaw (1961) felt that insecticide exposure "activated a tendency towards depression or schizophrenic reactions." They pointed to the early reports of activation of psychosis among schizophrenics and manic-depressive patients resulting from administration of diisopropyl fluorophosphonate (Dyflos), an irreversible cholinesterase inhibitor (Rowntree et al., 1950). Since that report, Janowsky et al. (1973) have shown that physostigmine (a centrally acting acetylcholinesterase inhibitor) produces definite effects in manic-depressive and schizophrenic patients. The effects, however, are in the direction of more inhibition, lethargy, and depression rather than psychosis activation. Gershon and Shaw wondered whether there was a higher incidence of psychiatric disorders in fruit-growing regions, but epidemiologic surveys have thus far failed to confirm this speculation (Stoller et al., 1965).

It is clear that acute organophosphate poisoning can cause giddiness, tension, anxiety, restlessness, and emotional lability, as well as insomnia and excessive dreaming (Biskind and Mobbs, 1972; Namba et al., 1971; Grob and Harvey, 1953). The use of dimpylate (Diazinon) by professional exterminators has led to outbreaks of nausea, vomiting, headache, respiratory distress, visual disturbances, extreme lethargy, myalgias, and mental confusion among hospital personnel. Extensive exposure can precipitate depression, impairment of concentration, and confusion. All of these changes have been experimentally produced in normal subjects by administration of anticholinesterase agents (Bowers et al., 1964; Janowsky et al., 1973; Janowsky et al., 1972).

Confusion is a common manifestation among the reported cases of organic-phosphorus poisoning. Patients may fail to seek medical help for a condition that might otherwise alarm them, may fail to take medical advice, or may be argumentative or passively euphoric. In one case, a pilot who lived through a crash reported that he had seen the obstacle he struck but just did not care (Durham et al., 1965). Redhead (1968) described a farm worker who had lost control of his tractor and ran into a dike, but who attributed the accident to a mechanical fault of the machine.

Impairment of memory appears to be common and occasionally dominates the clinical syndrome. In one well-described case of organophosphate-induced psychosis, the patient, a 43-year-old farm hand, displayed increasing difficulty in remembering minor events, such as where he had placed his boots the previous evening and which tasks he had or had not completed the day before (Conyers and Goldsmith, 1971). The patient became more irritable and memory difficulties increased until he was disoriented as to place and time. Hospitalization was followed by diagnosis of organophosphate poisoning on the basis of reduced serum cholinesterase content.

In this case of toxic psychosis, no other systemic signs were noted. This appears to be a rare occurrence. Although Redhead (1968) also reported a case in which only psychiatric symptoms were present, Durham et al. (1965), in a study of 187 cases of suspected organic-phosphorus poisoning, noted no cases in which mental symptoms were present in the complete absence of physical signs or symptoms of illness.

Despondency and depression with suicidal intent are common clinical findings that have also been precipitated experimentally. Taylor (1974) reported three suicides in 100 cases of pesticide poisoning. The number of suicide and homicide cases among figures reported at a national level is particularly striking. In Finland, (Toivonen et al., 1959) over a six-year period, organophosphate-insecticide poisoning was associated with 237 suicides and 7 homicides; in Denmark (Frost and Paulsen, 1964), during a six-year period with 263 suicides and 4 homicides; and in Japan, over a 17-year period (1953 to 1969), 9405 suicides or homicides as well as 10,031 accidents were reported. In Dade County, Florida, between 1956 and 1967, 27 suicides, 24 accidents, and 11 homicides were reported associated with pesticide poisoning (Reich et al., 1968).

The psychiatric effects of organophosphate poisoning appear to be transient if there is no continued exposure, though some complaints may persist for prolonged periods. The most common complaints are irritability, nervousness, fatigue, lethargy, and some memory impairment for several weeks following termination of exposure. Tabershaw and Cooper (1966) reported that 10 of 114 subjects experienced neuropsychiatric manifestations lasting more than six months. Only one of these had to be hospitalized for psychiatric reasons.

The question of the psychiatric status of workers chronically exposed to organophosphate compounds has also been addressed. Dille and Smith (1964) reported two cases, both aerial applicator pilots, who seemed to present typical chronic psychiatric symptoms. They maintain that chronic exposure is associated with anxiety, uneasiness, giddiness, insomnia, somnabulism, lassitude, drowsiness, emotional lability, depressive feelings, poor work performance, and a variety of minor neurologic symptoms such as paresthesias and muscle weakness. Levin et al. (1976) in assessing psychiatric manifestations of organophosphate compounds, found that commercial sprayers showed higher levels of anxiety and lower plasma cholinesterase than did control subjects; however, exposed farmers did not show these effects.

Findings on groups examined for mental alertness have been mixed. Durham et al. (1965) found evidence of decreased mental alertness in patients with varying degrees of chronic exposure to pesticides, but did not find mental alertness affected in any patients who did not show physical signs or symptoms of illness. In an early study, Metcalf and Holmes (1969) found that 53% of chronically exposed workers complained of forgetfulness and 60% complained of irritability and impatience. Later, they found clear dysfunctions consisting of disturbed memory, difficulty in maintaining alertness, and inappropriate focusing of attention, in an exposed group compared to a control group. They found that their subjects used a variety of compensations, such as delay, avoidance, inappropriate giving up, and slowing down when taking the psychological tests. It was their impression that the exposed men showed more so called "soft" neurologic signs, such as minor coordination deficits and ocular motor imbalance. However, Rodnitzky et al. (1975) tested 23 similar subjects for abnormalities in memory, signal processing, vigilance, language, and proprioceptive feedback performance, and were unable to document differences between these subjects and a control group matched for age and educational background.

REFERENCES

Adamson JS, Flanigan WJ, Ackerman GL: Treatment of bromide intoxication with ethacrynic acid and mannitol diuresis. Ann Intern Med 65:749–752, 1966.

Agate JN, Buchnell M: Mercury poisoning from fingerprint photography; An occupational hazard of policemen. Lancet 2:451–454, 1949.

Baloh R, Sturm R, Green B, Glesen G: Neuropsychological effect of chronic asymptomatic increased lead absorption. Arch Neurol 32:326–330, 1975.

Benning D: Outbreak of mercury poisoning in Ohio. *Ind Med Surg* 27:354–363, 1958.

Biskind MS, Mobbs RE: Psychiatric manifestations from insecticide exposure. *JAMA* 220:1248–1250, 1972.

Blench TH, Brindle H: Fingerprint detection and mercury poisoning. *Lancet* 1:378–380, 1951.

Blume RS, MacLowry JD, Wolff SM: Limitations of chloride determination in the diagnosis of bromism. *N Eng J Med* 279:593–595, 1968.

Bowers MB, Goodman E, Sim VM: Some behavioral changes in man following anticholinesterase administration. *J Nerv Ment Dis* 138:383–389, 1964.

Browne DC, McHardy G, Edwards EW: Amebiasis: A clinical evaluation. *New Orleans Med Surg J* 102:475–481, 1950.

Buge A, Pancurel G, Poisson M, et al: Twenty cases of acute encephalopathy with myoclonia during treatment with oral bismuth salts. *Ann Med Interne* (Paris) 125:877–888, 1974.

Burns R, Thomas DW, Barron VJ: Reversal encephalopathy possibly associated with bismuth subgallate ingestion. *Br Med J* 1:220–223, 1974.

Carney MWP: Five cases of bromism. *Lancet* 2:523–524, 1971.

Carney MWP: Bromism—A clinical chameleon. *Nursing Times* 69:859–860, 1973.

Cassells DK, Dodds EC: Tetra-ethyl lead poisoning. *Br Med J* 2:681–685, 1946.

Cheatham JS, Chobot EF: The clinical diagnosis and treatment of lead encephalopathy. *South Med J* 61:529–531, 1968.

Cole M, Scheulein M, Kerwin DM: Arsenical encephalopathy due to the use of milibis. *Arch Intern Med* 117:706–711, 1966.

Conyers RJ, Goldsmith LE: A case of organophosphorus-induced psychosis. *Med J Aust* 58:27–29, 1971.

Crutcher JC: Clincial manifestations and therapy of acute lead intoxication due to the ingestion of illicitly distilled alcohol. *Ann Intern Med* 59:707–715, 1963.

Dille JR, Smith TW: Central nervous system effects of chronic exposure to organophosphate insecticides. *Aerosp Med* 35:475–478, 1964.

Durham WF, Wolfe HR, Quinby GE: Organophosphorus insecticides and mental alertness. *Arch Environ Health* 10:55–66, 1965.

Ewing JA, Grant WJ: The bromide hazard. *South Med J* 58:148–152, 1965.

Felton JS, Kahn E, Salick B, et al. Heavy metal poisoning: Mercury and lead. *Ann Intern Med* 76:779–792, 1972.

Fischbein A, Rice C, Sarkozi L, Kon SH, Petrocci M, Selikoff IJ: Exposure to lead in firing ranges. *JAMA* 241:1141–1144, 1979.

Frank G: Neurologische und psychiarische folgesymptomie bei akuter arsen-wasserstoff-vergiftung. *J Neurol* 70:213–259, 1976.

Freeman JA: Mercurial disease among hatters. *Trans NJ State Med Soc* 61:64, 1860.

Freeman JW, Couch JR: Prolonged encephalopathy with arsenic poisoning. *Neurology* 28:853–855, 1978.

Frost J, Paulsen E: Poisoning due to parathion and other organophosphorous insecticides in Denmark. *Dan Med Bull* 11:169–173, 1964.

Gastaut JL, Tassinari CA, Terzano G, et al: Etude polygraphique de l'ence thalopathie myoclonique bismuthique. *Revue EEG at Neurophysiologie Clinique* 3:295–302, 1975.

Gershon S, Shaw FH: Psychiatric sequelae of chronic exposure to organophosphorus insecticides. *Lancet* 1:1371–1374, 1961.

Gowdy JM, Demers FX: Whole blood mercury levels in mental hospital patients. *Am J Psychiatry* 135:115–117, 1978.

Gowdy JM, Demers FX, Yates RL: Blood mercury levels in a hospitalized urban population. *J Sci Total Environ* (in press).

Grob D, Harvey A: The effects and treatment of nerve gas poisoning. *Am J Med* 14:52–63, 1953.

Hanes FM, Yates A: An analysis of four hundred instances of chronic bromide intoxication. *South Med J* 31:667–671, 1938.

Harvey SC: Heavy metals, in Goodman LS, Gilman W (eds): *The Pharmacological Basis of Therapeutics*, ed 4. New York, MacMillan Co., 1970, p 967.

Harvey SC: Heavy metals, in Goodman LS, Gilman W (eds): *The Pharmacological Basis of Therapeutics*, ed 5. New York, MacMillan Co., 1975, pp 924–928.

Hunter D: Industrial poisoning: V. Mercury. *Brit Encyclopedia of Medical Practice* 12:139–140, London, Butterworth, 1939.

Janowsky DS, El-Yousef MK, Davis JM, et al: A cholinergic–adrenergic hypothesis of mania and depression. *Lancet* 2:632–635, 1972.

Janowsky DS, El-Yousef MK, Davis JM, et al. Antagonistic effects of physostigmine and methylphenidate in man. *Am J Psychiatry* 130:1370–1376, 1973.

Jenkins RB: Inorganic arsenic and the nervous system. *Brain* 89:479–498, 1966.

Krüger G, Thomas DJ: Disturbed oxidative metabolism in organic brain syndrome caused by bismuth in skin creams. *Lancet* 4:485–487, 1976.

Law WR, Nelson ER: Gasoline sniffing by an adult: Report of a case with the unusual complication of lead encephalopathy. *JAMA* 204:1002–1004, 1968.

Levin HS, Rodnitzky RL, Mick DL: Anxiety associated with exposure to organophosphate compounds. *Arch Gen Psychiatry* 33:225–228, 1976.

Levin M: Bromide psychosis: Four varieties. *Am J Psychiatry* 104:798–800, 1948.

McDanal CE, Owens D, Bolman WM: Bromide abuse: A continuing problem. *Am J Psychiatry* 131:913–915, 1974.

Maghazaji HI: Psychiatric aspects of methyl mercury poisoning. *J Neurol Neurosurg Psychiatry* 37:954–958, 1974.

Metcalf DR, Holmes JH: EEG, psychological and neurological alterations in humans with organophosphate exposure. *Ann NY Acad Sci* 160:357–365, 1969.

Miller G, Chamberlain R, McCormack WM: An outbreak of neuromyasthenia in a Kentucky factory—the possible role of a brief exposure to organic mercury. *Am J Epidemiol* 86:756–764, 1967.

Monseu G, Struelens M, Roland M: Bismuth encephalopathy. *Acta Neurol Belg* 76:301–308, 1976.

Morgan JM, Oh Sj, Linn GE: Lead neuropathy in alcoholics. *Ala J Med Sci* 8:67–74, 1971.

Morris CE, Heyman A, Pozefsky T: Lead encephalopathy caused by ingestion of illicitly distilled whiskey. *Neurology* 14:493–499, 1964.

Muller DJ: Bromide intoxication continues to occur. *Tex Med* 64:72–73, 1968.

Namba T, Nolte CT, Jackrel J, et al: Poisoning due to organophosphate insecticides: Acute and chronic manifestations. *Am J Med* 50:475–492, 1971.

Neal PA, Jones RR: Chronic mercurialism in the hatters' fur-cutting industry. *JAMA* 110:337–342, 1938.

Needleman HL, Scanlon J: Getting the lead out. *N Engl J Med* 288:466–467, 1973.

Okinaka S, Yoshikawa M, Mozai T, et al: Encephalomyelopathy due to an organic mercury compound. *Neurology* 14:69–76, 1964.

Palatucci DM: Paradoxical halide levels in bromide intoxication. *Neurology* 28:1189–1191, 1978.

Pearlstein MA, Attala R: Neurologic sequelae of plumbism in children. *Clin Pediatr* 5:292–294, 1966.

Perkins HA: Bromide intoxication. *Arch Intern Med* 85:783–794, 1950.

Pleasure JR, Blackburn MG: Neonatal bromide intoxication: Prenatal ingestion of a large quantity of bromides with transplacental accumulation in the fetus. *Pediatrics* 55:503–506, 1975.

Poskanzer DC: Heavy metals, in Thorn GW, Adams RD, Braunwald E, et al (eds): *Harrison's Principles of Internal Medicine*, ed 8. New York, McGraw–Hill, 1977, p 706.

Raskind MA, Kitchell M, Alvarez C: Bromide intoxication in the elderly. *J Am Geriatr Soc* 26:222–224, 1978.

RedHead IH: Poisoning on the farm. *Lancet* 1:686–687, 1968.

Reich GA, Davis JH, Davis JE: Pesticide poisoning in South Florida. *Arch Environ Health (Chicago)* 17:768–771, 1968.

Reick RR: Chronic bromide intoxication. *Minn Med* 54:995–996, 1971.

Repko JD, Corum CR: Critical review and evaluation of the neurologic behavioral sequelae of inorganic lead absorption. *Crit Rev Toxicol* 6:135–187, 1979.

Robertson JF: Mental illness or metal illness? Bismuth subgallate. *Med J Aust* 1:887–888, 1974a.

Robertson JF: Comments: Bismuth subgallate poisoning. *Med J Aust* 2:648–649, 1974b.

Rodnitzky RL, Levin MS, Mick DL: Occupational exposure to organophosphate pesticides. *Arch Environ Health* 30:98–103, 1975.

Rollins RL, Cefalu SJ: Bromide ingestion in alcoholics. *NC Med J* 29:342–343, 1968.

Ross WD, Gechman AS, Sholiton MC, et al: Need for alertness to neuropsychiatric manifestations of inorganic mercury poisoning. *Compr Psychiatry* 18:595–599, 1977.

Rowntree DW, Nevin S, Wilson A: The effects of diisopropylfluorophosphonate in schizophrenia and manic-depressive psychosis. *J Neurol Neurosurg Psychiatry* 13:472–478, 1950.

Sanders LW: Tetraethyl lead intoxication. *Arch Environ Health* 8:270–277, 1964.

Schenk VW, Stolk PJ: Psychosis following arsenic (possible thallium) poisoning. *Psychiatr Neurol Neurochir* 70:31–37, 1967.

Segal I, Saffer D, Segal F: Diverse neurologic manifestations of lead encephalopathy. *S Afr Med J* 48:1721–1722, 1974.

Serpe SJ: Bromide intoxication. *New York State J Med* 72:2086–2088, 1972. Sharpless SK: Hypnotics and sedatives. II. Miscellaneous agents, in Goodman LS, Gilman A (eds): *The Pharmacological Basis of Therapeutics*, ed 4. New York, Macmillan Co., 1970, pp 121–123.

Snyder RD: The involuntary movements of chronic mercury poisoning. *Arch Neurol* 26:379–381, 1972.

Stoller A, Krupinski J, Christophers AJ, et al: Organophosphorus insecticides and major mental illness. *Lancet* 1:1387–1388, 1965.

Study Group of Minamata Disease: *Minamata Disease*, Kumamoto University, Kumamoto, Japan, 1968.

Supino-Viterbo V, Sicard C, Riszegliato M, et al: Toxic encephalopathy due to ingestion of bismuth salts: Clinical and EEG studies of 45 patients. *J Neurol Neurosurg Psychiatry* 40:748–752, 1977.

Tabershaw JR, Cooper WC: Sequelae of acute organic phosphate poisoning. *J Occup Med* 8:5–8, 1966.

Taylor CC: Chemical toxicity in mental disorder. *Am J Psychiatry* 131:609, 1974.

Toivonen T, Ohela K, Kaipain WJ: Parathion poisoning. Increasing frequently in Finland. *Lancet* 2:175, 1959.

Trump DL, Hochberg MC: Bromide intoxication. *Johns Hopkins Med J* 138:119–123, 1976.

Victor M, Adams RD, Collins GH: *The Wernicke–Korsakoff Syndrome*. Philadelphia, Davis, 1971.

Wilkinson P, Horvath TB, Santamaria JN, et al: Bromism in association with alcoholism: A report of 5 cases. *Med J Aust* 1:1352–1355, 1969.

Wuth O: Rational bromide treatment. *JAMA* 88:2013–2017, 1927.

14

Skin Disorders

There is no substantial body of literature describing dermatologic conditions with neuropsychiatric manifestations that could lead to misdiagnosis. Much has been written, however, about psychosomatic skin disorders in which authors espouse emotional *etiologies* for these conditions. It is important that physicians maintain a balanced perspective when dealing with disorders that have no readily apparent etiology, especially if they occur in emotionally unstable patients.

In his book, *Psychophysiological Aspects of Skin Disease*, Whitlock (1976) pleads for a more objective and rigorously controlled approach to the study of "psychosomatic" cutaneous disorders. He is justifiably critical of writers who "were content to indulge in generalizations, to draw rather far-reaching conclusions from a limited number of cases, or to make dogmatic statements unsupported by tested and testable investigations." He further cautions psychiatrists and psychologists that unless they keep abreast of recent advances in dermatology they will continue to make statements and draw conclusions that are at variance with the facts. It is refreshing to read his comment that one author "who contributed heavily to writings on psychosomatic dermatology, seems to have proceeded on the basis that controls to establish the validity of claims are little more than a passing fancy of experimental purists."

On the other hand, it is quite clear that the skin can be altered in response to emotional factors—blushing and sweating are obvious examples—and that emotional events can trigger exacerbations of a number of dermatologic conditions. It would be presumptuous, however, to assume that a rash is of "psychological" etiology merely because no readily apparent "organic" cause can be found.

Finally, it is well to remember that at least one aspect of beauty *is* only skin deep and that physical appearance is often a major source of self-esteem. Disfigurement can certainly *cause* a wide variety of severe emotional reactions that may be further compounded by the associated discomfort from pain and/or itching.

BURN DELIRIUM

A serious burn is a major injury that involves not only the skin but also alters fluid–electrolyte balance, predisposes to sepsis, and causes respiratory, cardiac, renal, gastrointestinal, and central nervous system dysfunction. Although the reported incidence of neuropsychiatric burn complications varies widely, their occurrence is felt to be common. Andreasen (1974) reports that of all adults with burns, 20% develop severe depression, 30% delirium, and 20% severe regression. On the other hand, Sevitt (in Haynes and Bright, 1967) found only one case of "encephalitis" among several thousand burn patients. Factors accounting for this variability include (1) the definition of neuropsychiatric complications, (2) frequency, duration, and depth of evaluation, and (3) patient variables.

Individuals predisposed to burns are likely to have one or more of the following characteristics: Drug abuse (especially alcohol), advanced age, chronic neurological disease, chronic mental illness, and degenerative vascular disease (MacArthur and Moore, 1975). Given such factors, it is apparent that "the soil is fertile" for the development of postburn neuropsychiatric complications.

Clinical Findings

The burn patient can manifest a spectrum of neuropsychiatric difficulties that range from unequivocally neurological (seizures, coma, hemiplegia) to those that are generally considered psychological (anxiety, depression, hostility). There is a broad middle ground, however, where no clear-cut distinction can be made, owing to a blending of the "organic" and "psychological." Andreasen et al. (1972) describe two forms of initial emotional response to burns, both of which suggest such a blend. The first is a "calm, dream-like state" in which the patient may talk lucidly but later have no recall of the conversation. The other is an "acute traumatic reaction" consisting of insomnia, emotional lability, exaggerated startle response, and nightmares.

Terms which have been used to describe central nervous system manifestations of burns include, (1) burn coma, (2) burn encephalopathy, and (3) burn delirium (all of which seem to represent the same entity). Haynes and Bright (1967) reported 10 cases of "burn coma" which were characterized by varying severity of coma, slurred speech, muscular incoordination, nystagmus, and ataxia. Symptoms began with lethargy between postburn day 9 and 23, and were associated with extensive burns (21–54% second and third degree). Generalized rather than focal findings were present on neurological examination, and the electroencephalogram (EEG) showed diffuse slowing compatible with a "toxic metabolic encephalopathy." Onset of the syndrome correlated with gram-negative sepsis and recovery was complete without neurological residua.

Andreasen et al. (1977) studied 10 severely burned patients and found a 70% incidence of cognitive and neurological abnormalities (burn delirium) and 90% incidence of EEG abnormalities. The EEG was usually abnormal prior to the appearance of clinical symptoms of delirium and was felt to be possibly of predictive value.

Electroencephalogram

The most common EEG abnormality found in the burn patient is diffuse nonspecific slow waves. In 49 recordings done in 40 acutely burned patients, Hughes et al. (1975) found slow wave abnormalities in 88%. Epileptiform activity was present in 8.2% (but only one of these four patients had seizures). They found a relationship between EEG abnormality and total body surface burned and time after burn. The EEG abnormalities were maximal 3–11 days after the injury.

When EEGs were done on 27 chronic burn patients (following discharge from the burn unit) who had been selected on the basis of persistent seizures (17 patients) or persistent cognitive behavioral disturbances (10 patients), all had abnormal tracings (82% slow wave, 41% epileptiform activity).

Petersén et al (1965) studied 58 acute and chronic burn patients and found a 67% incidence of EEG abnormality. If the total body surface burned was greater than 40%, all EEGs were abnormal.

While the EEG appears to have merit in the evaluation of neuropsychiatric burn complications, prospective studies are not yet available. Smith (in Haynes and Bright, 1967) mentioned that doing an EEG during the first 24 to 72 hr was routine in all his burn patients, and that of the first 27, 7 were abnormal. Whether the detection of an abnormal EEG in the acute phase of a burn will alter the treatment regimen or whether it will be of long-term prognostic value remain to be determined. It should be useful in differentiating between the restlessness of an anxiety reaction and that of an emerging delirium.

Relationship of Delirium to Severity of Burn

In general, there is a direct correlation between the extent and severity of burn, the severity of the neuropsychiatric disturbance, and the EEG abnormality. A patient with a less serious burn does not appear to be immune, however, as there have been reports of neurological complications following "trivial" burns (Emery and Reid, 1962).

Onset of Symptoms

Although neuropsychiatric manifestations tend to be more common during the first days following injury, they can appear at almost any time.

Emery and Reid (1962) described symptoms of burn encephalitis first appearing between postburn days 10–30 and, as mentioned earlier, Haynes and Bright (1967) noted the onset of "burn coma" between days 9–23. In fact, Lindsay et al. (1965) mentioned one severely burned pateint who developed seizures 33 days later and subsequently lapsed into a coma and died.

Significance of Burn Delirium

Although burn delirium has been described as a benign condition, with full recovery of cognitive function after physical recovery (Andreasen et al., 1972), this is not always the case (Antoon et al., 1972; Hughes et al., 1975; Andreasen et al., 1977). Andreasen et al. (1974) described two severely burned patients with residual CNS deficits. The first patient had persistent memory problems with associated EEG abnormalities and psychometric testing indicative of an organic brain syndrome. One year postburn, the second patient had complaints of "apathy, excessive drowsiness, anxiety, depression, irritability, sexual impotence, and memory disturbance." Both EEG and psychometric testing were indicative of an organic brain syndrome. The authors concluded that "burn encephalopathy may persist in mild form after full physical recovery of patients who survive massive burns." The more subtle forms of these persistent deficits may easily be mistaken for emotional reactivity, and it is suggested that the EEG and psychometric testing be employed to aid in the differential diagnosis. Confirming the persistence of organicity will have major implications regarding course of treatment, prognosis, and economic settlement.

Etiology of Burn Delirium

Although a burn is primarily an insult to the body surface, other organ systems may be directly or indirectly involved, and it is this secondary involvement that is responsible for the delirium.

The concept that burned tissue produces a toxic substance ("burn toxin") which circulates throughout the body causing widespread damage remains controversial. The early experiments of Hughes and Cayaffa (1973), showing that healthy dogs died after cross-circulation with burned dogs, suggested the presence of a "toxin," but such a substance has not yet been identified.

It is unrealistic to expect a single factor to be responsible for all the cases of burn delirium. In fact, even in individual cases, there are usually a number of factors that can be incriminated; hence, a multifactorial etiology seems the rule rather than the exception.

Complications of burns that might play a role in the etiology of burn delirium are shown in Table 14-1.

TABLE 14-1.   Factors which May Play a Role in Burn Delirium

1. Burn "toxin"
2. Hemoconcentration or hemodilution
3. Electrolyte imbalance
4. Cerebral edema
5. Respiratory insufficiency (airway burn; carbon monoxide poisoning)
6. Infection (especially gram negative)
7. Fever
8. Renal failure
9. Cardiovascular insufficiency
10. Drug toxicity (analgesics, antibiotics, etc.)
11. Pre-existing medical or psychiatric disorders

Treatment

As with any delirium, treatment is directed at correcting causative factors. If these cannot be identified or are not correctable, then treatment must be symptomatic, using appropriate psychotropic drugs and supportive measures.

In a series of ten patients, Haynes and Bright (1967) found that skin homografting played a major role in the reversal of burn coma, and Andreasen et al. (1972) felt that delirium was uncommon after grafting was complete. Restoration of body surface integrity appears to be quite important in the prevention or correction of burn delirium.

PSYCHOTROPIC DRUG-INDUCED DERMATOLOGIC DISORDERS

Quite a variety of cutaneous reactions have been reported in association with the use of psychiatric drugs. It is fortunate that such reactions are relatively uncommon. In addition, it is often not possible to establish a firm cause-and-effect relationship between the drug and cutaneous change so that the true incidence of such reactions cannot be accurately determined. Table 14-2 is based, to a large extent, on information provided by Bruinsma (1973), but with modifications dictated by a review of more recent literature. It is important that this table serve as a guide rather than as a source of absolutes, and that it not be a substitute for applying keen clinical judgment to individual cases.

There is a rough relationship between the extent of a drug's use and the number of reported side effects. Consequently, only time can resolve the issue of whether a low incidence of cutaneous reactions in the newer drugs is an inherent characteristic of the drugs or due to their more limited use.

Cross-reactivity among psychotropic drugs within the same chemical class is a subject that has not been widely studied. It is generally accepted that the more similar in structure, the more likely drugs are to cross-react.

TABLE 14-2. Cutaneous Reactions to Psychotropic Drugs[a,b]

	Rash	Urticaria	Alopecia	Pigmentation	Acne or acne-like	Fixed drug eruption	Increased sweating	Toxic epidermal necrolysis	Erythema multiforme Stevens–Johnson syndrome	Paresthesias, Pruritus	Eczematous eruption	Purpura	Edema	Photosensitivity
Antipsychotics														
Phenothiazines[c]	+	+	√	√					√?	√	√	√	√	√
Thioxanthenes	+	+								√				√
Butyrophenones	+	+			√					√			√	√
Dibenzoxazepines[c]	+													
Dihydroindolones	+													
Antidepressants—Tricyclic														
Amitriptyline	+	+					√			√			√	√
Imipramine	+	+					√			√				√
Doxepin	+	+					√			√			√	√
Desipramine	+	+					√			√			√	√
Nortriptyline	+						√			√				
Protriptyline	+	+					√			√				√

Antidepressants—MAOI
  Isocarboxizid
  Phenelzine
  Tranylcypromine
Antianxiety—Benzodiazepine
  Chlordiazepoxide
  Diazepam
  Oxazepam
Sedative—Hypnotic
  Barbiturates
  Chloralhydrate
  Glutethimide
  Meprobamate
Other
  Lithium[d]
  Amphetamines

[a] Modified from Bruinsma (1973) with permission of author and publisher.
[b] ++++, Common; +++, may occur; ++, unusual; +, rare.
[c] Also seborrheic dermatitis.
[d] May aggravate psoriasis.

Consequently, in the event of an allergic reaction, especially if it is severe, substituting a structurally dissimilar drug is advised. This option, fortunately, is becoming more and more available with the continued development of newer psychotropic agents.

REFERENCES

Andreasen NJC: Neuropsychiatric complications in burn patients. Int J Psychiatr Med 5:161–171, 1974.

Andreasen NJC, Hartford CE, Knott JR, et al: Cerebral deficits after burn encephalopathy. N Engl J Med 290:1487–1488, 1974.

Andreasen NJC, Hartford CE, Knott JR, et al: EEG changes associated with burn delirium. Dis Nerv Syst 38:27–31, 1977.

Andreasen NJC, Noyes R, Hartford CE, et al: Management of emotional reactions in seriously burned adults. N Engl J Med 286:65–69, 1972.

Antoon AY, Volpe JJ, Crawford JD: Burn encephalopathy in children. Pediatrics 50: 609–616, 1972.

Bruinsma W: A Guide to Drug Eruptions. Amsterdam, Excerpta Medica, 1973.

Emery JL, Reid DAC: Cerebral oedema and spastic hemiplegia following minor burns in young children. Br J Surg 50:53–56, 1962.

Haynes BW, Bright R: Burn coma: A syndrome associated with severe burn wound infection. J Trauma 7:464–475, 1967.

Hughes JR, Cayaffa JJ: Seizures following burns of the skin. Dis Nerv Syst 34:203–211, 1973.

Hughes JR, Cayaffa JJ, Boswick JA: Seizures following burns of the skin: III. Electroencephalographic recordings. Dis Nerv Syst 36:443–447, 1975.

Lindsay WK, Murphy EG, Birdsell DC: Thermal burn encephalopathy. Can J Surg 8:165–171, 1965.

MacArthur JD, Moore FD: Epidemiology of burns, the burn-prone patient. JAMA 231:259–263, 1975.

Petersén I, Sorbye R, Johanson B, et al: An electroencephalographic and psychiatric study of burn cases. Acta Chir Scand 129:359–366, 1965.

Whitlock FA: Psychophysiological Aspects of Skin Disease. London, WB Saunders, 1976.

Reproductive and Sexual Function Disorders

PREMENSTRUAL SYNDROME

Women and clinicians have long been aware of changes in mental and physical states related to the menstrual cycle. These changes, first described by Frank (1931) as premenstrual feelings consisting of "indescribable tension, irritability," and "a desire to find relief by foolish and ill-considered actions," came to be called the premenstrual tension syndrome. Since tension is only one of the components occurring during this period, the term "premenstrual syndrome" is currently preferred, since it more completely encompasses somatic and psychological components. A recent review (Steiner and Carroll, 1977) offers "premenstrual dysphoria" as an alternative term.

Menstrual Cycle Hormonal Changes

The recurrent cyclical processes of ovulation and menstruation are caused by a complex interaction of the hypothalamus, pituitary gland, ovary, and adrenal cortex. Broadly, the process is as follows. During the preovulatory phase of the menstrual cycle, hypothalamic releasing factor causes the anterior pituitary to produce follicle-stimulating hormone (FSH). FSH causes development of the ovarian follicles, which produce constant estrogen secretion during this phase. Estrogen secretion rises to a peak at midcycle when, through a hypothalamic feedback mechanism, luteinizing hormone (LH) is released together with a peak of FSH release. The ovum is released from the follicle, which under the influence of LH, is then converted to a corpus luteum, which secretes progesterone. This is termed the luteal phase of the cycle. If fertilization of the ovum has not occurred, progesterone secretion begins to decrease about six days prior to menstruation. Estrogen secretion also falls at approximately the same time. Prolactin is felt to be important in this process, but the exact mechanism is not understood. Evidence at this time seems to indicate that at least some women have higher plasma prolactin levels during the luteal phase of the cycle than during the follicular phase and that these high levels are maintained until the onset of menstruation. During the menstrual cycle, there are phasic changes also in the secretions of ACTH and cortisol, mineralocorticoids, and androgens from the adrenal gland and the ovary.

Clinical Features

The incidence of the syndrome depends, to a large extent, on the definition used. Reports have varied from finding 25–100% of women experiencing some symptoms (Coppen and Kessel, 1963; Brown-Parlee, 1973). Symptoms usually begin 2–12 days before menstruation; although most symptoms commonly occur in the premenstrual phase, they may occur with ovulation, in the early part of the menstrual phase, or even 1–2 days after flow has ceased (Greene and Dalton, 1953). Rees (1953) found that in 85% of his patients the symptoms were relieved by menstruation. Most authors feel that the symptoms making up the premenstrual syndrome can be readily distinguished from dysmenorrhea (painful menses). The two conditions may occur together but are not strongly associated.

The clinical dimensions of the syndrome have always been broad. It is considered among the commonest of the minor endocrine disorders, and a large number of women suffer many of the symptoms, which are unpleasant in the mildest forms and near incapacitating at worst. A commonly used description is that of Rees (1953), and includes "nervous tension, irritability, anxiety, depression, bloated feeling of the abdomen, swelling of the fingers and legs, itching and tightness of the skin, headaches, dizziness, and palpitations." Less common symptoms noted by Rees were hypersomnia, excessive thirst, increased appetite, and increased sexual desire. He also described an increased tendency for psychosomatic disorders, such as asthma, migraine, rhinitis, and angioneurotic edema to occur during this period. Dalton, in 1964, listed an equally wide range of symptoms and emphasized the major psychological symptoms of irritability, depression, and lethargy. In a large study, Moos (1969b) attempted to bring more order to the group of commonly reported symptoms by identifying eight major clusters: pain, inability to concentrate, behavior change, autonomic reactions, water retention, negative affect, arousal, and one group of nonspecific symptoms. He suggests that the syndrome might more appropriately be labeled the "premenstrual syndromes."

Neuropsychiatric Features

From a neuropsychiatric viewpoint, the negative affects associated with the premenstrual syndrome may be of most interest. They have been variously described as irritability, depression, sadness, anxiety, lethargy, tear-fulness, impatience, restlessness, and tension, and are lumped together in most studies (Sletten and Gershon, 1966; Morton, 1950; Janowsky et al., 1967; Gregory, 1957; Dalton, 1964). Smith (1975) felt that "the totality of the literature leaves it beyond doubt that there exists in many women (probably between one-third and three-fourths) the tendency to suffer negative affective changes." Cullberg (1972) felt that two groups could be defined, one with premenstrual irritability and one with depression.

From a clinical standpoint, the depressive component is often more prominent. Perhaps Dalton's (1971) description of premenstrual depression is most striking.

> The mood changes are short lived, the depression lasting only a few days at a time with improvement, often abrupt, occurring during menstruation. But the depth of depression may be extreme, reaching suicidal level, or a temporary psychosis may develop. Depression is accompanied by tension, irritability with aggression which may result in a battered baby or bruised husband, and lethargy, both mental and physical.

Smith (1975) summed up the studies that have specifically examined depression by stating that premenstrual depression does not now fit accurately into any of the current depressive classifications. In general, there seem to be fewer vegetative signs, and less likelihood of early morning sleep disturbance and diurnal mood variation. It more closely resembles a neurotic depressive picture.

The line between "normal" and pathological is, of course, vague and arbitrary. Wetzel et al. (1975), in a followup study of females with premenstrual affective symptoms, found that 18% sought help for affective disorders during a four year period. Supporting this, Kashiwagi et al. (1976), found a definitely increased prevalence of premenstrual mood change in women with primary affective disorders compared to a control group of women with hysteria or anxiety neuroses. A number of authors have described cases of recurrent severe depression exacerbated during the premenstrual period (Heggarty, 1955; Dalton, 1959; Janowsky et al. 1966). McClure et al. (1971) noted that a number of females with premenstrual mood elevations were found to have personal and family histories of bipolar affective disorders. He also noted bipolar symptoms in some women with premenstrual mood changes. Williams and Weekes (1952) related premenstrual symptoms to manic and catatonic states.

Because negative affect changes are extensive for some women in the late luteal phase of the menstrual cycle, some attention has been paid to the effect of these changes on cognitive functioning. Studies indicate that a small percentage (8–16%) of women (by self report) feel that their judgmental or mental faculties are impaired to some extent in the premenstrual phase of their menstrual cycle (Morton et al., 1953; Moos, 1968b). However, Sommer (1973), in a comprehensive review, pointed out that objective performance measures in most studies failed to demonstrate changes related to the menses cycle. As Smith (1975) noted, "the performance-versus-affect distinction is vital, since the existence of premenstrual negative affect can be and has been used to disparage women as a group and deny equal opportunity to females."

The same caution is necessary in interpreting the many studies showing that social behaviors are also influenced by menstrual periodicity. In one study, 45% of females reporting sick in a factory were one to three days premenstrual or were menstruating (Dalton, 1964). Others found an increased incidence of crimes of violence committed during the premenstrual week (Ribeiro, 1962; Cooke, 1945; Morton, 1950). Dalton (1961) reported 49% of the crimes for which women had been imprisoned had occurred in either the four days premenstrually or within four days after the onset of menstrual flow. Other behaviors, such as taking a child to a medical clinic, loss of control of an aircraft, and increased frequency of accidents, have been reported as linked to the premenstrual period, but are rather poorly substantiated (Dalton, 1966; Whitehead, 1934; MacKinnon et al., 1959). As with the studies having to do with cognitive ability, these may all be criticized from a methodologic standpoint. Brown-Parlee (1973), in an extensive article, emphasizes the poor quality of most studies in this area, particularly those suggesting irrationality, impulsivity, or criminality to be the mark of a premenstrual or menstruating women.

In addition to the previously mentioned studies on affect, interest has focused on psychopathology that may accompany or be intensified by the premenstrual phase. Studies using indirect measurements of psychopathology include those that found increased visits to psychiatric emergency rooms during the premenstrual and early menstrual periods (Glass et al., 1971; Dalton, 1959; Jacobs and Charles, 1970) and increased admissions to a psychiatric hospital during the first four days of menstruation (Dalton, 1964). Mandell and Mandell (1967) reported increased use of a suicide prevention center phone service by women in the premenstrual and early menstrual phases. Suicide attempts and suicides have also been reported as occurring more often during these phases than would be expected statistically (Ribeiro, 1962; MacKinnon et al., 1959; Tonks et al., 1967; Mandell and Mandell, 1967).

The psychiatric literature contains scattered reports of patients with psychoses characterized by periodic exacerbation of symptoms during the premenstrual or menstrual phases (Endo et al., 1978). Although the relationship to the menstrual cycle is poorly documented in some of these cases, Endo et al. (1978) reported seven patients with psychoses regularly occurring in close association with their menstrual cycles. The psychoses began acutely during the premenstrual period and subsided rapidly after menstruation. These episodes seemed to be self-limiting, with cessation of symptoms after three to four periods of exacerbation and no residual signs, even upon extended follow up. They were characterized by marked psychomotor changes, excitement or retardation, ideas of reference or persecution, and delusions or hallucinations of an illusory, fantastic, or dreamlike nature. Although autonomic symptoms such as flushing, anorexia, and nausea were occasionally present, the authors felt that they were dealing with a primary mental illness aligned with the menstrual cycle, rather than a premenstrual tension phenomenon. Kramer (1977) added a report of a case of a menstrual psychosis in an adolescent girl with a background of temporal lobe seizures that would begin several days prior to her menstrual period and abate shortly thereafter. It is interesting to note that these patients and five others in the literature were all young, unmarried women (Ota et al., 1954; Takagi, 1959; Altschule and Brem, 1963). Endo et al. (1978), tentatively advanced the explanation that in predisposed women (teenagers with EEG abnormalities) monoamine metabolism in the CNS, fluctuating in connection with the menstrual cycle, becomes disturbed by unknown causes. These disturbances derange CNS activity, producing psychotic symptoms in the sphere of emotion and behavior.

There is also a well known correlation of menstrual periods with migraine headaches and epileptic seizures. In the former, patients appear to have characteristic migraines with a striking relationship to the premenstrual period or menstrual onset. The patients do not suggest that the relationship to menses is exclusive, but rather facilitatory. Somerville (1972) successfully treated six patients suffering from menstrually related migraines with estradiol (an estrogen), implying that an estrogen withdrawal mechanism may be significant in the etiology.

Premenstrual epilepsy is a well known condition that has been documented extensively (Laidlow, 1956; Dalton, 1964; Logothetics et al., 1959). It has been shown that epileptic seizures of all types are more frequent during the premenstrual and menstrual phases of the cycle. Though the mechanism is not known, it is tempting to speculate about increases of neuronal excitability as a possible dramatic reflection of other premenstrual phenomena.

Etiology

Thus far, a convincing explanation of premenstrual physiologic and psychologic symptoms is lacking. A detailed exploration of the various hypotheses is beyond the scope of this discussion. Two recent excellent reviews are available (Smith, 1975; Steiner and Carroll, 1977). Psychosocial factors felt to be important include individual, social, and cultural attitudes toward menses (Novell, 1965), childhood experiences, traumatic menarche (Shainess, 1962), mother–daughter relationships (Deutsch, 1944), poor self-esteem (Frank, 1931), and general neuroticism (Coppen and Kessel, 1963; Rees, 1953).

Many theories and variations of physiologic functioning have been proposed. Most of the work has focused on the ovarian hormones estrogen and progesterone. Benedek and Rubenstein (1939a,b) felt that they could demonstrate tendencies toward assertiveness in the estrogenic phase and passivity in the luteal phase (progesterone). Benedek and Rubenstein and others have postulated that these hormones cause trends that interact with existing personality traits, producing varying symptomatology. Overall, behavioral changes have been ascribed to (1) a relative deficiency of estrogens, (2) a relative deficiency of progesterones, (3) idiosyncratic sensitivity to estrogens, or (4) a withdrawal reaction to either estrogen or progesterone (Steiner and Carroll, 1977). All of these theories have advocates and some supportive laboratory evidence. There is, however, no general agreement about these basic changes. It is possible that definitional difficulties have resulted in the study of patients who constitute different subgroups of the premenstrual syndrome.

The renin–angiotensin–aldosterone system has received recent attention. Janowsky et al. (1973) suggested that emotional upheaval is caused by a complex interaction of these components with ovarian hormones that ultimately affect central nervous transmitters. However, doubt is cast on this view by the observation that premenstrual dysphoria occurs in menstrual cycles that are anovulatory, during which changes in the renin–angiotensin–aldosterone system do not occur. (This observation also tends to rule out progesterone as a major factor.)

Some workers point to high levels of plasma monoamine oxidase (MAO) action in premenstrual women, and speculate that progesterone stimulation may cause changes in MAO activity that might lead to depression in susceptible females (Claiber et al., 1971; Grant and Pryse-Davies, 1968). Several studies, however, found no significant relationship between platelet MAO activity and premenstrual mood variations (Gilmore et al., 1971; Belmaker et al., 1974). Others have suggested that the depressed affect occasionally found with oral contraceptive treatment may be related to a functional deficiency of pyridoxine, and that a similar mechanism could be the basis for premenstrual dysphoria (Rose, 1969; Winston, 1973; Herzberg et al., 1971).

Carroll and Steiner (1978) recently reviewed a number of studies providing direct and indirect evidence for an important role of prolactin in premenstrual dysphorias. Included are studies reporting occurrence of premenstrual symptoms coinciding with the late luteal elevation of plasma prolactin levels and reports that women with high premenstrual ratings of dysphoria have significantly elevated prolactin levels during the premenstruum.

Treatment

Since the interaction of the physiologic and psychologic components of the premenstrual syndrome has failed to be convincingly explained, it is not surprising that a large number of treatments have been applied, with varying effectiveness. Smith (1975) makes two important points in his review of treatments. First, no matter how incorrect the etiologic hypotheses have proven to be, most treatments have universally been claimed to work. Second, whereas uncontrolled studies have virtually all shown positive results, no matter what the treatment, adequately controlled double-blind studies frequently show negative findings.

Oral Contraceptives

Several studies have reported that women taking oral contraceptives generally have fewer premenstrual symptoms than nonusers (Paige, 1971; Moos, 1969; Kutner and Brown, 1972). Other workers have found less depression and irritability occurring in the 7- to 10-day period prior to menstruation among oral contraceptive users (Herzberg and Coppen, 1970; Herzberg et al., 1970). In a controlled study, Silbergeld et al. (1971), found premenstrual anxiety was lessened when an oral contraceptive rather than a placebo was administered.

Among studies in which women were specifically treated for premenstrual tension symptoms with oral contraceptives, the results are less clear. Hood and Bond (1959) found that premenstrual tension was relieved temporarily by oral contraceptives but not significantly relieved over a prolonged period. Cullberg (1972), in a well controlled study, felt that he had identified a small subgroup of patients with premenstrual dysphoria who were "clearly hormone dependent." Oral contraceptives that were highly estrogenic made these patients worse, whereas progestogenic oral contraceptives improved their symptoms. In summary, the administration of oral contraceptives to patients with premenstrual symptomatology is probably worth trying. If depressive side effects occur as a result of the medication, a more progestogenic oral contraceptive could be tried prior to abandoning this approach.

There have also been efforts to treat symptoms of mental illness that appear to be premenstrually exacerbated. One uncontrolled study found that 80% of psychiatric patients were improved while on an oral contraceptive (Kramp, 1968). Other, more careful studies have shown negative results (Simpson et al., 1962; Simpson et al., 1964). Kane and Keeler (1965) reported excellent results treating five postpartum psychotic patients with Enovid (norethynodrel with mestranol). Three of the five patients relapsed when a placebo was substituted for the active medication. Swanson et al. (1964) also reported using Enovid successfully in the treatment of schizophrenic patients. Janowsky et al. (1973) reported two cases of using Ortho-novum for menses suppression, with successful treatment of aggressive and assaultive psychotic features.

Synthetic and natural progestogens (progesterone) have also been claimed effective in treating the premenstrual syndrome. Controlled studies, however, have shown unimpressive results, particularly for the progestogens (Swyer, 1955; Coppen et al., 1969; Jordheim, 1972). The case for progesterone has been pushed for many years by Dalton (1964) and Rees (1953), who claim dramatic results. However, there are no carefully done supportive studies available. Several recent reports of vigorously controlled double-blind studies with patients specifically selected for premenstrual depression have found no beneficial effects attributable to progesterone treatment (Smith, 1975).

Bromocriptine

A new drug that suppresses the secretion of prolactin from the anterior pituitary has recently been developed and is being studied. Called bromocriptine, it has previously been shown to be a specific antigalactic (inhibitor of milk production) in animals and puerperal women (Billetiere and Fluckiger, 1971; Varga et al., 1972). In both open and double-blind evaluations, this drug has been shown to produce dramatic relief of several types of premenstrual symptoms—breast symptoms, edema, weight gain, and mood (Benedek-Jaszmann and Hearn-Sturtevant, 1976). The success of this drug suggests that high prolactin levels are involved in the etiology of the premenstrual tension syndrome, but further exploratory work is needed.

Lithium

Given the cyclic nature of the syndrome of premenstrual tension and the association of affective symptoms, a number of workers have attempted to treat the syndrome with lithium carbonate. Initial reports were optimistic; several different studies indicated partial to complete success (Sletten and Gershon, 1966; Fries, 1969; Tupin, 1972; Horrobin et al., 1973). Subsequent controlled studies, however, have failed to demonstrate a significant effectiveness of lithium (Mattsson and von Schoultz, 1974).

Miscellaneous

Throughout the years, a variety of other treatments have been tried, including aldosterone antagonists, diuretics, minor tranquilizers, testosterone, radiation of the ovaries, and pyridoxine as well as virtually every other vitamin (Smith, 1975). Psychotherapy has also been both praised and specifically disclaimed by numerous authors. At this point, a conjoint or adjunctive role for psychotherapy is most highly recommended.

ORAL CONTRACEPTIVES

The utilization of a drug (oral contraceptive) that could interfere with fertility became widespread in the early 1960's. The discovery of these agents came about as a result of an investigation of inhibition of ovulation by the use of progestational agents in women who failed to conceive. It was later found that estrogen enhanced the suppressive effect of progestin, which led to a mixture of these two agents (in most oral contraceptives). Many different progestins have been used; the most common estrogens used are mestranol and ethinyl estradiol. Surprisingly, the exact mechanism by which these mixtures of hormones inhibit ovulation has not been defined. In part, this is due to the diverse action of the components. For example, the orally active progestins differ from progesterone because some are inherently estrogenic, some slightly androgenic, and some purely progestational. They may also have different biologic activity at different sites, thus mediating their ovulation-inhibitory action in different manners.

Depression

Depression or dysphoric effects are common complaints among women who are taking oral contraceptives, but the contribution of these compounds to these complaints remains unclear. Astwood (1970) noted that complaints of mood and behavioral disturbance are "not surprising when one counts millions of women whose lives are punctuated daily by the taking of a medium for a condition from which they do not suffer for a contingency that may not materialize." Different mechanisms may lead to a final complaint of depressive symptomatology. Scapegoating "the pill" for emotional distress, fears of side effects or complications, and responses to symbolic meaning cannot easily be separated from effects due to the hormonal content of the medication. Research in this area is problematic. Comparison studies examining different hormonal combinations may include women who experience relief from premenstrual depressive symptoms, thus hiding subgroups of patients who have adverse reactions. Often the studies deal with samples from which women unable to tolerate drug effects have already been self removed.

A number of articles show no relationship of contraceptives to depression. In one of the larger studies, Kutner and Brown (1972) "cast doubt on the hypothesis that oral contraceptives cause depression," and found no evidence for aggravation among those with a history of depression. They did note that patients with histories of depression often tend to discontinue the drug. Goldzieher et al. (1971), in a placebo-controlled double-blind examination of various oral contraceptives, found that the placebo group did not differ from the contraceptive group in frequency of complaints of nervousness or depression. However, they did not examine the severity of the complaints. Several other studies, including those by Bakker and Dightman (1966), Murawaski (1969), Murawaski et al. (1968), and Fleming and Seager (1978), also could not find mental status changes attributable to oral contraceptives. Murawaski's group felt that women who became depressed on oral contraceptives did not do so through a direct pharmacologic effect. They suggested that the sedative-like effects often associated with a progestational component of contraceptives could be highly distressing to women with particular defense mechanisms and life styles, especially those who use compulsive activity for control and management of their lives.

The preponderance of evidence does, however, suggest a relationship between oral contraceptives and depression. Cullberg (1972), studying 320 subjects in a double-blind design, noted two separate but related factors, best called "irritability" and "insecurity." His results indicated that significantly more patients showed dysphoric responses to oral contraceptives than to the placebo. Moos (1968a) found that, although the majority of females experienced slight decreases in menstrual symptomatology, a group of approximately 10% experienced a significant increase in menstrual symptomatology, including "negative affects." Other studies noted that an overall incidence of approximately 6% of females on oral contraceptives had moderate to severe depression, while the control group figures were in the 1–2% range (Herzberg et al., 1970; Herzberg and Coppen, 1970; Lewis and Hoghughi, 1969; Glick, 1967; Nilsson and Almgren, 1968; Leeton, 1973). Kane (1968) reported a surprisingly higher figure of 34% experiencing depression in the drug group.

Several authors have commented that females taking oral contraceptives who had a prior history of depression were more likely to become depressed than a random group (Lewis and Hoghughi, 1969; Ayd, 1966). This may be a contraindication to the administration of oral contraceptives. There appears to be a trend toward more severe and lengthening periods of depression the longer the patient has been on the drug (Lewis and Hoghughi, 1969; Wearing, 1963).

There is conflicting evidence over whether predominantly progestogenic or estrogenic medications are more likely to produce dysphoric affects. Cullberg (1972) noted that the most severe responses occurred with highly estrogenic medications. The converse finding has been reported by others (Lewis and Hoghughi, 1969; Grant and Pryse-Davies, 1968). Thus, it appears that when individual susceptibility and the differing makeup of oral contraceptive medications are considered, a poor response to one medication does not necessarily mean the same response will occur with another. When contraception is desirable, a switch to a medication with a different mixture or to a lower dose drug may alleviate the problem. Occasionally, a change from the combined to the sequential variety may be helpful.

It has been speculated that depression might be caused by oral contraceptives interfering with tryptophan metabolism, with a resulting decrease in the amount of serotonin produced (Rose, 1969). It is hypothesized that this may occur by diminishing the availability of pyridoxine (vitamin B_6), a necessary component in the manufacture of serotonin. Studies which have tried to demonstrate an absolute deficiency of vitamin B_6 are conflicting (Adams et al., 1973; Davis and Smith, 1973). The use of oral pyridoxine to combat the depressive side effects of oral contraceptives is also inconclusive (Baumblatt and Winston, 1970; Stokes and Mendels, 1972). Those who do advocate the use of pyridoxine suggest daily oral administration in the 50 mg range (Winston, 1973; Malek-Ahmadi and Behrmann, 1976). The idea that neurotransmitter levels are altered in one direction in all depressions is not tenable, thus, explanations are not likely to be simple ones (Bunney et al., 1971).

In summary, there is probably insufficient evidence to label depression secondary to oral contraceptives as a separate and specific clinical entity. The clinician must be aware that some women, particularly those who may have been depressed prior to oral contraceptive administration and those with positive depressive histories, probably will respond with increased depressive symptomatology. Change of type of drug, or, if possible, discontinuance for several cycles, are useful diagnostic practices. Pyridoxine supplementation may be considered.

Psychotic Reactions

There have been scattered reports of psychoses occurring in close temporal association with oral contraceptive use. In one case, the psychosis followed withdrawal of 30 mg/day of Enovid (norethynodrel with mestranol) given for endometriosis (Keeler et al., 1964). Restarting the drug appeared to alleviate the psychosis, and substitution of a placebo intensified it. Four additional patients were reported who suffered psychotic episodes coincident with the use of oral contraceptive agents (Kane, 1968). In two instances, these were associated with the use of combined agents; the others used sequential hormone combinations. Of seven women reported as experiencing a psychosis while on oral contraceptives, four had a history of severe postpartum disturbance, and two others had had previous psychiatric illness (Marcotte et al., 1970). It is not clear whether the symptoms associated with oral contraceptive use are direct pharmacologic effects or related to psychological factors. In any case, in these situations a switch to nonhormonal methods of contraception seems indicated.

SEXUAL DYSFUNCTION (IMPOTENCE)

Tradition holds that erectile dysfunction has a psychological cause in 90% of cases. The source of this figure is unclear, and its clinical usefulness has been challenged for a number of reasons. Even if diagnosis could be known with absolute certainty, prevalence figures would have to be determined for a population that was not distorted by preselection. For example "psychogenic" impotence would be found more frequently in a sexual dysfunction clinic and "organic" impotence more often in a diabetic clinic.

In addition, one suspects that the diagnosis of psychogenic impotence is often made by the process of elimination without also establishing clear psychological determinants. The fallacy of this approach can be shown by the following illustration: Dr. A screens patients for organicity by physical examination alone; Dr. B, in addition, takes a thorough drug and alcohol history; Dr. C does all of this plus laboratory work to screen for diabetes and androgen deficiency while Dr. D is even more comprehensive. The likelihood of finding an organic cause increases with the thoroughness of the evaluation, and the incidence of "psychogenic" impotence would shrink, to approximate more closely the true incidence.

Even the most comprehensive evaluation, however, is limited by the state of knowledge extant at the time it is done. Both psychiatric and medical diagnosis were less refined in 1950 than in 1980, and prospects for further improvements in the future are bright. The goals, of course, are to minimize the likelihood of misdiagnosis, to enhance diagnostic specificity (impotence due to diabetic neuropathy is more specific than impotence found in association with diabetes), and to utilize these diagnostic refinements to develop specific, effective treatments.

Although diagnosis does serve a number of functions, clinicians and patients most highly value diagnosis for its ability to lead to appropriate treatment. The absolute incidence of "psychogenic" versus "organic" impotence in the general population is far less important than an accurate diagnosis in a particular patient. The tendency to diagnose "psychogenic" merely because "all the tests are negative" is to be condemned.

This section has two purposes. The first is to discuss the state of the art with regard to evaluating a complaint of impotence, with the hope that greater awareness of modern diagnostic techniques will decrease the incidence of presumptive diagnoses. The second is to present new findings in the area of etiology and treatment of impotence that portend an encouraging trend toward greater diagnostic specificity and treatment efficacy.

Diagnostic Evaluation of Impotence

The importance of a thorough evaluation cannot be overstated, although few centers have the time, interest, or facilities to provide one. The program developed at Baylor College of Medicine is an exception, and it is described here to provide a standard against which other programs should be compared.

As reported by Karacan et al. (1978a) and Kaya et al. (1979) an evaluation takes place over a three-day period and includes monitoring of nocturnal penile tumescence (NPT) in the Sleep Disorders Center. During a comprehensive initial interview, the presenting complaint is carefully defined; sexual, marital, family, and social history obtained; and possible medical, psychiatric, and drug-related etiologies considered. In addition to a thorough general physical examination, emphasis is placed on neurological and vascular evaluation. Penile blood pressures and pulses are recorded using special instruments and compared with findings elsewhere in the body. Finally, the external genitalia are carefully examined and measurements of the flaccid penis are recorded. When indicated, a more extensive urological examination is performed, which may include urodynamic studies to evaluate bladder function.

The patient is interviewed by a psychiatrist for several reasons: (1) to provide an independent evaluation of the cause of the impotence, (2) to evaluate psychological stresses occurring secondary to the impotence, (3) to assess for intrapersonal, marital, or social psychopathology, and (4) to assess for suitability for various treatment approaches. The patient also undergoes a battery of psychological tests, and when indicated, an interview by a psychologist. Finally the psychiatric evaluation may be extended to include the patient's wife or partner, either independently or together with the patient.

In addition to routine screening for disorders such as diabetes, more extensive laboratory studies are dictated by the history obtained. For example, a more detailed endocrine evaluation would include measurement of testosterone and prolactin levels.

Finally, a three-night sleep laboratory study of NPT is an essential part of the evaluation. Studies have established that nocturnal erections are a normal sleep-related occurrence, usually in association with the rapid eye movement (REM) stage of sleep. For example, between the ages of 20–29, approximately one third of sleep time is spent erect (even at ages 70–79 the figure is reduced to only 22%). Evidence to date suggests that normal NPT in an indication of physiologically intact daytime erectile capacity and, alternatively, that impaired NPT is a reliable confirmation that impaired daytime erectile ability is of an organic nature. Karacan et al. (1978a) discuss the possibility of psychological factors inhibiting nighttime erections (perhaps through affectively charged dream content) but have been unable to find supporting evidence and conclude that *properly performed* NPT studies will accurately reflect organic erectile capacity. In the exceptionally rare instance of a patient whose organic impotence is due to loss of penile sensation, relying only on the presence of normal NPT could lead to the false conclusion that the problem was psychogenic.

It is important to stress that NPT studies must be performed properly to avoid both false-positive and false-negative results. With the progressively greater emphasis being placed on NPT as the ultimate diagnostic technique, misdiagnosis due to improper use of the procedure can have grave results. The Baylor Group monitors penile circumference using strain gauges located at the tip and base of the penis together with electroencephalogram, and electrooculogram. They feel that sleep pattern must be assessed, since NPT recordings are valid only in the presence of normal sleep. The first night of recording allows the patient to become familiar with the procedure and to adjust to the setting. In this way, atypical sleep and NPT patterns due to "first-night effect" will not be misinterpreted as abnormal. On the second night, a full set of NPT recordings is obtained and on the third night an additional series of special evaluations are performed. These evaluations involve awakening the patient during a period of maximum erection and include the following: (1) both patient and examiner estimate the degree of erection, (2) the erect penis is photographed, and (3) penile rigidity is measured (buckling pressure) to assess for ability to achieve successful vaginal penetration.

In at least 90% of cases, Karacan et al. (1978a) found that an increase in penile circumference at the tip of 16–20 mm provides an erection sufficiently rigid for penetration. The other 10% illustrates the need for a more direct measurement of rigidity (for instance a 10-mm increase in circumference can be associated with adequate rigidity, while a 30-mm increase may not).

This multidisciplinary approach to the evaluation of impotence is to be commended. It will do much toward eliminating diagnoses based on assumption rather than "hard" data and assuring appropriate treatment. Traditionally accepted symptoms of "psychogenic" impotence such as selectivity (with a particular partner), abrupt onset, and ability to have erections under certain circumstances may not be as reliable as once expected. For example, a patient with organic impotence may be able to have successful intercourse with one partner but not another because of differences in vaginal wall support, while a patient with psychogenic impotence may be ineffective with all partners. In addition, NPT studies have shown that psychologically impotent men may be unable to achieve full erection during masturbation, while organically impotent men may be capable of occasional brief yet full erection (Fisher et al., 1979).

Work by Fisher et al. (1979) illustrates the value of NPT recording in confirming or correcting clinical diagnostic impressions. Of 14 patients initially diagnosed as having psychogenic impotence, 7 had the diagnosis confirmed while 7 were finally diagnosed as organic. A more specific example is given by Barry and Hodges (1978) who described a 48-year-old man with a 12-year history of progressive impotence that had been evaluated by "a general practitioner, an internist, several urologists, two psychiatrists, and a hypnotist" and diagnosed as "psychogenic." The absence of erections during three consecutive nights of NPT recording resulted in a revised diagnosis and referral for more appropriate treatment. Alternatively, since diabetes is associated with a high incidence of vascular or neuropathic impotence there is a tendency to forget that psychogenic impotence is just as likely to occur in diabetics as in anyone else. The diagnostic value of NPT recording is again obvious.

Despite great progress in recent years, there is much to be learned about the diagnosis of impotence. As this work unfolds, it is imperative that the clinician be attentive to these developments so that his patients are afforded every possibility of being accurately diagnosed and properly treated.

Recent Developments in the Diagnosis and Treatment of Organic Impotence

Endocrine

Testosterone injections have been a traditional, yet largely unproven and often unsuccessful treatment for impotence. All too commonly, the treatment is empirically applied without evaluation for or documentation of a hormone deficiency. It is likely that when potency returns in association with such injections that the response is a placebo effect associated with return of confidence that allows one to overcome psychogenic factors. In general, the indiscriminate use of testosterone is to be condemned.

When serum testosterone levels are found to be low in impotent patients, the likelihood of a causal relationship increases, but is far from certain. For example, low circulating testosterone levels are found in uremia, yet when exogenous testosterone is given to dialysis patients, there is often no improvement in potency. In fact, two uremic patients had a return of potency when androgen use was discontinued, suggesting that high testosterone levels may have adversely affected sexual functioning (Chopp and Mendez, 1978).

Recently, 105 consecutive impotent patients were evaluated for hypothalamic-pituitary-gonadal dysfunction and abnormalities were found in 37 of them (Spark et al., 1980). The authors state that "twenty patients had hypogonadotropic-hypogonadism, seven had hypergonadotropic-hypogonadism, eight had hyperprolactinemia, and two had occult hyperthyroidism. Once the specific defect was defined, appropriate therapy was instituted, and potency was restored in 33 patients."

Thirty-six of the 37 patients had abnormal serum testosterone levels when a single screening determination was performed (by a specific radioimmunoassay). The disorders were then more specifically defined by additional endocrinological evaluation. While the population studied was not a random sample of impotent men, the findings strongly suggest that impotence secondary to hormonal dysfunction has been greatly underdiagnosed.

Chronic alcohol administration to animals, normal men, and alcoholic men has been shown to cause a dose-dependent decrease in serum testosterone levels (Mendelson and Mello, 1979). This effect, apparently, is due to inhibition of testicular biosynthesis of testosterone. While these findings allow greater explanation of the association of sexual dysfunction with excessive alcohol use, treatment would best be directed at the elimination of alcohol rather than the addition of exogenous testosterone, which has not been shown to be of value.

The possible role of prolactin in sexual dysfunction is an area of great clinical interest. Such work has been fostered by developments in the 1970's that include the confirmation that prolactin is a distinct hormone in man, the development of a radioimmunoassay for measuring it, and a drug (bromocriptine) for blocking its release.

Hyperprolactinemia in men has been associated with decreased libido, galactorrhea, and, especially, impotence. While acknowledging that it is an uncommon cause of impotence, investigators have cited a double misfortune resulting from misdiagnosis. First, these patients may be assumed to have psychogenic impotence and therefore be subjected to inappropriate psychological treatments. Second, the elevated prolactin level is quite likely due to a pituitary adenoma which will become progressively more symptomatic and more difficult to treat as it enlarges. There is some evidence to suggest that potency will return if such a tumor is surgically removed or if prolactin secretion is inhibited by treatment with bromocriptine (González, 1979).

Whether *all* patients with impotence should be routinely evaluated for hyperprolactinemia has not yet been resolved (Anonymous, 1978). Since this is a promising area for clinical study, more definitive guidelines should be forthcoming. According to Thorner (see González, 1979), although the incidence of prolactin-induced impotence is low, the risks of misdiagnosis are sufficient to warrant serum prolactin determination in all suggestive cases.

Vascular

The hemodynamic changes necessary for the process of erection and detumescence are reasonably well understood (Weiss, 1972). Continuous high-volume blood flow to the erectile tissue is necessary to maintain an erection (as can be nicely demonstrated in animals by aortic constriction, which promptly results in detumescence). While it has been long known that atherosclerotic obstruction of the aorta and iliac vessels is often associated with impotence, the role of small vessel occlusive disease is not widely appreciated (see Impotence section in the chapter on Cardiovascular Disease).

Techniques are now available to measure penile blood pressure and pulse volume, and preliminary studies suggest that up to 10% of impotent men have abnormally low penile pressures (Anonymous, 1979a). That such abnromalities can occur selectively (in the absence of other findings of vascular disorder) has led Karacan et al. (1978b) to state that "since the penis can apparently be a target organ for vascular pathophysiology in otherwise healthy males, an incorrect diagnosis of psychogenic impotence is quite likely in those patients if they are not evaluated properly with NPT and blood pressure measurements."

When diabetics with abnormally diminished NPT were compared with nondiabetics with normal NPT, their systolic penile blood pressure was found to be significantly lower (Karacan et al., 1978b). At least some of the impotence associated with the use of antihypertensive drugs may be due to abnormally low-penile blood pressure.

Once impotence is diagnosed as vasculogenic and easily reversible causes such as drugs are excluded, further consideration can be given to surgical revascularization procedures. Arteriography is an important technique that allows better definition of the abnormalities and helps determine whether a shunting procedure will be useful. While the treatment of impotence by arterial bypass surgery must still be considered experimental, the subject is of sufficient interest to have resulted in an international conference in 1979 (First International Conference on Corpus Cavernosum Revascularization—New York) (Albertson, 1979). Current surgical techniques include anastomosing the inferior epigastric artery to the dorsal artery of the penis and saphenous vein bypass graft from the inferior epigastric artery to the corpus carvernosum.

Zinc

Studies in both Egypt and Iran have shown that malnourished, sexually retarded dwarfs show a striking response in sexual maturation when zinc is added to an otherwise balanced diet (Prasad, 1966).

Low plasma zinc levels have been found in uremic patients (both dialyzed and nondialyzed) and may contribute to the high prevalence of sexual dysfunction in this group. When supplemental zinc chloride was added to the dialysis bath of four uremic patients, low plasma zinc levels were corrected and sexual function improved considerably (only to deteriorate when the supplement was discontinued) (Antoniou et al., 1977). Although the authors state: "We conclude that zinc deficiency is a major, reversible cause of impotence in some haemodialysed men," they also recognize the need for further experimental support and advise a cautious approach to zinc therapy in uremic patients.

There is also some evidence that low zinc levels are associated with oligospermia and infertility in nonuremic men. Hartoma et al. (1977) found a correlation between low serum zinc and low dihydrotestosterone (but not testosterone) levels and noted an increase in sperm count following oral zinc supplementation. In an experimental study of dietary zinc restriction, marked reductions in sperm counts were noted after several months of deficiency (Anonymous, 1979b).

At the present time, the role zinc plays in both the etiology and treatment of sexual dysfunction is not well established. It is a promising research area, which should be followed with interest, since confirmation of these preliminary findings would define a specifically treatable entity in the presently ambiguous area of sexual dysfunction. It has been speculated that marginal zinc deficiency may be the cause of impotence in a substantial number of men that have previously been diagnosed as psychogenic. In the presence of impotence of unknown etiology and chronically low plasma zinc or dihy-drotestosterone levels, consideration should be given to a trial of long-term supplemental treatment with low doses of zinc.

Parathyroid Hormone

Another perspective of impotence in uremic patients on maintenance hemodialysis is presented by Massry et al. (1977). They suggest that in-creased levels of parathyroid hormone are involved in at least some patients. They cite evidence that includes: (1) a correlation between degree of im-potence and magnitude of secondary hyperparathyroidism, (2) finding that 70% of parathyroidectomized, nephrectomized dogs develop permanent erections, and (3) improved sexual potency in some dialysis patients when hyperparathyroidism is chemically suppressed.

Further work with uremic patients is necessary before definitive state-ments can be made. Whether any of these findings can be generalized to the nonuremic, impotent population is unknown.

Drug-Induced

An extensive review of this topic was done by Segraves (1977) who concluded: "Because of the paucity of adequately designed studies using adequate numbers of subjects and reasonable controls, few definitive state-ments can be made about pharmacological effects on the human sexual response."

For most physicians, the double-blind, placebo-controlled study is not a practical approach to clinical medicine, and they must rely on careful history and keen clinical judgment to assess and treat drug side effects. A thorough pretreatment sexual history, however, is often neglected by psy-chiatrists and is rarely obtained by nonpsychiatric physicians. Patients tak-ing medications are often reluctant to volunteer information about sexual dysfunction, especially to physicians who appear unreceptive to or uncom-fortable with this line of inquiry.

In addition to the likelihood of underdiagnosing drug-induced sexual dysfunction because of incomplete, superficial, insensitive, or nonexistent history taking, the possibility of misdiagnosis is often great. Controlled stud-ies have shown a substantial incidence of placebo-associated sexual dys-function, which in an open setting might have been erroneously attributed to active drug. A medication may become a scapegoat in a setting of inter-personal discord allowing one or both parties to avoid focusing on more central issues. Finally, drug-induced sexual dysfunction can be an iatrogenic problem created by a physician who erroneously assumes that a preexistent sexual problem is drug related because his first history is taken after the drug was started.

Assuming that a thorough and sensitive history uncovers a sexual dysfunction that has developed in association with the use of a drug or drugs, how should this problem be addressed? Whether the drug should be discontinued must be assessed in the context of the "whole" patient and, when indicated, should involve the patient's partner. For example, depressive symptoms (including decreased libido) were responding well to a tricyclic antidepressant when the patient developed erectile dysfunction. This latter problem was diagnosed as a drug side effect, which, in view of the therapeutic effectiveness of the drug, the patient and his wife felt could be tolerated. When the antidepressant was eventually discontinued, sexual function returned to normal.

The prompt and accurate recognition of drug-induced sexual dysfunction will help prevent secondary interpersonal complications which may arise due to performance anxiety, guilt, and misunderstanding by both partners. For example, a patient with asymptomatic hypertension developed erectile dysfunction from antihypertensive drugs. This led to progressive anxiety, which he coped with by avoiding sexual encounters with his wife. She interpreted this as "he must be seeing someone else," "he doesn't love me anymore," and "there must be something wrong with me." The situation became progressively worse owing to these secondary sexual complications.

On the other hand, if the patient recognizes the problem as drug-related, he may drop out of treatment and again be at high risk for hypertensive complications. A well established doctor–patient relationship is necessary to work out a treatment program that maximizes benefit and minimizes adverse effects (Murphy, 1978).

Cardiovascular drug-induced sexual dysfunction is discussed in the chapter on Cardiovascular Disease (also see Segraves, 1977; and Horowitz and Goble, 1979, for a critical evaluation). Psychotropic drugs are the other group associated with a high incidence of sexual dysfunction. A comparison of dysfunction in patients taking thioridazine or other neuroleptic drugs is outlined in Table 15-1 (Kotin et al., 1976). This study suggests not only that thioridazine is associated with a high incidence of sexual dysfunction but also that sexual dysfunction is a common finding with other antipsychotic drugs.

There have also been many reports of erectile dysfunction occurring in

TABLE 15-1. Sexual Dysfunction in Patients Taking Thioridazine or Other Neuroleptic Drugs

	Thioridazine (%)	Other neuroleptics (%)
Overall incidence of sexual dysfunction	60	25
Difficulty achieving erection	44	19
Difficulty maintaining erection	35	11
Changes in ejaculation	49	0

association with the use of tricyclic and monoamine oxidase inhibitor antidepressants (Segraves, 1977). Drug discontinuation was associated with the return of normal functioning.

Although lithium is generally felt not to cause sexual dysfunction, one double-blind, placebo-controlled study found that two of ten patients became impotent on active drug but not on placebo (Vinarova et al., 1972).

The role of benzodiazepines in causing sexual dysfunction has not been adequately studied, but clinical experience does not suggest that these drugs are major offenders.

An area that should not be overlooked is the association of illicit drug use and sexual dysfunction (Piemme, 1976). Unfortunately, rigorously controlled scientific studies are lacking, information is often difficult to obtain from patients, and therapeutic interventions that threaten certain life styles are likely to be resisted. Erectile dysfunction related to heroin use does appear to be a well established association.

Overall, it seems wise to assume that any drug can be associated with sexual dysfunction; the association may be entirely coincidental or there may be a more causal relationship through pharmacologic or psychologic mechanisms. In most cases, a clinical trial of drug discontinuation will be both practical and safe and should be one of the first treatment considerations. If the problem appears owing to a particular drug, switching to a structurally unrelated drug may be an effective intervention.

Surgical Treatment of Erectile Dysfunction

In addition to the above-mentioned revascularization procedures, erectile dysfunction has also been treated by the surgical implantation of semirigid or inflatible penile prostheses (Small, 1978; Scott et al., 1979; Renshaw, 1979). Results have been gratifying in many patients, but surgery should be undertaken only after an exhaustive evaluation for more specifically treatable dysfunctions (see above) and only after careful psychological screening. While most appropriate for organic dysfunction, most centers that have done large series of implants feel that certain *carefully selected* patients with psychogenic impotence also benefit from the procedure. There is a need for more extensive followup studies of both patient *and partner* before the benefit of this procedure can be fully assessed.

REFERENCES

Adams PW, Rose DP, Folkard J, et al: Effects of vitamin B$_6$ upon depression associated with oral contraception. *Lancet* 1:897–900, 1973.

Albertson P: The new arterial bypass that reverses organic impotence. *Sexual Med Today* 3:8–13, January 29, 1979.

Altschule, MD, Brem J: Periodic psychoses of puberty. *Am J Psychiatry* 119:1176–1178, 1963.

Anonymous: Endocrine basis for sexual dysfunction in men. *Br Med J* 2:1516–1517, 1978.

Anonymous: Do drugs cause impotence by lowering penile blood flow? *Med World News* 20:85, February 19, 1979a.

Anonymous: VA study ties zinc deficiency to male infertility. *Med World News* 20:12, June 11, 1979b.

Antoniou LD, Shalhoub RJ, Sudhakar T, et al: Reversal of uraemic impotence by zinc. *Lancet* 2:895–898, 1977.

Astwood EB: Estrogens and progestins, in Goodman L, Gilman A (eds): *The Pharmacological Basis of Therapeutics*, ed 4. New York, Macmillan, 1970, pp 1550–1557.

Ayd F: Oral contraceptives—psychic effects. *Int Drug Ther News* 1:3–4, 1966.

Bakker CB, Dightman CR: Side effects of oral contraceptives. *Obstet Gynecol* 28:373–379, 1966.

Barry JM, Hodges CV: Impotence: A diagnostic approach. *J Urol* 119:575–578, 1978.

Baumblatt MJ, Winston F: Pyridoxine and the pill. *Lancet* 1:832–833, 1970.

Belmaker RH, Murphy DL, Wyatt RJ, et al: Human platelet monoamine oxidase changes during the menstrual cycle. *Arch Gen Psychiatry* 31:553–556, 1974.

Benedek T, Rubenstein B: The correlations between ovarian activity and psychodynamic processes: I. The ovulative phase. *Psychosom Med* 1:245–270, 1939a.

Benedek, T, Rubenstein B: The correlations between ovarian activity and psychodynamic processes: II. The menstrual phase. *Psychosom Med* 1:461–485, 1939b.

Benedek-Jaszmann LJ, Hearn-Sturtevant MD: Premenstrual tension and functional infertility. *Lancet* 1:1095–1098, 1976.

Billetiere E, Fluckiger E: Evidence for a luteolytic function intact cyclic rat using 2-BR-alpha-ergocryptine (B-154). *Experiencia* (Basel) 27:464–466, 1971.

Brown-Parlee M: The premenstrual syndrome. *Psychol Bull* 80:454–465, 1973.

Bunney WE, Brodie KH, Murphy DL, et al: Studies of alpha-methyl-para-tyrosine, L-dopa and L-tryptophan in depression and mania. *Am J Psychiatry* 127:872–881, 1971.

Carroll BJ, Steiner M: The psychobiology of premenstrual dysphoria: The role of prolactin. *Psychoneuroendocrinology* 3:171–180, 1978.

Chopp RT, Mendez R: Sexual function and hormonal abnormalities in uremic men on chronic dialysis and after renal transplantation. *Fertil Steril* 29:661–666, 1978.

Claiber EL, Kobayashi Y, Groverman DM, et al: Plasma monoamine oxidase activity in regularly menstruating women and in amenorrheic women receiving cyclic treatment with estrogens and a progestin. *J Clin Endocrinol Metab* 33:630–637, 1971.

Cooke WR: The differential psychology of the American woman. *Am J Obstet Gynecol* 49:457–460, 1945.

Coppen A, Kessel N: Menstruation and personality. *Br J Psychiatry* 109:711–721, 1963.

Coppen AJ, Milne HB, Autran DH, et al: Dytide, norethisterone and a placebo in the premenstrual syndrome—a double-blind comparison. *Clin Trials J* 6:33–36, 1969.

Cullberg J: Mood changes and menstrual symptoms with different progestagen/estrogen combinations. *Acta Psychiatr Scand* 236(suppl):1–84, 1972.

Dalton K: Menstruation and acute psychiatric illness. *Br Med J* 1:148–149, 1959.

Dalton K: Menstruation and crime. *Br Med J* 2:1752–1753, 1961.

Dalton K: *The Premenstrual Syndrome*. Springfield, Charles C Thomas, 1964.

Dalton K: The influence of a mother's menstruation on her child. *Proc R Soc Med* 59:1014–1015, 1966.

Dalton K: Prospective study into puerperal depression. *Br J Psychiatry* 118:689–692, 1971.

Davis RE, Smith BK: Pyridoxine and depression associated with oral contraception. *Lancet* 1:1245, 1973.

Deutsch H: *Psychology of Women*. London, Research Books, 1944, p 118.

Endo M, Daiguji M, Wytaka A, et al: Periodic psychoses reoccurring in association with menstrual cycle. *J Clin Psychiatry* 39:456–461, 465–466, 1978.

Fisher C, Schiavi RC, Edwards A, et al: Evaluation of nocturnal penile tumescence in the differential diagnosis of sexual impotence. *Arch Gen Psychiatry* 36:431–437, 1979.

Fleming O, Seager CP: Incidence of depressive symptoms in users of the oral contraceptive. *Br J Psychiatry* 132:431–440, 1978.

Frank RT: The hormonal causes of premenstrual tension. *Arch Neurol Psychiatry* (Chicago) 26:1053–1055, 1931.

Fries H: Experience with lithium carbonate treatment at a psychiatric department in the period 1964–1967. *Acta Psychiatr Scand* 207(suppl):41–43, 1969.

Gilmore NJ, Robinson DS, Nies A, et al: Monoamine oxidase levels in pregnancy and during the menstrual cycle. *J Psychosom Res* 15:215–220, 1971.

Glass JS, Heninger GR, Lansky N, et al: Psychiatric emergency related to the menstrual cycle. *Am J Psychiatry* 128:705–711, 1971.

Glick ID: Mood and behavioral changes associated with the use of the oral contraceptive agents: A review of the literature. *Psychopharmacologia* 10:363–374, 1967.

Goldzieher JW, Moses LE, Averkine E, et al: Nervousness and depression attributable to oral contraceptives: A double-blind placebo-controlled study. *Am J Obstet Gynecol* 111:1013–1020, 1971.

González ER: Hyperprolactinemia: Still perplexing but eminently treatable. *JAMA* 242:401–409, 1979.

Grant ECG, Pryse-Davies J: Effects of oral contraceptives on depressive mood changes and on endometrial monoamine oxidase and phosphatases. *Br Med J* 3:777–780, 1968.

Greene R, Dalton K: The premenstrual syndrome. *Br Med J* 1:1007–1008, 1953.

Gregory BAJC: The menstrual cycle and its disorders in psychiatric patients: I. Review of the literature. *J Psychosom Res* 2:61–66, 1957.

Hartoma TR, Nahoul K, Netter A: Zinc, plasma androgens and male sterility. *Lancet* 2:1125–1126, 1977.

Heggarty AB: Post-puerperal recurrent depression. *Br Med J* 1:637–640, 1955.

Herzberg B, Coppen A: Changes in psychological symptoms in women taking oral contraceptives. *Br J Psychiatry* 116:161–164, 1970.

Herzberg BN, Draper KC, Johnson AL, et al: Oral contraceptives, depression and libido. *Br Med J* 3:495–500, 1971.

Herzberg BN, Johnson AL, Brown S: Depressive symptoms in oral contraceptives. *Br Med J* 4:142–145, 1970.

Hood WE, Bond WL: Enovid therapy for premenstrual tension. *Obstet Gynecol* 14:239–241, 1959.

Horowitz JD, Goble AJ: Drugs and impaired male sexual function. *Drugs* 18:206–207, 1979.

Horrobin DF, Manku MF, Massar B, et al: Prolactin and fluid and electrolyte balance, in Pasteels JL, Robyn C (eds): *Human Prolactin*. Amsterdam, Excerpta Medica, 1973, pp 152–155.

Jacobs TI, Charles E: Correlation of psychiatric symptomatology in an outpatient population. *Am J Psychiatry* 126:1504–1508, 1970.

Janowsky DS, Berens S, Davis JM: Correlations between mood, weight and electrolytes during the menstrual cycle: A renin–angiotensin–aldosterone hypothesis of premenstrual tension. *Psychosom Med* 35:143–154, 1973.

Janowsky DS, Gorney R, Kelly B: "The Curse:" Vicissitudes and variations of the female fertility cycle. *Psychosomatics* 7:242–247, 1966.

Janowsky DS, Gorney R, Mandell AJ: The menstrual cycle. Psychiatric and ovarian–adrenocortical hormone correlates: Case study and literature review. *Arch Gen Psychiatry* 17:459–464, 1967.

Jordheim O: The premenstrual syndrome—clinical trials of treatment with a progesterone combined with a diuretic compared with both a progesterone and with a placebo. *Acta Obstet Gynecol Scand* 51:77–80, 1972.

Kane FJ: Psychiatric reactions to oral contraceptives. *Am J Obstet Gynecol* 102:1053–1063, 1968.

Kane FJ, Keeler MH: Use of Enovid in post-partum mental disorders. *South Med J* 58:1089–1092, 1965.

Karacan I, Salis PJ, Williams RL: The role of the sleep laboratory in diagnosis and treatment of impotence, in Williams RL, Karacan I (eds): *Sleep Disorders, Diagnosis and Treatment*. New York, John Wiley and Sons, 1978a, pp 353–382.

Karacan I, Ware JC, Dervent B, et al: Impotence and blood pressure in the flaccid penis: Relationship to nocturnal penile tumescence. *Sleep* 1:125–132, 1978b.

Kashiwagi T, McClure JN, Wetzel RD: Premenstrual affective syndrome and psychiatric disorder. *Dis Nerv Syst* 37:116–119, 1976.

Kaya N, Moore, Karacan I: Nocturnal penile tumescence and its role in impotence. *Psychiatr Ann* 9:426–431, 1979.

Keeler MH, Daly R, Kane FJ: An acute schizophrenic episode following the abrupt withdrawal of Enovid in a patient with previous post-partum psychiatric disorder. *Am J Psychiatry* 121:1123–1124, 1964.

Kotin J, Wilbert DE, Verburg D, et al: Thioridazine and sexual dysfunction. *Am J Psychiatry* 113:82–85, 1976.

Kramer MS: Menstrual epileptoid psychosis in an adolescent girl. *Am J Dis Child* 131:316–317, 1977.

Kramp JL: Studies of the premenstrual syndrome in relation to psychiatry. *Acta Psychiatr Scand* 203(suppl):261–267, 1968.

Kutner SJ, Brown WL: Types of oral contraceptives, depression and premenstrual symptoms. *J Nerv Ment Dis* 155:153–162, 1972a.

Kutner SJ, Brown WL: History of depression as a risk factor for depression with oral contraceptives and discontinuance. *J Nerv Ment Dis* 155:163–169, 1972b.

Laidlow J: Catamenial epilepsy. *Lancet* 2:1235–1237, 1956.

Leeton J: The relation between oral contraception and depression. *Aust N Z J Obstet Gynecol* 13:115–118, 1973.

Lewis A, Hoghughi M: An evaluation of depression as a side effect of oral contraceptives. *Br J Psychiatry* 115:697–701, 1969.

Logothetics J, Herner R, Morrell F, et al: The role of estrogen in catamenial exacerbation of epilepsy. *Neurology* 9:352–360, 1959.

McClure JN, Reich T, Wetzel RD: Premenstrual symptoms as indicator of bi-polar affective disorder. *Br J Psychiatry* 119:527–528, 1971.

MacKinnon IL, MacKinnon PC, Thompson A: Lethal hazards of the luteal phase of the menstrual cycle. *Br Med J* 1:1015–1017, 1959.

Malek-Ahmadi D, Behrmann PJ: Depressive syndrome induced by oral contraceptives *Dis Nerv Syst* 37:406–408, 1976.

Mandell A, Mandell M: Suicide in the menstrual cycle. *JAMA* 200:792–793, 1967.

Marcotte DB, Kane FG, Obrist P, et al: Psychophysiologic changes accompanying oral contraceptive use. *Br J Psychiatry* 116:165–167, 1970.

Massry SG, Goldstein DA, Procci WR, et al: Impotence in patients with uremia: A possible role for parathyroid hormone. *Nephron* 19:305–310, 1977.

Mattsson B, von Schoultz B: A comparison between lithium, placebo, and a diuretic in premenstrual tension. *Acta Psychiatr Scand* 255(suppl):75–84, 1974.

Mendelson JH, Mello NK: Biologic concomitants of alcoholism. *N Eng J Med* 301:912–921, 1979.

Moos RH: Psychological aspects of oral contraceptives. *Arch Gen Psychiatry* 19:87–94, 1968a.

Moos RH: The development of a menstrual distress questionnaire. *Psychosom Med* 30:853–867, 1968b.

Moos RH: Assessment of psychological concomitants of oral contraceptives, in *Metabolic Effects of Gonadal Hormones and Contraceptive Steroids.* New York, Plenum Press, 1969a, pp 676–705.

Moos RH: Typology of menstrual psychosymptoms. *Am J Obstet Gynecol* 103:390–402, 1969b.

Morton JH: Premenstrual tension. *Am J Obstet Gynecol* 60:343–352, 1950.

Morton JH, Addition H, Haddison RG, et al: Clinical study of premenstrual tension. *Am J Obstet Gynecol* 65:1182–1191, 1953.

Murawaski B: Psychologic considerations for the evaluation of long-term use of oral contraceptives. *J Reprod Med* 3:151–155, 1969.

Murawaski B, Sapir B, Shulman N, et al: Investigation of mood states in women taking oral contraceptives. *Fertil Steril* 19:50–63, 1968.

Murphy RJ: Compliance dilemma: Antihypertensives and sexual dysfunction. *Behav Med* 12:10–14, October 1978.

Nilsson A, Almgren PE: Psychiatric symptoms during the post-partum period as related to use of oral contraceptives. *Br Med J* 2:453–455, 1968.

Novell HA: Psychological factors in premenstrual tension in dysmenorrhea. *Clin Obstet Gynecol* 8:222–232, 1965.

Ota Y, Mukai T, Gotoda K: Studies on the relationship between psychotic symptoms and sexual cycle. *Folia Psychiatr Neurol Jpn* 8:207–217, 1954.

Paige KE: The effects of oral contraceptives on affective fluctuations associated with the menstrual cycle. *Psychosom Med* 33:515–517, 1971.

Piemme TE: Sexuality and illicit drugs. *Med Asp Hum Sexuality* 10:85–86, 1976.

Prasad AS: Metabolism of zinc and its deficiency in human subjects, in Prasad AS (ed): *Zinc Metabolism*. Springfield, Charles C Thomas, 1966, pp 250–303.

Rees L: Psychosomatic aspects of the premenstrual tension syndrome. *Br J Psychiatry* 99:162–173, 1953.

Renshaw DC: Inflatable penile prosthesis. *JAMA* 241:2637–2638, 1979.

Ribeiro AL: Menstruation and crime. *Br Med J* 1:640–641, 1962.

Rose DP: Oral contraceptives and depression. *Lancet* 2:321, 1969.

Scott FB, Byrd GJ, Karacan I, et al: Erectile impotence treated with an implantable, inflatable prosthesis. *JAMA* 241:2609–2612, 1979.

Segraves RT: Pharmacological agents causing sexual dysfunction. *J Sex Marit Ther* 3:157–176, 1977.

Shainess N: Psychiatric evaluation of premenstrual tension. *NY State J Med* 62:3573–3579, 1962.

Silbergeld S, Brast N, Nobel EP: The menstrual cycle—a double-blind study of symptoms, mood and behavior and biochemical variables, using Enovid and placebo. *Psychosom Med* 33:411–428, 1971.

Simpson GM, Badinger N, Rochlin D: Enovid in the treatment of psychic disturbances associated with menstruation. *Dis Nerv Syst* 23:589–590, 1962.

Simpson GM, Rochlin D, Kline NS: Further studies of Enovid in the treatment of psychiatric patients. *Dis Nerv Syst* 25:484–488, 1964.

Sletten IW, Gershon S: The premenstrual syndrome: A discussion of its pathophysiology and treatment with lithium ion. *Compr Psychiatry* 7:197–206, 1966.

Small MP: Small-Carrion penile prosthesis: A report on 160 cases and review of the literature. *J Urol* 119:365–368, 1978.

Smith SL: Mood and the menstrual cycle, in Sacher EJ (ed): *Topics in Psychoendocrinology*. New York, Grune & Stratton, 1975, pp 19–58.

Somerville BW: The influence of progesterone and estradiol upon migraine. *J Headache* 12:93–102, 1972.

Sommer B: The effect of menstruation on cognitive and perceptual–motor behavior: A review. *Psychosom Med* 35:515–534, 1973.

Spark RF, White RA, Connolly PB: Impotence is not always psychogenic: Newer insights into hypothalamic–pituitary–gonadal dysfunction. *JAMA* 243:750–755, 1980.

Steiner M, Carroll BJ: The psychobiology of premenstrual dysphoria: Review of theories and treatments. *J Psychoneuroendocrinol* 2:321–335, 1977.

Stokes J, Mendels J: Pyridoxine and premenstrual tension. *Lancet* 1:1177–1178, 1972.

Swanson DW, Burron A, Floren A, et al: The use of norethynodrel in psychotic females. *Am J Psychiatry* 120:1101–1103, 1964.

Swyer GIM: Treatment of the premenstrual syndrome—value of ethisterone, nephinesin and a placebo compared. *Br Med J* 1:1410–1414, 1955.

Takagi H: Periodic psychosis in preadolescence. *Psychiatr Neurol Jpn* 61:1194–1208, 1959.

Tonks CN, Rack PH, Rose MJ: Attempted suicide in the menstrual cycle. *J Psychosom Res* 11:319–323, 1967.

Tupin JP: Lithium use in non-manic depressive condition. *Compr Psychiatry* 13:209–214, 1972.

Varga L, Lutterbeck BM, Pryor JS, et al: Suppression of puerperal lactation with an ergot alkaloid: A double-blind study. *Br Med J* 2:743–744, 1972.

Vinarova E, Uhlir O, Stika L, et al: Side effects of lithium administration. *Activ Nerv Sup* 14:105–107, 1972.

Wearing MP: The use of norethindrone (2 mg) and mestranol (1 mg) in infertility control. *Can Med Assoc J* 89:239–241, 1963.

Weiss HD: The physiology of human penile erection. *Ann Intern Med* 76:793–799, 1972.

Wetzel RD, Reich T, McClure JN, et al: Premenstrual affective syndrome and affective disorder. *Br J Psychiatry* 127:219–221, 1975.

Whitehead RE: Women pilots. *J Aviat Med* 5:47–49, 1934.

Williams EY, Weekes LR: Premenstrual tension associated with psychotic episodes. *J Nerv Ment Dis* 116:321–329, 1952.

Winston F: Oral contraceptives, pyridoxine and depression. *Am J Psychiatry* 30:1217–1221, 1973.

16

Sleep and Arousal Disorders

Although the sleep disorder, narcolepsy, was first described in the medical literature a century ago, the modern era of sleep research did not begin until the 1950s when rapid eye movements (REMs) were discovered (Aserinsky and Kleitman, 1953). Since then, the field has expanded rapidly, with the development of specialized centers for the study of sleep which utilize all-night recordings of electroencephalogram (EEG), electrooculogram (EOG), electromyogram (EMG), and other physiological measurements. Organizations such as the American Association of Sleep Disorder Centers and the Association for Psychophysiological Study of Sleep have been working to bring better definition and standardization to the field and to provide a stage for the exchange of information and discussion of controversial areas. A publication explosion in the form of books, articles in medical and psychiatric journals, and specialized journals such as *Sleep, Sleep Research*, and *Waking and Sleeping* attest to the growing interest in the study of sleep disorders.

Most sleep disturbances have a readily apparent cause, the correction of which will lead to improved sleep. Examples of conditions which cause secondary insomnia include "organic" disorders such as heart failure (paroxsysmal nocturnal dyspnea), chronic obstructive pulmonary disease (cough), and prostatic hypertrophy (nocturia); and "psychiatric" disorders such as mania, depression, anxiety, and drug dependency.

In recent years, sleep researchers have identified an additional number of well delineated sleep disorders that hitherto had either been poorly defined or not recognized. In coming years, research can be expected to subdivide still further the broad and amorphous areas of insomnia and hypersomnia. As a result, fewer and fewer patients will be inappropriately placed in the category of sleep disorders secondary to psychological disturbances merely because "organic" causes have been excluded. In addition, clinicians will be better able to separate those disorders caused by underlying psychological difficulties from those in which psychological difficulties are secondary to the disorder. Finally, the definition of specific, well characterized sleep disorders will lead to the development of specific treatments that should reduce the need for symptomatic and often inappropriate and hazardous remedies such as sleeping pills. The overuse of the latter has recently come under progressively stronger and well justified scrutiny (Institute of Medicine, 1979).

This chapter is not intended to be an extensive review of sleep physiology, sleep disorders, and sleep research, but rather an overview of some of the better established sleep disorders. Hopefully, this will alert clinicians to the benefits of careful differential diagnosis and the risks of misdiagnosis and inappropriate treatment. Data presented by the Stanford University Sleep Disorders Clinic underscore the high incidence of nondiagnosis, misdiagnosis, and mistreatment (Guilleminault and Dement, 1978). Of 100 patients evaluated for excessive daytime sleepiness, 35% were symptomatic for *five years* before seeking medical help. Extensive medical workup included glucose tolerance tests in 92% (with 12% misdiagnosed as hypoglycemia) and thyroid function tests, as a result of which 32% of the women were treated with thyroid medication.

DIAGNOSTIC CLASSIFICATION

The current state of the art with regard to the classification of sleep and arousal disorders is summarized in Table 16-1, which was prepared by the Sleep Disorders Classification Committee of the Association of Sleep Disorder Centers and reprinted with their permission. It is presented here to give the reader some idea of the depth and breadth of the field. The classification reflects the newness of the field and the need for standardization of terminology, and, consequently, modifications and revisions should be frequent, as is befitting any new science.

SPECIFIC DISORDERS

Narcolepsy

The definition of narcolepsy given by Karacan et al. (1979) as having been accepted by the First International Symposium on Narcolepsy in 1975 is as follows:

> a syndrome of unknown origin that is characterized by abnormal sleep tendencies, including excessive daytime sleepiness and often disturbed nocturnal sleep, and pathological manifestations of REM (rapid-eye-movement) sleep. The REM sleep abnormalities include sleep-onset REM periods and the dissociated REM sleep inhibitory processes, cataplexy, and sleep paralysis. Excessive daytime sleepiness, cataplexy, and less often sleep paralysis and hynagogic hallucinations are the major symptoms of the disease.

TABLE 16-1. Outline of Diagnostic Classification of Sleep and Arousal Disorders

A. DIMS: Disorders of Initiating and Maintaining Sleep (Insomnias)
  1. Psychophysiological
      a. Transient and situational
      b. Persistent
  2. Associated with psychiatric disorders
      a. Symptom and personality disorders
      b. Affective disorders
      c. Other functional psychoses
  3. Associated with use of drugs and alcohol
      a. Tolerance to or withdrawal from CNS depressants
      b. Sustained use of CNS stimulants
      c. Sustained use of or withdrawal from other drugs
      d. Chronic alcoholism
  4. Associated with sleep-induced respiratory impairment
      a. Sleep apnea DIMS syndrome
      b. Alveolar hypoventilation DIMS syndrome
  5. Associated with sleep-related (nocturnal) myoclonus and "restless legs"
      a. Sleep-related (Nocturnal) myoclonus DIMS syndrome
      b. "Restless legs" DIMS syndrome
  6. Associated with other medical, toxic, and environmental conditions
  7. Childhood-onset DIMS
  8. Associated with other DIMS conditions
      a. Repeated REM sleep interruptions
      b. Atypical polysomnographic features
      c. Not otherwise specified[a]
  9. No DIMS abnormality
      a. Short sleeper
      b. Subjective DIMS complaint without objective findings
      c. Not otherwise specified[a]
B. DOES: disorders of excessive somnolence
  1. Psychophysiological
      a. Transient and situational
      b. Persistent
  2. Associated with psychiatric disorders
      a. Affective disorders
      b. Other functional disorders
  3. Associated with use of drugs and alcohol
      a. Tolerance to or withdrawl from CNS stimulants
      b. Sustained use of CNS depressants
  4. Associated with sleep-induced respiratory impairment
      a. Sleep apnea DOES syndrome
      b. Alveolar hypoventilation DOES syndrome
  5. Associated with sleep-related (nocturnal) myoclonus and "restless legs"
      a. Sleep-related (nocturnal) myoclonus DOES syndrome
      b. "Restless legs" DOES syndrome
  6. Narcolepsy
  7. Idiopathic CNS hypersomnolence
  8. Associated with other medical, toxic, and environmental conditions

(Continued)

TABLE 16-1. (*Continued*)

9. Associated with other DOES conditions
    a. Intermittent DOES (periodic) syndromes
        i. Kleine-Levin syndrome
        ii. Menstrual-associated syndrome
    b. Insufficient sleep
    c. Sleep drunkenness
    d. Not otherwise specified[a]
10. No DOES Abnormality
    a. Long sleeper
    b. Subjective DOES complaint without objective findings
    c. Not otherwise specified[a]
C. Disorders of the sleep-wake schedule
    1. Transient
        a. Rapid time zone change ("jet lag") syndrome
        b. "Work shift" change in conventional sleep-wake schedule
    2. Persistent
        a. Frequently changing sleep-wake schedule
        b. Delayed sleep phase syndrome
        c. Advanced sleep phase syndrome
        d. Non-24-hour sleep-wake syndrome
        e. Irregular sleep-wake pattern
        f. Not otherwise specified[a]
D. Dysfunctions associated with sleep, sleep stages, or partial arousals (parasomnias)
    1. Sleepwalking (somnambulism)
    2. Sleep terror (pavor nocturnus, incubus)
    3. Sleep-related enuresis
    4. Other dysfunctions
        a. Dream anxiety attacks (nightmares)
        b. Sleep-related epileptic seizures
        c. Sleep-related bruxism
        d. Sleep-related headbanging (jactatio capitis nocturnus)
        e. Familial sleep paralysis
        f. Impaired sleep-related penile tumescence
        g. Sleep-related painful erections
        h. Sleep-related cluster headaches and chronic paroxysmal hemicrania
        i. Sleep-related abnormal swallowing syndrome
        j. Sleep-related asthma
        k. Sleep-related cardiovascular symptoms
        l. Sleep-related gastroesophageal reflux
        m. Sleep-related hemolysis (paroxysmal nocturnal hemoglobinuria)
        n. Asymptomatic polysomnographic finding
        o. Not otherwise specified[a]

[a] This entry is intended to leave place in the classification for both undiagnosed ("don't know") conditions and additional (as yet undocumented) conditions that may be described in the future. Reproduced with permission from *Sleep* 2:17–19, 1979.

The Narcoleptic Tetrad (Pentad?)

Narcoleptic sleep attacks tend to be brief, usually lasting no more than 15–20 min. While episodes are more likely to occur in conductive settings (after meals, in warm rooms, in monotonous surroundings), they can also happen under quite inappropriate circumstances (while driving, talking, teaching, or engaging in athletic or even sexual activities) (Karacan et al., 1979). Although the urge to sleep tends to be irresistible, after a short sleep the individual awakes refreshed—until the next attack, which occurs with a frequency ranging from only a few to over a hundred per day. In addition, many narcoleptic individuals feel generally sleepy throughout the course of the day.

Automatic behavior is commonly found in narcoleptics who describe blackout periods for which they have no recall but during which they may engage in complex but usually inappropriate behaviors. For example, Dement et al. (1976) described a patient who was planning to do the dishes but had an episode during which the dishes were put in the clothes dryer and the dryer turned on. Automatic behavior may represent repetitive microsleep episodes (Karacan et al., 1979).

Cataplexy refers to the sudden and reversible loss of skeletal muscle tone, which may be generalized or restricted to certain muscle groups. The episodes are precipitated particularly by strong emotion such as laughter, fright, or anger, or by exercise; last from seconds to minutes; and may be complete (patient falls to the ground) or incomplete (a sense of weakness in the knees). During an episode, the patient may be totally unable to move, yet remain conscious.

Sleep paralysis occurs in association with falling asleep or awakening and is characterized by the inability to move. Although readily reversible and of short duration (seconds to minutes), this period of muscular flaccidity may be quite frightening to the patient.

Hypnagogic hallucinations complete the narcoleptic tetrad. These are vivid, often frightening, visual, auditory, or tactile hallucinations that occur during the period of falling asleep or awakening (those occurring during awakening are sometimes referred to as hypnapompic).

Disturbed nocturnal sleep is found in 60–70% of narcoleptic patients and, hence, is sometimes included as the fifth member of the narcoleptic pentad. Characteristically, patients fall asleep without difficulty but wake frequently during the night.

Various Forms of Narcolepsy

According to Roth (1978), 25–35% of patients with narcolepsy have only narcoleptic sleep attacks (isolated narcolepsy). Dement et al., 1976), on the other hand, state that with rare exceptions, "a history of cataplexy is absolutely necessary to establish a diagnosis of narcolepsy in a sleepy patient."

To further summarize the review by Roth, 65–75% of all cases of narcolepsy are associated with cataplexy, while sleep paralysis and hypnagogic hallucinations occur in 20–30%. The complete tetrad is uncommon, being found in only 11–14% of patients.

Sleep Laboratory Findings

According to Dement et al. (1976), under proper conditions *every* patient with narcolepsy–cataplexy will have sleep onset REM periods during daytime recording or at the onset of nocturnal sleep (normal adults first enter non-REM sleep and pass into the first REM sleep period only after about an hour.)

Other authorities (Roth, 1978) feel that sleep attacks in narcolepsy–cataplexy patients may be associated with either REM or non-REM sleep, while nocturnal sleep is characterized by sleep onset REM periods. On the other hand, the sleep attacks in patients with isolated narcolepsy are associated with non-REM sleep and nocturnal sleep tends to be normal.

Missing the diagnosis of narcolepsy can occur if one depends on the finding of sleep onset REM periods to make the diagnosis. In addition to those patients whose narcoleptic attacks are associated with non-REM sleep, narcoleptics with sleep onset REM episodes may also have normal sleep onsets. If a single or limited number of nap-time recordings are too heavily relied upon, sleep onset REM periods may be missed and false negative diagnoses may be made. The more extensive the polysomnographic study, the more likely the sleep disturbance will be detected. Clinical history should be the foremost aspect of diagnosis, and overreliance on sleep laboratory findings is ill-advised.

Etiology

While the cause of narcolepsy is not known, there is general agreement that is *not* a psychogenic illness. Dement et al. (1976) considered it a "neurological disease involving impairment of brain mechanisms that regulate REM and non-REM sleep and wakefulness."

Diagnostic Difficulties

According to Dement and Baird (1977)

the average patient who is ultimately diagnosed as suffering from narcolepsy has consulted at least 3 to 5 physicians about their symptoms over a period of ten to fifteen years before receiving the correct diagnosis! Many have spent years misdiagnosed as schizophrenics, thyroid cases, or malingerers. Inappropriate, unsuccessful and sometimes dangerous treatments are frequent. When questioned carefully, patients with narcolepsy almost universally recount instances of negligence, misinformation, ineptness, and apparent lack of concern on the part of physicians they have consulted.

Friends, relatives, employers, and even the patient may come to think of himself as lazy, disinterested, and unmotivated, unless the organic nature of the illness is recognized. In the occupational arena, narcolepsy has reduced job performance, prevented promotion, reduced earning capacity, and led to job dismissal (Dement and Baird, 1977).

Although most cases of idiopathic narcolepsy begin during adolescence or early adulthood, symptoms may develop before puberty. Children with undiagnosed narcolepsy have been misdiagnosed as hyperactive or schizophrenic, and, even without such diagnoses, the misunderstandings engendered by inappropriate sleepiness can have a devastating effect on development.

An association between depression, especially endogenous, and narcolepsy has been noted, with depression being found in 28.6% of patients with isolated narcolepsy and in 17.2% with narcolepsy–cataplexy (Roth, 1978). The reason for this greater than anticipated incidence of depression is unclear.

Other aspects of the differential diagnosis require exclusion of other sleep–arousal disorders such as the hypersomnias and sleep apnea; medical and neurological disorders such as hypothyroidism, hypoglycemia, epilepsy, myasthenia gravis, and multiple sclerosis; and psychiatric disorders such as fugue state, dissociative reaction, and psychoneurosis.

Treatment

While no ideal treatment exists, appropriate intervention can have a dramatic impact on the life of a narcoleptic. Frequent, scheduled naps may help minimize daytime sleepiness and inappropriate sleep attacks. Avoiding a sleep-conducive environment may also be helpful. Finally, drug therapy will be necessary in many, if not all cases. Stimulants such as amphetamines or methylphenidate can be quite effective in preventing narcoleptic attacks and attenuating daytime drowsiness. Side effects, tolerance, and abuse potential make these agents less than ideal.

Cataplexy, sleep paralysis, and hypnagogic hallucinations are less responsive to stimulants but may successfully respond to imipramine or chlorimipramine. Commonly, both a stimulant and one of these latter drugs must be used in combination to get optimal results.

Education is also an essential aspect of treatment. Not only the patient but all others influenced by his illness must understand its nature, realize that there is no evidence that its cause is psychogenic, and be aware that it can have grave secondary psychological consequences. As aptly said by Dement et al. (1976): "For example, a man whose wife falls asleep each time he talks to her may assume that the sleep is a hostile response."

Sleep Apnea Syndrome

Introduction

Apnea has been defined as a cessation of breathing lasting at least 10 sec. The criteria for the diagnosis of a **sleep apnea syndrome** require at least 30 apneic episodes during both REM and non-REM sleep during seven hours of nocturnal sleep (Derman and Karacan, 1979).

Of 85 patients diagnosed at the Stanford University Sleep Disorders Clinic as having the sleep apnea syndrome, 78% complained of excessive daytime sleepiness, while 19% were troubled by insomnia (Guilleminault and Dement, 1978). Twenty-three percent of 235 consecutive patients complaining of excessive daytime sleepiness had sleep apnea, and all but two of them (52/54) were male (Guilleminault and Dement, 1977). The incidence in patients with insomnia varied from none in 150 patients (Soldatos et al., 1979) to 5–7% in other series (Derman and Karacan, 1979). The ratio of males to females is greater than 20 to 1. While the incidence of this syndrome in the general population requires further definition, conservative estimates suggest that there are more than 50,000 sleep apnea patients in the United States.

Types of Sleep Apnea Syndromes

Central sleep apnea has been defined as the "cessation of nasal and oral airflow for more than 10 sec, accompanied by the absence of respiratory efforts as measured by nasal/oral thermistors, abdominal and thoracic strain gauges, intercostal electromyocardiograms, and esophogeal pressure transducers" (Derman and Karacan, 1979).

Obstructive sleep apnea is characterized by upper airway air flow obstruction despite persistent respiratory muscle effort in the intercostals and diaphragm.

Mixed sleep apnea begins with a central sleep apnea followed by an obstructive phase. Thus, there is initial cessation of both air flow and respiratory effort followed by progressive respiratory muscle activity until the obstruction is overcome.

All three types can occur in the same patient, but one type usually predominates. Patients with the obstructive or mixed type tend to complain of excessive daytime sleepiness, while insomnia is likely to be the main complaint in those with the central type.

Clinical Features

Obstructive Sleep Apnea   (from Guilleminault and Dement, 1978).

1. Snoring—A characteristic snoring pattern is found, in which each apneic episode is ended by loud, forceful snores as the obstruction

is overcome. Apparently, such snoring can be so noisy and disruptive as to cause spouses to move to other rooms and neighbors to complain.

2. Abnormal motor activity during sleep—Patients may flail about the bed, sleepwalk, sleep in unusual positions, and, in general, leave the sleeping area quite disorganized.

3. Excessive daytime sleepiness and inappropriate sleep episodes—Patients have histories of excessive sleepiness of many years' duration with adverse social consequences similar to those seen in narcoleptics.

4. Automatic behavior syndrome—Periods lasting minutes to hours are associated with marked deterioration in overall performance and appear related to repetitive daytime microsleep episodes.

5. Intellectual deterioration—Even when awake, patients often have difficulty with alertness, concentration, memory, and judgment.

6. Hypnagogic hallucinations—These tend to occur when the patient is fighting sleep, and may result in brief periods during which the patient responds to the images as though they were real.

7. Morning headaches—These frontal headaches tend to be present on awakening and gradually resolve as the day progresses. They may recur following a long daytime nap.

8. Personality changes and behavioral outbursts—Commonly found are symptoms such as anxiety and depression, which in some patients lead to psychiatric consultation. Less common are confusion, irritability, and aggressiveness. Spouses often comment on uncharacteristic outbursts of anger, suspicion, jealousy, or irrationality directed at family members. When compared to narcoleptics, these patients are found to be more neurotic, hysterical, and hypochondriacal (Derman and Karacan, 1979).

9. Sexual behavior—Diminished libido and erectile dysfunction are not infrequent findings and are sometimes, but not always, related to the degree of depression present.

Although no single patient is likely to have all of these manifestations, many of them will coexist in the same patient. No single manifestation is pathognomonic of the sleep apnea syndrome.

Obstructive sleep apnea in children was described in 14 patients (ages 5–14 years) who had a mean number of 345 apneic periods per night. Symptoms included loud snoring, excessive daytime sleepiness, poor school performance, nocturnal enuresis, morning headache, and personality change (Guilleminault and Dement, 1978).

Central Sleep Apnea. Insomnia at night (frequent awakening but no difficulty falling asleep) and tiredness during the day are the most common complaints, while excessive daytime sleepiness is not usually found. Morning headaches and sexual dysfunction may also occur, but, in contrast to the obstructive apneics, psychiatric evaluation tends to be normal.

Diagnosis

The definitive diagnosis of sleep apnea is made by polysomnography (all night polygraphic monitoring). In a series of 30 patients with obstructive or mixed sleep apnea, a mean of 57% of total sleep time was spent without air exchange. This figure, coupled with an average of 371 apnea periods during an 8-hr recording period, helps one appreciate the magnitude of this disorder (Guilleminault and Dement, 1978). A thorough history taken from both patient and spouse, with close attention to the above-mentioned clinical manifestations, should raise a high index of suspicion and prompt a referral to a sleep laboratory.

Since sleep disorder centers are not readily accessible to the majority of physicians, Riedy et al. (1979) have described a diagnostic method utilizing the thermistor in a Swan–Ganz thermodilution catheter to measure airflow, and modified electrocardiogram electrodes to record chest wall movement that is applicable to use in community hospitals.

Associated Cardiovascular Findings

Obstructive sleep apnea is associated with a high incidence of pulmonary and systemic hypertension during sleep. In addition, nocturnal cardiac arrhythmias are the rule and consist of extreme sinus bradycardia, sinus arrhythmia, asystole, heart block, and ventricular arrhythmia. Bradyarrhythmias occur so consistently that all-night Holter electrocardiography may be a useful screening procedure (Tilkian et al., 1977).

In central sleep apnea, less marked elevations in pulmonary artery pressure occur, while systemic pressure remains normal. Studies of arrhythmia have been quite limited, but both sinus arrhythmias and asystole have been reported.

Treatment

Obstructive Sleep Apnea. A diet for weight reduction may occasionally be of value. Medication such as theophylline, aminophylline, progesterone, chlorimipramine, pemoline, and thioridazine have either been ineffective or have had such limited use that firm conclusions cannot be drawn. There is, however, some evidence that protriptyline may be of major benefit in carefully selected cases (Clark et al., 1979). The most dramatic treatment is tracheostomy, which allows airflow to bypass the area of intermittent obstruction. Symptoms are likely to totally resolve following this procedure (Guilleminault and Dement, 1978).

Central Sleep Apnea. A well established, effective treatment for central sleep apnea has not been developed. Therapy with drugs such as respiratory stimulants and electrical pacing of the diagram are experimental approaches which have been tried.

MISCELLANEOUS CONDITIONS

Delayed Sleep Phase Syndrome (Sleep Onset Insomnia)

Because of postulated abnormalities of the circadian pacemaker governing sleep, certain people ("night people") are unable to fall asleep at conventional times—instead, lying awake for hours. Once asleep, they sleep well, and, if undisturbed, will get a full allotment of sleep. Occupational or educational obligations, however, usually demand arising at more conventional times, resulting in sleep lack, daytime drowsiness, and tardiness. This condition is not responsive to drugs, psychotherapy, or behavioral therapy, and is likely to be misdiagnosed as emotional in origin. Preliminary studies suggest that the patient's biological clock can be reset by delaying sleep by about 3 hr on successive nights until the sleep cycle is rotated ahead into a more conventional time frame (Weitzman, 1979).

Noctural Myoclonus

This disorder is characterized by intermittent, pronounced jerking of the legs associated with EEG and behavioral arousals. Movements may be severe enough to wake the patient or disturb the bed partner. Nocturnal myoclonus has been reported as causative in 10–20% of insomnia cases, yet other investigators found that a large group of insomniacs and controls did not differ in the amount of nocturnal myoclonic activity (discussed in Soldatos et al., 1979).

CONCLUSION

Disorders such as narcolepsy, sleep apnea, delayed sleep phase syndrome, and nocturnal myoclonus are illustrations of the rich, complex, and fascinating area of sleep and arousal disorders. They emphasize the need for the current awareness of this rapidly expanding field to avoid summarily assigning psychological diagnoses to patients complaining of chronic insomnia or excessive daytime sleepiness. This is not to suggest that a large proportion of these complaints are not of emotional etiology, but rather to reenforce the need for comprehensive and unbiased differential diagnosis.

REFERENCES

Aserinsky E, Kleitman N: Regularly occurring periods of eye motility and concomitant phenomena, during sleep. *Science* 118:273–274, 1953.
Clark RW, Schmidt HS, Schaal SF, et al: Sleep apnea: Treatment with protriptyline. *Neurology* 29:1287–1292, 1979.

Dement WC, Baird WP: *Narcolepsy: Care and Treatment.* Stanford, The American Narcolepsy Association, 1977.

Dement WC, Carskadon MA, Guilleminault C, et al: Narcolepsy: Diagnosis and treatment. *Primary Care* 3:609–623, 1976.

Derman S, Karacan I: Sleep-induced respiratory disorders. *Psychiatr Ann* 9:411–425, 1979.

Guilleminault C, Dement WC: 235 cases of excessive daytime sleepiness. *J. Neurol Sci* 31:13–27, 1977.

Guilleminault C, Dement WC: Sleep apnea syndromes and related sleep disorders, in Williams RL, Karacan I (eds): *Sleep Disorders: Diagnosis and Treatment.* New York, John Wiley and Sons, 1978, pp. 9–28.

Institute of Medicine: *Sleeping Pills, Insomnia, and Medical Practice.* Washington DC, National Academy of Sciences, 1979.

Karacan I, Moore CA, Williams RL: The narcoleptic syndrome. *Psychiatr Ann* 9:377–381, 1979.

Riedy RM, Hulsey R, Bachus BF, et al: Sleep apnea syndrome, practical diagnostic method. *Chest* 75:81–83, 1979.

Roth B: Narcolepsy and hypersomnia, in Williams RL, Karacan I (eds): *Sleep Disorders: Diagnosis and Treatment.* New York, John Wiley and Sons, 1978, pp. 29–59.

Soldatos CR, Kales A, Kales JD: Management of insomnia. *Ann Rev Med* 30:301–312, 1979.

Tilkian AG, Guilleminault C, Schroeder JS: Sleep-induced apnea syndrome: Prevalence of cardiac arrhythmias and their reversal after tracheostomy. *Am J Medicine* 63:348–358, 1977.

Weitzman E: "Night people" who have trouble sleeping helped by resetting their biological clocks. *Clin Psychiatr News* 7:3, 35, 1979.

17

Substance Abuse Disorders

CAFFEINE

Introduction

The fact that caffeine in the form of coffee, tea, cocoa, cola beverages, and over-the-counter medications is probably the most widely used psychoactive substance helps account for its neglect as the cause of a variety of psychiatric symptoms. Caffeine is such an integral part of our society that its use (and abuse) is not associated with the stigma attached to other substances of abuse such as alcohol, opioids, and barbiturates. Unlike even tobacco, the use of caffeine in children in the form of colas, cocoa, and chocolate is almost universally accepted.

For the most part, caffeine-containing substances are well tolerated and quite safe, and, while there have been suggestions that caffeine use is associated with heart attacks, hypertension, cancer, fibrocystic disease of the breast and birth defects, a cause and effect relationship has yet to be firmly established (Garfield, 1980). On the other hand, it is reasonably well established that excessive caffeine intake or caffeine withdrawal can be associated with symptoms of a psychiatric nature that are prone to frequent misdiagnosis.

Pharmacology

Caffeine, together with theophylline and theobromine, are methylated xanthines that occur naturally and can also be synthesized. Caffeine is rapidly absorbed orally (in about 1 hr), is distributed throughout body water (reaching both placenta and fetus), and is excreted almost entirely by the kidney. A pharmacological half-life of about 3 hr insures that it does not accumulate in the body. It causes central nervous system stimulation, with increased wakefulness, alertness, concentration ability, and work capacity. Other effects include stimulation of gastric secretion, diuresis, and cardiac stimulation.

Typical pharmacological effects are produced by 50–200 mg of caffeine, although there is a wide variation in dose-response owing to body size, habituation, and other factors. The caffeine content of various beverages and over-the-counter drugs is such that large doses are easily consumed in the course of a day (Gilbert et al., 1976; Mikkelsen, 1978; Bunker and Mc-Williams, 1979). For example, representative caffeine contents include:

12 oz can of cola	30–65 mg
cup of coffee	29–176 mg (one study showed that the caffeine content of a cup of coffee could be as high as 333 mg)
cup of tea	150 mg
tablet of caffeine-containing analgesic	15–100 mg
small bar of chocolate	25 mg

While these figures are approximations and vary considerably from source to source (due to factors such as brand, container size, and brewing method), they can be used to get a rough estimate of daily intake. Calculated on the basis of body weight, it has been stated that a single can of cola will provide a very young child with the caffeine equivalent of four cups of instant coffee in an adult.

Manifestations of Caffeine Use, Abuse, and Withdrawal

Caffeine Use and Overuse

In nonusers, relatively modest doses of caffeine will produce nervousness, irritability, headache, anxiety, dysphoria, and sleep disturbance. Toxicity associated with prolonged heavy use ($\geq$600–1000 mg/day) are similar, consisting of headache, sleep disturbance, restlessness, irritability, anxiety, agitation, tremor, palpitations, muscle twitching, and gastrointestinal distress. Chronic tinnitus has also been reported.

In 1892, Kraeplin reported:

> Large quantities of caffeine often cause headaches and some confusion and in rare cases of special susceptibility a mild form of delirium may be elicited, or noises in the ears and flashes of light may indicate derangement of special senses (from Mikkelsen, 1978).

Greden (1974) called attention to the long neglected syndrome of "caffeinism," noting that this is a common cause of psychiatric referral with tentative diagnoses such as "anxiety reaction," "chronic anxiety," "anxiety neurosis," and "psychophysiologic disturbance." He also found that while 42% of psychiatric outpatient records referred to anxiety symptoms, none mentioned caffeine ingestion pattern—small wonder that the diagnosis is often missed!

Especially high doses of caffeine over short periods of time can produce a delirium and, again, a thorough drug history is necessary if the cause is to be recognized. At least one patient was initially misdiagnosed as "hysteria without question" (McManamy and Schube, 1936).

Caffeine Withdrawal

In a questionnaire survey of housewives, Goldstein and Kaizer (1969) found a characteristic set of dysphoric symptoms in heavy coffee users (five or more cups per day) who omitted their morning coffee. These included headache, irritability, inability to work effectively, nervousness, restlessness, and lethargy.

Caffeine-withdrawal headache was produced experimentally in 1943 (Dreisbach and Pfeiffer) and has a fairly consistent clinical picture. It tends to occur in association with a fairly high daily caffeine intake (usually in excess of 500 mg/day) and the development of tolerance followed by abrupt discontinuation of caffeine intake (this may simply involve missing one's morning coffee). The syndrome begins with a feeling of fullness in the head followed by a diffuse, throbbing headache which reaches maximum intensity in 3–6 hr. Symptom relief is afforded, of course, by "a cup of coffee to settle the nerves" or by the use of caffeine-containing analgesics. It has been suggested that many chronic tension headaches are actually due to caffeine withdrawal but are not properly diagnosed because of the failure to take an adequate caffeine history (Greden et al., 1980). The extent to which physicians are willing to pursue an incorrect diagnosis is illustrated in one patient in whom "tension was suspected, but when the psychiatrist failed to find tension in her homelife, he suggested that the headaches might have been caused by too much serenity in the home" (Harrie, 1970).

Use of Caffeine in Psychiatric Patients

Winstead (1976) found that in hospitalized psychiatric patients heavy coffee drinkers had higher scores on anxiety tests and were more often diagnosed as psychotic. Greden et al. (1978) found that psychiatric inpatients who consumed greater than 750 mg of caffeine daily had higher anxiety and depression scores, more clinical symptoms, used more sedative hypnotics and minor tranquilizers, and felt that their health was not as good. When a hospital ward was switched, in double-blind fashion, to decaffeinated coffee for three weeks, a statistically significant reduction was noted in anxiety, irritability, and hostility, suggesting that unregulated caffeine intake may have an adverse effect on psychiatric inpatients (De Freitas and Schwartz, 1979).

In addition, it has been suggested that self medication with large doses of caffeine-containing substances may cause diagnostic difficulties in patients who have hypersomnic depression that would otherwise be easily recognized (Neil et al., 1978). Finally, excessive coffee ingestion can apparently cause exacerbation of an underlying schizophrenic disorder (Mikkelsen, 1978). Whether this was due to the stimulant effect of caffeine or to an interaction between caffeine and antipsychotic drugs (see below) is not clear.

Caffeine and Psychiatric Drugs

When many antipsychotic drugs are in contact with coffee or tea, a milky, flaky precipitate is formed, a precipitate which has been shown to contain the antipsychotic drug (Kulhanek et al., 1979; Hirsch, 1979). This interaction has, thus far, been demonstrated in vitro with the liquid forms of fluphenazine, chlorpromazine, promethazine, prochlorperazine, haloperidol, and droperidol, but not with trifluoperazine or propranolol. The clinical implications of this interaction are profound but remain to be established.

Caffeine-containing beverages may also be used (intentially or not) to counteract the sedative side effects of a variety of psychiatric drugs (antipsychotics, antidepressants, anxiolytics, and sedative–hypnotics). It is also likely that excessive caffeine intake interferes with the expected therapeutic effect of antianxiety or sedative–hypnotic agents.

Conclusion

A thorough caffeine ingestion history should be taken from all patients. This will increase the likelihood of correctly diagnosing caffeine toxicity, caffeine withdrawal, and caffeine-induced complications of preexisting psychiatric disorders. Interactions between caffeine-containing beverages and psychiatric drugs may have an adverse effect on treatment outcome and should be further investigated.

ALCOHOL

Introduction

While the percentage of our adult population felt to show alcohol abuse or alcoholism behavior in 1971 was small (7%), the absolute number of people involved (9 million) indicates that these are problems of major proportion (in Victor and Adams, 1980a). Alcohol misuse is associated with accidents and crime, with over half of all motor vehicle deaths involving a driver or pedestrian who has been drinking, and over half of all murders associated with an intoxicated murderer or victim (DSM III, 1980). Alcoholism can have profound effects on individual psychological and physical well being, interpersonal relationships, economic productivity, and social functioning.

According to *The Diagnostic and Statistical Manual of Mental Disorders* (*DSM III*, 1980), the essential feature of *Alcohol Abuse* is "a pattern of psychological use for at least a month that causes impairment in social or occupational functioning" and the essential features of *Alcohol Dependence* are "either a pattern of pathological alcohol use or impairment of social or occupational functioning due to alcohol, and either tolerance or withdrawal." Chronic pathological alcohol use is likely to follow one of three patterns: (1) regular daily intake of large amounts, (2) regular heavy weekend drinking, or (3) binges of heavy drinking lasting for weeks or months interspaced with long periods of sobriety (*DSM III*, 1980).

Complications of alcohol abuse and dependence have profound medical, psychological, and social consequences that are not restricted to any particular segment of our population. Although Schuckit (1979) notes that the highest alcoholism rates are likely to be found in lower socioeconomic strata, lower income, less educated, 30–50 year old, French and Irish-Catholic men, he also cautions that "it is important to recognize that alcoholism is a problem of all socioeconomic strata, all ages, all religions, all parts of the country, and both sexes." Although the stereotypic skid row alcoholic is easily recognized, it is important to realize that many people with alcohol-related problems (1) do not recognize or acknowledge the problem, (2) withhold information that would allow a proper diagnosis, and (3) do not realize that medical and psychological difficulties are complications of alcohol use. Consequently, clinicians must maintain high indices of suspicion and be adept at obtaining comprehensive histories.

Pharmacology

Alcohol is rapidly absorbed from the gastrointestinal tract (stomach—20%; small intestine—80%) with detectable levels appearing in the blood in five minutes and maximum concentrations reached in 30–90 minutes. Susceptibility to intoxication from alcohol varies considerably. Chronic users metabolize alcohol faster and tolerate equivalent blood levels better than normal individuals. Metabolism occurs mainly in the liver, utilizing the enzymes alcohol dehydrogenase and acetaldehyde dehydrogenase to ultimately form carbon dioxide and water. A small percentage (2–10%) is excreted unchanged by lung, kidney, and skin.

Metabolic effects of alcohol are widespread. It is a central nervous system depressant that causes behavioral disinhibition at lower doses and general anesthesia, respiratory depression, coma, and death if consumption is excessive. Other effects include alteration of lipid and carbohydrate metabolism, sometimes complicated by hypoglycemia and lactic acidosis; stimulation of gastric acid secretion; and inhibition of hypothalamic release of antidiuretic hormone. Organ systems adversely effected by alcohol include gastrointestinal (gastritis, peptic ulcer, pancreatitis, fatty liver and cirrhosis), cardiovascular (myocardiopathy), skeletal muscle (myopathy), blood (anemia and thrombocytopenia) and, of course, the nervous system (peripheral neuropathy, seizures, dementias, cerebellar degeneration, etc.) (Schuckit, 1979; Victor and Adams, 1980a).

Manifestations of Alcohol Abuse and Withdrawal

There are two broad areas of potential diagnostic difficulty faced by the clinician dealing with alcohol-related problems. The first relates to the failure to recognize secondary complications of alcoholism or unrelated medical problems occurring in the obviously intoxicated patient. These include traumatic injuries (such as subdural hematoma), infections, hypoglycemia, hepatic encephalopathy, and vitamin deficiency states. To blithely assume that a patient is "just drunk" can have grave consequences that can be avoided if the clinician looks beyond the obvious.

The second area of diagnostic difficulty is failing to recognize that alcohol is the cause of a variety of organic mental disorders. Critical to such a diagnosis, of course, is an accurate history of alcohol intake which, unfortunately, is not easily obtained. Alcohol withdrawal delirium (delirium tremens), for example, is easily recognized in an alcoholic detoxification center but may be misdiagnosed if it occurs in a "closet" alcoholic who is hospitalized for unrelated reasons. The various alcohol abuse and withdrawal disorders will be summarized. It is important to realize that the ease with which a proper diagnosis is made will depend on both setting and available history.

Alcohol intoxication produces a characteristic constellation of psychological (mood change, irritability, loquacity, impaired attention) and physiological (slurred speech, incoordination, flushed face) findings such that diagnosis is seldom difficult. Nonetheless, even when a patient smells of alcohol and has a confirmatory blood-alcohol level, it is important to exclude the associated use of other drugs. While the clinical presentation of alcohol intoxication is characteristic, it is by no means diagnostic, and it is important to remember that disorders and toxins other than alcohol can cause a similar picture. For example, slurred speech and an unsteady gait are commonly found in lithium intoxication.

Alcohol idiosyncratic intoxication (pathological intoxication) is a syndrome in which amounts of alcohol insufficient to intoxicate most people cause an extreme reaction, usually one of aggressive, assaultive, destructive behavior. Although this disorder is included in *DSM III*, whether it exists as a well-defined entity is still open to question (Hollender, 1979). To consider such a diagnosis, it is important to exclude malingering, and also other disorders such as temporal lobe seizures and the use of drugs such as barbiturates or amphetamines.

Alcoholic blackouts are not periods of unconsciousness, but, rather, are episodes of amnesia occurring following alcohol ingestion. A person having blackouts is generally heavily intoxicated but still able to function, and later, when sober, has little or no recall for events which occurred during that time. The cause of blackouts is unknown, although they are more likely to occur in people with a history of head trauma and in people who are "gulpers" rather than "sippers" of alcohol (Goodwin, 1974).

Alcohol withdrawal symptoms vary considerably in character and severity. They generally follow alcohol discontinuation, although a relative decrease in alcohol intake may also result in a similar syndrome. In its milder form, alcohol withdrawal occurs after several days of heavy, prolonged drinking and manifests as tremulousness (the shakes), irritability, autonomic hyperactivity, and gastrointestinal symptoms such as nausea and vomiting. Alcohol intake will suppress the symptoms, or, with continued abstinence, they will gradually resolve over a period of days. Patients with essential, action, or senile tremor have been misdiagnosed as alcoholics, despite the fact that they lack the other characteristics of the syndrome. The fact that alcohol is often effective in suppressing this type of tremor may dispose these people to eventually becoming alcoholic.

Alcoholic hallucinosis is sometimes misdiagnosed as paranoid schizophrenia. It tends to occur during alcohol withdrawal or during a period of reduced consumption in an alcohol-dependent individual, and is characterized by vivid auditory hallucinations occurring in the presence of a clear sensorium. The hallucinations are often unpleasant, threatening, and disturbing to the patient, who is quite convinced of their reality. Associated findings of alcohol withdrawal, such as tremulousness, visual hallucinations, seizures, and delirium, may also be present. Generally, alcoholic hallucinosis resolves over a period of hours to days. Occasionally (10%) a chronic form develops, in which the patient becomes quite resigned to the hallucinations and also develops ideas of reference and persecutory delusions. At this point, distinction from chronic schizophrenia may not be possible, although it does not seem that the chronic form of alcoholic hallucinosis represents an unmasking of latent schizophrenia (*DSM III*, 1980; Victor and Adams, 1980a).

Alcohol delirium (delirium tremens) is essentially a delirium occurring 2–4 days after stopping or rapidly reducing alcohol consumption. It is characterized by "profound confusion, delusions, vivid hallucinations, tremors, agitation, and sleeplessness, as well as by increased activity of the autonomic nervous system, i.e., dilated pupils, fever, tachycardia, and profuse perspiration" (Victor and Adams, 1980). Although the syndrome resolves favorably in most cases, it must be taken seriously, since a mortality of 5–15% has been reported.

While a combination of delirium, coarse tremors, and vivid visual hallucinations is suggestive of alcohol withdrawal delirium, it is not specific for this entity, and diagnostic consideration must be given to other possible causes of delirium.

Chronic abuse of alcohol, with associated nutritional and vitamin deficiencies can lead to Wernicke disease, alcohol amnestic disorder (Korsakoff syndrome), and alcoholic dementia. Less common alcohol-associated disorders include cerebellar degeneration, Marchiafava-Bignami disease, and central pontine myelosis (Victor and Adams, 1980a).

Use of Alcohol in Psychiatric Patients

The treatment of preexisting psychiatric disorders is clearly complicated by alcohol abuse, such that prognosis becomes considerably less favorable. The extensive use of alcohol may also be consequent to a preexisting disorder, such that successful treatment of the latter will favorably resolve the former. For example, a depressed person may drink to modulate the depression, while a manic individual may consume excessive amounts during periods of increased sociability or to attentuate the mania. Consequently, all patients presenting with an alcohol abuse or withdrawal disorder should be carefully evaluated for an underlying primary psychiatric disorder (Schuckit, 1979).

Alcohol and Psychiatric Drugs

Alcohol can interact adversely with psychiatric drugs by potentiating central nervous system side effects. Fatalities from benzodiazepine overdose are rare, unless those drugs are taken in combination with alcohol. The ability to drive can be greatly compromised by a combination of alcohol with psychiatric drugs. Alcohol may increase metabolism of other drugs by inducing hepatic microsomal enzymes, or reduce drug metabolism by causing extensive damage to liver tissue. Given the widespread and often erratic use of alcohol, a physician prescribing any medication must be aware of the possibility of adverse interactions (Rosenberg, 1975; Buckman, 1976; Seixas, 1979; Anonymous, 1979).

The use of psychiatric drugs in the treatment of alcoholism and its complications is beyond the scope of this book. Interested readers are referred to an excellent review by Rada and Kellner (1979). These authors, incidentally, point out the need to approach alcohol–drug interactions in a "reasonable and sensitive manner," since a patient may respond to an order to abstain from alcohol by choosing to abstain, instead, from the prescribed medication.

Conclusion

Alcohol is probably the most widely abused drug in the United States. Familiarity with the psychiatric syndromes produced by alcohol abuse and withdrawal is important to insure accurate diagnosis, especially in settings in which a reliable history of alcohol intake is not available. It is also important to realize that these syndromes are not specific to alcohol, so as to avoid assuming etiology in situations in which alcohol use is only coincidental.

AMPHETAMINES AND AMPHETAMINE-LIKE DRUGS

Introduction

Although amphetamine was first synthesized in 1887, its medical uses were not explored until the early 1930s. It was initially used as a nasal decongestant and a bronchodilator and, shortly thereafter, as a central nervous system stimulant. Other amphetamines were developed, and uses grew to include the treatment of narcolepsy, minimal brain dysfunction, obesity, fatigue, depression, parkinsonism, and poisoning by central nervous system depressants. During World War II, the amphetamines were widely used to combat fatigue and to promote alertness and endurance, and were preferable to cocaine for these purposes because of oral effectiveness and longer duration of action. After the war, these drugs were widely prescribed for the treatment of depression both alone and in combination with barbiturates (Angrist and Sudilovsky, 1978).

In the late 1960's and throughout the 1970's, abuse became a progressively bigger problem not only with the oral amphetamines but also with parenterally administered forms. The "speed freak" would use intravenous amphetamines many times a day in doses of hundreds of milligrams, remaining continuously awake for days on end and becoming progressively more restless, agitated, and paranoid until "crashing" into a period of profound sleep and depression. In recent years, progressively greater restrictions have been placed on the legal manufacture and medical use of amphetamines, yet black market sources continue to provide a ready availability of often impure drugs.

Pharmacology

Amphetamines are readily absorbed from the gastrointestinal tract and are found in high concentration in brain and cerebrospinal fluid. They are metabolized in the liver but are also excreted in substantial amounts in the urine. Plasma half-life is greatly influenced by urinary pH. With acid urine,

67–73% of amphetamine is excreted unchanged with a plasma half-life of 7–14 hr, while with alkaline urine, plasma half-life increases to 18–34 hr, with metabolism being the main route of elimination. For this reason, acidification of the urine is an important part of treating amphetamine toxicity (Änggård et al., 1973).

The predominant pharmacological action of amphetamine is central nervous system stimulation. A moderate oral dose is likely to produce "wakefulness, alertness, and a decreased sense of fatigue; elevation of mood, with increased initiative, confidence, and ability to concentrate; often elation and euphoria; increase in motor and speech activity" (Innes and Nickerson, 1975). Performance that has been reduced by fatigue and sleep lack is often markedly improved. In addition, amphetamines stimulate the respiratory center and have hypothalamic activity that suppresses appetite. Other effects include blood pressure elevation and bronchial smooth muscle relaxation.

Manifestations of Amphetamine Abuse and Withdrawal

Amphetamine Abuse

The neuropsychiatric symptoms produced by amphetamines depend, in part, on the particular pattern of use. Types of abuse have been divided by Cohen (1975) into (1) sporadic use of average amounts, (2) average oral doses, (3) large oral doses, (4) large inhaled or ingested doses, and (5) in combination with other drugs.

The acute toxic effects are dose dependent and range from restlessness, jitteriness, irritability, insomnia, and tremulousness to confusion, delirium, hallucinations, paranoia, and assaultiveness. In cases of fatal overdose, convulsions, coma, and cerebral hemorrhage are common findings.

Psychiatric reactions to high dose methamphetamine use were divided into five categories (Smith and Fischer, 1970): (1) anxiety reactions characterized by fear, tremor, and somatic concern, (2) psychosis (see below), (3) exhaustion syndrome, (4) prolonged depression, (5) prolonged hallucinosis (with preexisting psychopathology felt to be a factor).

In the absence of a history of amphetamine use, symptoms produced by the drug can easily be misdiagnosed. Euphoria, and an increased sense of well being, initiative, and confidence suggest hypomania; anxiety, restlessness, fear, and tremors suggest an anxiety disorder; paranoia, delusions, and hallucinations suggest a schizophrenic, paranoid, or manic disorder; and confusion, disorientation, and impaired attention span suggest delirium of unknown etiology.

Amphetamine Psychosis

It was not long after its introduction into medicine that amphetamine was recognized as a cause of paranoid psychosis (Young and Scoville, 1938).

Because of the frequent surreptitious use of amphetamine and because of the similarity of symptoms to paranoid schizophrenia, many patients have been erroneously diagnosed and mistreated. Beamish and Kiloh (1960) described hospitalized patients who secretly ingested amphetamines and who were misdiagnosed as schizophrenic for as long as three years, during which time they were treated with electroconvulsive and insulin-coma therapies.

Amphetamine psychosis is characterized by paranoid ideation with well-formed delusions, stereotyped compulsive behavior, auditory, visual, tactile, and olfactory hallucinations, and the retention of clear consciousness and correct orientation (Snyder, 1973). Features felt to be helpful in distinguishing this disorder from paranoid schizophrenia are the absence of a formal thought disorder, a high incidence of visual hallucinations, a relatively appropriate affect, and a rapid remission following drug withdrawal (Siomopoulos, 1975). In clinical settings, such distinctions are not always easily made, a drug history may not be available, and urinary screening for amphetamines is often neglected. The diagnosis of amphetamine psychosis should be considered with any patient presenting with a paranoid psychosis or a paranoid schizophreniform illness, and appropriate toxicologic screening should be performed.

The psychosis produced by amphetamine does not seem to be owing to sleep deprivation nor to the activation of a preexisting schizophrenic disorder. It has been reliably produced in subjects with no prior schizophrenic or drug psychosis history by the regular oral administration of dextroamphetamine at hourly intervals in total doses ranging from 120–700 mg (Griffith et al., 1970).

Amphetamine psychoses are treated by:

1. Drug discontinuation
2. Acidification of urine to enhance renal elimination
3. Use of a dopamine antagonist such as haloperidol or droperidol to control symptoms and behavior (Gary and Saidi, 1978). The psychosis should clear completely within 1–$1\frac{1}{2}$ weeks.

Amphetamine Abstinence Psychosis

While amphetamine use psychosis is a well established entity, controversy still surrounds the possibility of an amphetamine withdrawal psychosis. Two psychotic withdrawal syndromes have been described in a limited number of patients—the first a delirium and the second a paranoid reaction in the presence of a clear sensorium (Streltzer and Leigh, 1977). These reports have been criticized on grounds such as (1) psychotic symptoms actually began prior to drug withdrawal, (2) a preexisting latent-schizophrenic process was unmasked, and (3) other drugs such as alcohol, benzodiazepines, and barbiturates were also involved.

Amphetamine Withdrawal

Abrupt discontinuation of amphetamines, especially following high doses and intravenous use, can result in an exhaustion syndrome associated with severe fatigue and need for sleep. Intense depressive symptoms have also been described during this period, and at least some clinicians feel that "amphetamine withdrawal causes apathy, psychomotor retardation, and sleep disturbances that may last for weeks or even months" (Wesson and Smith, 1973). Although depression is considered the major symptom associated with amphetamine withdrawal, its incidence, clinical course, and treatment require further definition.

Amphetamine-like Drugs

Although less extensively studied than the amphetamines, related drugs such as cocaine, ephedrine, methylphenidate, fenfluramine, diethylpropion, and phenmetrazine have been reported to cause psychoses in certain users (Angrist and Sudilovsky, 1978).

Use of Amphetamines in Psychiatric Patients

Under double-blind conditions, methylphenidate has been shown to aggravate symptoms of acute schizophrenia (Janowsky et al., 1973). There have also been case reports of schizophrenic relapse associated with the use of amphetamines for weight reduction (West, 1974). Amphetamine-induced activation or aggravation of manic symptoms in bipolar patients is also a possibility.

Amphetamines and Psychiatric Drugs

Amphetamines have direct sympathomimetic activity, cause catecholamine release, block catecholamine reuptake inactivation, and inhibit monoamine oxidase. Their use is contraindicated in patients who are being treated with **monoamine oxidase inhibitors** such as phenelzine, tranylcypromine, isocarboxazid, and pargyline.

Both amphetamines and methylphenidate have been used to predict clinical response to **tricyclic antidepressants**. Although not firmly established, there is some support for patients who experience a euphoric response to these drugs having a positive response to treatment with imipramine or desipramine (Stern et al., 1980). Also, the stimulants inhibit the hepatic metabolism of tricyclics, leading to correspondingly higher tricyclic blood levels (Wharton et al., 1971).

There is some evidence that **lithium** attenuates both the activation and euphoriant responses to amphetamines in man (Van Kammen and Murphy, 1975) although lithium is not an accepted treatment for amphetamine abuse.

Antipsychotic drugs are the drugs of choice for treating amphetamine psychoses. There appears to be no therapeutic use for a combination of antipsychotics and amphetamines.

Conclusion

The major psychiatric syndrome associated with amphetamine use is a paranoid psychosis that is often misdiagnosed as paranoid schizophrenia. Amphetamines may also uncover or aggravate symptoms in patients with preexisting schizophrenic or manic disorders.

CANNABIS (MARIJUANA)

Introduction

Cannabis is a drug obtained from the hemp plant, *Cannabis sativa*, which, depending on locale and method of preparation, is known by names such as hashish, charas, bhang, kif, ganja, dagga, and marijuana (Pillard, 1970). It is one of the oldest and most widely used drugs and is currently used throughout the world by hundreds of millions of people. It is also a highly controversial substance about which much has been written in social, political, economic, legal, and medical arenas. Many of these issues are not yet resolved.

The hemp plant manufactures a number of closely related cannabinoids, which include cannabinol, cannabinolic acid, cannabigerol, cannabicyclol, and several isomers of tetrahydrocannabinol (THC). The major psychoactive component is felt to be Δ^9-THC and to a lesser extent Δ^8-THC. The concentration of Δ^9-THC in the various natural preparations is quite variable and accounts for their differing potencies. The synthesis of Δ^9-THC has allowed a more standardized approach to the study of the pharmacological effects of cannabis.

Pharmacology

While cannabis in high doses can cause hallucinations, there are sufficient differences from true hallucinogens such as LSD, mescaline, and peyote to consider it pharmacologically distinct.

Although no more than half the THC in a marijuana cigarette is absorbed, absorption through the lungs is rapid, with pharmacological effects occurring in minutes, and peak plasma concentrations being reached in 10–30 min. The effect of a single cigarette lasts about 2–3 hr. Oral absorption is slow and uneven, with peak effects occurring after 2–3 hours and lasting 3–5 hr. The drug is lipid soluble and distributes to lipid rich tissues such as the central nervous system. Traces of THC and its metabolites can be detected in the plasma and urine for days after administration of even a single dose (Jaffe, 1975).

In animals, cannabis causes sedation and a decrease in spontaneous behavior and motivation, although a paradoxical prolongation of amphetamine stimulation has also been noted. In man, reports have differed owing to dose, preparation, route of administration, setting, subject expectation, and prior experience. Central nervous system effects from modest doses include alterations of mood, memory, motor coordination, cognition, sensorium, time sense, and self-perception. Cardiovascular changes include an increase in heart rate and conjunctival reddening.

Cannabis is an extremely safe substance, with lethal doses in animals being quite high and reports of death in man limited to sporadic case reports of questionable reliability (Nahas, 1974). Considering its widespread use, the incidence of adverse reactions to cannabis is quite low.

Manifestations of Cannabis Use and Withdrawal

Cannabis Use

Evaluation of cannabis toxicity is often made difficult by its ocurrence in a setting of multiple drug abuse and by the reluctance or inability of many patients to provide an accurate drug history.

A nonpsychotic **anxiety or panic reaction** is the most common adverse effect, occurring more often in the naive user. Symptoms which include apprehension, agitation, paranoia, fear of insanity or loss of control or death generally respond well to firm reassurance and seldom require hospitalization or pharmacotherapy.

Toxic psychoses from cannabis have no unique characteristics and consist of symptoms such as confusion, disorientation, altered attention, excitement, paranoia, and visual and auditory hallucinations. Resolution tends to occur promptly following discontinuation of the drug, and in those cases of prolonged disability a preexisting psychiatric disorder has usually been present.

Acute schizophreniform psychoses from cannabis have been distinguished from toxic psychoses by their occurrence in the presence of a clear sensorium. These reactions were found more often with multiple drug abuse in patients with preexisting psychiatric illness who later developed a characteristic schizophrenic syndrome (Tennant and Groesbeck, 1972).

Long-term, heavy cannabis use has been associated with what has been termed the **"amotivational syndrome"** which was described by Tennant and Groesbeck (1972) as follows:

> Major manifestations were apathy, dullness, and lethargy with mild-to-severe impairment of judgment, concentration, and memory. Intermittent episodes of confusion and inability to calculate occurred with high levels of chronic intoxication. Physical appearance was stereotyped in that all patients appeared dull, exhibited poor hygiene, and had slightly slowed speech. So apathetic were many patients that they lost interest in cosmetic appearance, proper diet, and personal affairs such as paying debts, job performance, etc. Although violence or overt acts of crime were rare in these patients, they were frequently in social and legal difficulties due to failure to care for their personal affairs.

Discontinuation of cannabis tends to result in resolution of these symptoms although there have been some reports of residual disability which raised the issue, as yet unresolved, of cannabis-induced brain damage (Kolansky and Moore, 1972; Maugh, 1974).

The effects of cannabis on sexual functioning have not been fully resolved. One report showed that plasma testosterone levels were lower in marijuana smokers than in nonsmokers, raising the issue of a possible relationship to **impotence** (Kolodny et al., 1974).

Cannabis Withdrawal

Although tolerance to cannabis has been demonstrated in both animal and man (Nahas, 1974), a well developed withdrawal syndrome has not been observed. Nonetheless, some heavy users have great difficulty giving up the drug.

Use of Cannabis in Psychiatric Patients

Like other psychoactive drugs, cannabis has been associated with exacerbation of preexisting psychiatric disorders. Even in this patient population, however, the incidence of adverse reactions appears to be quite low. Despite widespread medicinal use in the 19th and early 20th century, cannabis has no established value in the treatment of psychiatric disorders.

Cannabis and Psychiatric Drugs

In animals, THC potentiates both the depressant effects of barbiturates and alcohol and the stimulant effects of amphetamines and caffeine. In man, similar effects have been shown with alcohol, but adequate studies with most classes of psychiatric drugs have not been done (Nahas, 1974).

Conclusion

Cannabis (marijuana) can cause anxiety reactions and toxic psychoses. Other possible reactions include a schizophreniform psychosis and the "amotivational syndrome." Correct diagnosis depends on the history of cannabis use and is supported by resolution of symptoms upon drug discontinuation.

OPIATES AND SYNTHETIC ANALGESICS (OPIOIDS)

Introduction

Poppy juice was used by ancient Greek and Arabian physicians to treat medical ills of those times; in fact, the word **opium** is derived from the Greek name for juice. Opium smoking has been popular in the Orient for hundreds of years, and opium was an indispensible part of many over-the-counter medicines used during the 19th century in the United States. The isolation of morphine (in 1803) and codeine (in 1832) from opium was followed by the invention of the hypodermic syringe, which greatly facilitated both the medical and illicit use of the narcotic analogesics (Jaffe and Martin, 1975).

The main medical uses of the opioids are the treatment of pain, cough, diarrhea, and pulmonary edema due to left ventricular failure. The abuse potential for these drugs is high, with users somewhat arbitrarily classified as either medical abusers (patients who misuse prescribed drugs and health-care professionals who have access to medical sources) and street abusers (those whose source of opiate is primarily nonmedical).

In general, the therapeutic effects and addiction and abstinence characteristics of the opiates and synthetic analgesics are qualitatively similar, with quantitative differences being determined by dose, duration of use, duration of drug action, and potency. In addition to codeine, other opioids chemically related to morphine include diacetylmorphine (heroin), hydromorphone (Dilaudid), oxymorphone, hydrocodone, and oxycodone (Percodan). Synthetic analgesics which are structurally dissimilar yet pharmacologically similar to morphine include meperidine (Demerol), methodone (Dolophine), fentanyl, diphenoxylate (in Lomotil), propoxyphene (Darvon), and pentazocine (Talwin).

Pharmacology

The opioids exert their predominant effects on the central nervous system and gastrointestinal tract. Morphine produces analgesia, mood change, drowsiness, and a clouding of mental function. Other central effects include pupillary constriction, respiratory depression, nausea, and vomiting. A spasmogenic effect on the bowel wall results in the effective treatment of diarrhea and dysentery, as well as the side effect of constipation.

Opioids can be administered via the gastrointestinal tract, nasal mucosa (heroin snorting), and lungs (opium smoking), as well as by subcutaneous, intramuscular, and intravenous routes. They vary greatly in terms of overall potency (etorphine is 1000 times more potent than morphine), individual oral-parenteral potency (high for codeine, low for morphine), duration of action (hydrocodone—4–8 hr; meperidine—2–4 hr, propensity for causing constipation (meperidine—little or none; morphine—marked), and withdrawal syndrome (methadone withdrawal, while qualitatively similar to that of morphine, is less severe, slower to develop, and more prolonged) (Jaffe and Martin, 1975).

Tolerance, physical dependency, and withdrawal symptoms can readily develop from use of the opioids. Apparently, narcotic antagonists can cause mild abstinence symptoms in subjects who have taken as little as 15 mg of morphine thrice daily for three days (Victor and Adams, 1980b). A high degree of cross-tolerance exists between almost all of the opioids, such that a person tolerant to high doses of one will be tolerant to high doses of another. Once withdrawal is complete, however, tolerance is lost, and a previously well tolerated dose may become a fatal overdose.

The discovery of endogenous opiate receptors in man has been a recent major medical advance, and studies of endogenous peptides (endorphins, enkephalins) and their antagonists are providing a better understanding of pain, addiction, and psychiatric disorders such as schizophrenia.

Manifestations of Opioid Use, Abuse, and Withdrawal

The degree of euphoria or dysphoria from various opioids depends on dose, route of administration, individual predisposition, pattern of use, and a variety of other factors. While some addicts describe a "rush" or "thrill" or "kick" from the intravenous injection of an opioid, they often develop tolerance to this effect, and then maintain their drug habit primarily to avoid withdrawal symptoms. If an adequate supply of drug is always available, some addicts are able to live productive, respectable lives (Brecher, 1972).

Opioid intoxication is suggested by the presence of pupillary constriction, together with either euphoria, dysphoria, apathy, or psychomotor retardation, and either drowsiness, slurred speech, or impaired attention or memory (DSM III, 1980). Less frequently, opioids can cause a delirium, with confusion, disorientation, and hallucinations. In severely ill patients (trauma, myocardial infarction, or postoperative), these drugs may be one of a number of factors contributing to a delirium.

Opioid poisoning should be the primary consideration in a patient with respiratory depression, coma, and pinpoint pupils (although dilated pupils can occur in the presence of severe hypoxia). The presence of needle marks further supports a diagnosis of opioid abuse. These drugs can be detected in the urine, but in cases of suspected severe overdose, the use of a narcotic antagonist such as naloxone (Narcan) can not only be rapidly diagnostic but may also be life saving.

The toxic effects of meperidine can differ from those of morphine since meperidine can cause central nervous system excitation, with tremors, muscle twitches, and seizures.

The diagnosis of **opioid abuse** and **opioid dependence** may be difficult if the addict conceals his drug use history. One should be alert for physical signs of opioid use such as needle marks, thrombosed veins, constricted pupils (although meperidine addicts may have dilated pupils), cutaneous abscesses, and hepatitis. Drug seeking behaviors such as repeated emergency room visits with difficult to diagnose pain complaints, or visits to multiple physicians for analgesics should be viewed with suspicion. Often addicts have developed most convincing presentations of what appear to be legitimate pain syndromes (renal colic, myocardial infarction, migraine headache, etc.) in order to obtain narcotics from medical sources.

Opioid withdrawal or abstinence syndrome is diagnosed by a history of heavy, prolonged use (or the use of a narcotic antagonist after a briefer period of use) and the finding of symptoms such as the following after rapid cessation or reduction of use: Lacrimation, rhinorrhea, pupillary dilatation, piloerection, sweating, diarrhea, yawning, mild hypertension, tachycardia, fever, and insomnia (*DSM III*, 1980). For morphine and heroin, symptoms begin 8–12 hr after the last dose, and consist of yawning, sweating, watery eyes, and runny nose, and peak after 48–72 hr, with insomnia, restlessness, irritability, weakness, piloerection, nausea, vomiting, diarrhea, muscle cramps, chills, and sweating being prominent features. According to *DSM III* (1980), the symptoms of influenza and opioid withdrawal are quite similar and should be considered as part of the differential diagnosis.

Untreated, the acute withdrawal syndrome resolves clinically in 7–10 days, but a period of **protracted abstinence** may persist for many months (Jaffe, 1975; Schuckit, 1979). During this period, subtle physiological abnormalities can be demonstrated, and these, together with persistent behavioral alterations, may be responsible for the tendency of addicts to relapse.

Use of Opioids in Psychiatric Patients

Patients with preexisting psychiatric disorders appear to tolerate and respond appropriately to opioids when used for short-term, medically appropriate indications. Those individuals who meet diagnostic criteria for antisocial personality are at high risk for developing and maintaining patterns of substance abuse.

Opioids and Psychiatric Drugs

The depressant effects of opioids may be both exaggerated and prolonged by phenothiazines, tricyclic antidepressants, and monoamine oxidase inhibitors. Some phenothiazines appear to increase the analgesic potency of opioids, while others appear antianalgesic while at the same time enhancing sedative effects (Jaffe and Martin, 1975). The antipsychotic, antidepressant, and antianxiety drugs have no established role in the treatment of opioid intoxication, dependence, or withdrawal. A high incidence of depression has been reported among addicts on methadone maintenance, but the role of antidepressant drugs in their treatment is not well established (Weissman et al., 1976).

The use of meperidine (Demerol) in patients receiving monoamine oxidase inhibitors has been associated with reactions characterized by excitation, delirium, seizures, and hyperthermia or central nervous system depression, and, consequently, the combined use of these drugs is now contraindicated.

There is no evidence suggesting either adverse reactions or reduced effectiveness if narcotics are used in patients receiving lithium. Likewise, lithium is not a useful drug for treating opiate dependence or withdrawal.

Conclusion

The diagnosis of opiate and synthetic analgesic abuse and dependence may be quite difficult if the individual chooses to conceal his drug history. Both overdose and abstinence syndromes are quite characteristic, and if one is familiar with the symptoms, diagnosis should not be a problem.

The opioids have no role in the treatment of psychiatric disorders and, conversely, psychiatric drugs play no major role in the treatment of opioid disorders. Nonetheless, the discovery of endogenous opiate receptors and opioid peptides has produced a promising area of psychiatric research.

HALLUCINOGENS AND PHENCYCLIDINE

Introduction

Natural substances have been used for their hallucinatory properties for hundreds of years and have been an integral part of certain cultures and religions. Prominent examples include the peyotl cactus (peyote—mescaline), the sacred mushroom (Psilocybe mexicana—psilocybin and psilocin), and ololiuqui (the seeds of Rivea corymbosa or morning glory—lysergic acid-1-

hydroxyethylamide) (Hofmann, 1970). The modern era of hallucinogens began with the synthesis of lysergic acid diethylamine (LSD) in 1938 and the discovery of its psychoactive properties in 1943. It was not until the 1960's, however, that the abuse of these drugs became widespread and that various adverse psychotoxic reactions were identified. The clinical symptoms produced by hallucinogens such as LSD, mescaline, psilocybin, dimethyltryptamine (DMT), 2,5-dimethoxy-4-methyl-amphetamine (DOM; also called STP), and others, vary in duration of action but are sufficiently similar to be discussed as a group (Schuckit, 1979).

Phencyclidine (PCP) has sufficient differences from the more classic hallucinogens to be considered separately, although its abuse patterns as a "hallucinogen" have led to its inclusion in this section. Synthesized in 1957, PCP was briefly used as a general anesthetic in man until a high incidence of adverse reactions led to its withdrawal. It is still used in veterinary medicine as an immobilizing agent for subhuman primates. In 1967, PCP began its history as a street drug, but a reputation for unpleasant effects made it unpopular. In the 1970's, however, it made a comeback in epidemic proportion both in its own right and also misrepresented as THC, LSD, and other hallucinogens. Synthesis by clandestine laboratories was both easy and profitable (one pound of PCP, made from about $75 in raw materials, can bring in over $20,000 in street sales) so that supplies were readily available (Showalter and Thornton, 1977).

Pharmacology

The hallucinogens are well absorbed orally and are effective at relatively low doses. LSD is distributed throughout the body, with highest concentrations in lungs, liver, kidney, and brain. It is metabolized in the liver to 2-oxy-LSD and excreted in the feces. Its half-life in man is about 3 hr. In addition to central nervous system effects, LSD also causes pupillary dilatation, increased blood pressure, tachycardia, tremor, increased body temperature, antidiuresis, and elevated blood levels of free fatty acids (Byck, 1975).

PCP can be swallowed, snorted, smoked, or injected. Onset of action is rapid, and while plasma half-life is about 11 hr, the duration of action can be considerably longer. The prolonged effect may be due to factors such as lipid solubility, recycling through the gastrointestinal tract, and active metabolites (although pharmacological activity in the metabolites has been questioned) (Hollister, 1979). The drug can be measured in serum and urine, although there is often not a good correlation between drug level and symptoms. PCP has central nervous system depressant, sympathomimetic, and weak anticholinergic properties.

Manifestations of Hallucinogen and PCP Use

The profound psychedelic effects of the hallucinogens are well known, and because of differences in individual predisposition can be quite variable. The most common adverse effect is a **panic reaction** associated with a high level of stimulation, fright, fear of insanity, and terrifying hallucinations, which is generally responsive to reassurance in a nonthreatening environment. A more extreme reaction is a **toxic psychosis**, manifested by exaggerated panic reaction symptoms together with loss of contact with reality, depersonalization, paranoia, and confusion. Physical findings of sympathetic overstimulation are often present. Improvement generally occurs within hours or days. **Prolonged psychoses** have occurred in association with LSD use, but whether these represent the unmasking of latent schizophrenia or whether they can arise de novo in otherwise healthy individuals is not clear. **Flashbacks** (recurrences of hallucinatory experiences in the absence of further drug ingestion) may occur over a period of months but eventually decrease in frequency and intensity and eventually disappear (Louria, 1968; Schuckit, 1979).

The clinical spectrum of PCP symptoms is dose-dependent. Low doses (5–10 mg) can cause euphoria, agitation, paranoia, disorientation, confusion, depersonalization, and bizarre behavior, associated with ataxia, drowsiness, horizontal and vertical nystagmus, muscle rigidity, elevated blood pressure, and midsize to constricted pupils (Sioris and Krenzelok, 1978; Morgan and Solomon, 1978; Petersen and Stillman, 1979). According to Morgan and Solomon (1978), "The presence of horizontal or vertical nystagmus, muscular rigidity, and hypertension in a patient who is agitated, psychotic, or comatose and whose respiration is not depressed is diagnostic for PCP intoxication." Unless such diagnostic distinctions are made, the toxic syndrome can be mistaken for schizophrenia (Cohen, 1977). The value of blood and urine screening in such situations should be quite apparent.

High-dose intoxication is characterized by prolonged coma (days) and can be associated with hypertensive crises, seizures, renal failure, cardiovascular collapse, and death. Recovery may take weeks, during which time the patient may experience those symptoms found with low-dose intoxication.

Chronic use of PCP has been associated with persistent memory problems, speech difficulties, disordered mood, social deterioration, and periods of violent behavior. Whether PCP causes irreversible brain damage or can cause chronic psychoses in otherwise healthy individuals has not been resolved (Cohen, 1977; Petersen and Stillman, 1979).

Use of Hallucinogens and PCP in Psychiatric Patients

Although hallucinogens have been employed experimentally in a variety of psychiatric disorders, Schuckit (1979), quite appropriately, states:

"Hallucinogens have no medical uses in which their assets are known to outweigh their liabilities." The incidence of untoward reactions is many times higher in a psychotic population than in normals (Louria, 1968).

Hallucinogens and PCP and Psychiatric Drugs

Little is known about the potential or real adverse reactions between these classes of drugs. Both benzodiazepines and antipsychotic agents have been used to treat hallucinogen and PCP toxicity, although firm reassurance in an appropriate setting is often all that is necessary. Because adulterants with anticholinergic properties often contribute to hallucinogen toxicity and because STP (DOM) has intrinsic anticholinergic activity, treatment with antipsychotic drugs could conceivably aggravate certain toxic syndromes.

Conclusion

Hallucinogens and PCP have profound psychotoxic effects and can produce clinical states varying from panic attacks to toxic psychoses to schizophreniform psychoses. Diagnostic difficulties are likely, especially if the patient is unable or unwilling to give a history of drug ingestion, and also because the contents of street drugs are often impure and misrepresented.

REFERENCES

Änggård E, Jönsson L-E, Hogmark A-L, et al: Amphetamine metabolism in amphetamine psychosis. *Clin Pharmacol Ther* 14:870–880, 1973.

Angrist B, Sudilovsky A: Central nervous system stimulants: Historical aspects and clinical effects, in Iverson LL, Iverson SD, Snyder SH (eds): *Handbook of Psychopharmacology*. New York, Plenum Press, 1978, pp 99–165.

Anonymous: Alcohol-drug interactions. *FDA Drug Bull* 9:10–12, 1979.

Beamish P, Kiloh LG: Psychoses due to amphetamine consumption. *J Ment Sci* 106:337–343, 1960.

Brecher EM: *Licit and Illicit Drugs*. Mount Vernon, New York, Consumers Union, 1972, pp 33–41.

Buckman RW: Drug interactions and the practice of psychiatry. *Current Concepts Psychiatry* 2:1–12, January and April, 1976.

Bunker ML, McWilliams M: Caffeine content of common beverages. *J Am Dietetic Assoc* 74:28–32, 1979.

Byck R: Drugs and the treatment of psychiatric disorders, in Goodman LS, Gilman A (eds): *The Pharmacological Basis of Therapeutics*. New York, Macmillan, 1975, pp 152–200.

Cohen S: Amphetamine abuse. *JAMA* 231:414–415, 1975.

Cohen S: Angel dust. *JAMA* 238:515–516, 1977.

De Freitas B, Schwartz G: Effects of caffeine in chronic psychiatric patients. *Am J Psychiatry* 136:1337–1338, 1979.

Diagnostic and Statistical Manual of Mental Disorders, ed 3. Washington, American Psychiatric Association, 1980.

Dreisbach RH, Pfeiffer C: Caffeine-withdrawal headache. *J Lab Clin Med* 28:1212–1219, 1943.

Garfield E: Should we kick the caffeine habit? *Curr Contents* 23:5–9, February 18, 1980.

Gary NE, Saidi P: Methamphetamine intoxication, a speedy new treatment. *Am J Med* 64:537–540, 1978.

Gilbert RM, Marshman JA, Schwieder M, et al: Caffeine content of beverages as consumed. *J Can Med Assoc* 114:205–208, 1976.

Goldstein A, Kaizer S: Psychotropic effects of caffeine in man: III. A questionnaire survey of coffee drinking and its effects in a group of housewives. *Clin Pharmacol Ther* 10:477–488, 1969.

Goodwin DW: Alcoholic blackout and state-dependent learning. *Fed Proc* 33:1833–1835, 1974.

Greden JF: Anxiety or caffeinism: A diagnostic dilemma. *Am J Psychiatry* 131:1089–1092, 1974.

Greden JF, Fontaine P, Lubetsky M, et al: Anxiety and depression associated with caffeinism among psychiatric inpatients. *Am J Psychiatry* 135:963–966, 1978.

Greden JF, Victor BS, Fontaine P, et al: Caffeine-withdrawal headache: A clinical profile. *Psychosomatics* 21:411–418, 1980.

Griffith JD, Cavanaugh JH, Held J, et al: Experimental psychosis induced by the administration of d-amphetamine, in Costa E, Garattini S (eds): *Amphetamines and Related Compounds.* New York, Raven Press, 1970, pp 897–904.

Harrie JR: Caffeine and headache. *JAMA* 213:628, 1970.

Hirsch SR: Precipitation of antipsychotic drugs in interaction with coffee or tea. *Lancet* 2:1130–1131, 1979.

Hofmann A: The discovery of LSD and subsequent investigations on naturally occurring hallucinogens, in Ayd FJ, Blackwell B (eds): *Discoveries in Biological Psychiatry.* Philadelphia, Lippincott, 1970, pp 91–106.

Hollender MH: Pathological intoxication—is there such an entity? *J Clin Psychiatry* 40:424–426, 1979.

Hollister LE: Phencyclidine (PCP) use: Current problems. *Int Drug Ther News* 14:17–20, 1979.

Innes IR, Nickerson M: Norepinephrine, epinephrine, and the sympathomimetic amines, in Goodman LS, Gilman A (eds): *The Pharmacological Basis of Therapeutics.* New York, Macmillan, 1975, pp 477–513.

Jaffe JH: Drug addiction and drug abuse, in Goodman LS, Gilman A (eds): *The Pharmacological Basis of Therapeutics.* New York, Macmillan, 1975, pp 284–324.

Jaffe JH, Martin WR: Narcotic analgesics and antagonists, in Goodman LS, Gilman A (eds): *The Pharmacological Basis of Therapeutics.* New York, Macmillan, 1975, pp 245–283.

Janowsky DS, El-Yousef MK, Davis JM, et al: Provocation of schizophrenic symptoms by intravenous administration of methylphenidate. *Arch Gen Psychiatry* 28:185–191, 1973.

Kolansky H, Moore WT: Toxic effects of chronic marihuana use. *JAMA* 222:35–41, 1972.

Kolodny RC, Masters WH, Kolodner RM, et al: Depression of plasma testosterone levels after chronic intensive marihuana use. *N Eng J Med* 290:872–874, 1974.

Kulhanek F, Linde OK, Meisenberg G: Precipitation of antipsychotic drugs in interaction with coffee or tea. *Lancet* 2:1130, 1979.

Louria DB: Lysergic acid diethylamide. *N Eng J Med* 278:435–438, 1968.

McManamy MC, Schube PG: Caffeine intoxication: Report of a case the symptoms of which amounted to a psychosis. *N Eng J Med* 215:616–620, 1936.

Maugh TH: Marihuana: II. Does it damage the brain? *Science* 185:775–776, 1974.

Mikkelsen EJ: Caffeine and schizophrenia. *J Clin Psychiatry* 39:732–736, 1978.

Morgan JP, Solomon JL: Phencyclidine: Clinical pharmacology and toxicity. *NY State J Med* 78:2035–2038, 1978.

Nahas GG: Marihuana: Toxicity, tolerance, and therapeutic efficacy. *Drug Ther* 4:33–47, January 1974.

Neil JF, Himmelhoch JM, Mallinger AG, et al: Caffeinism complicating hypersomnic depressive episodes. *Comp Psychiatry* 19:377–385, 1978.

Petersen RC, Stillman RC: Phencyclidine: A review. *Hosp Formul* 14:334–344, 1979.

Pillard RC: Marihuana. *N Eng J Med* 283:294–303, 1970.

Rada RT, Kellner R: Drug treatment in alcoholism, in Davis JM, Greenblatt D (eds): *Psycho-pharmacology Update: New and Neglected Areas*. New York, Grune & Stratton, 1979, pp 105–144.

Rosenberg JM: Alcohol, your toughest prescribing problem. *Curr Prescribing* 1:40–43, 1975.

Schuckit MA: *Drug and Alcohol Abuse*. New York, Plenum Press, 1979.

Seixas FA: Drug/alcohol interactions: Avert potential dangers. *Geriatrics* 34:89–102, 1979.

Showalter CV, Thornton WE: Clinical pharmacology of phencyclidine toxicity. *Am J Psychiatry* 134:1234–1237, 1977.

Siomopoulos V: Amphetamine psychosis: Overview and a hypothesis. *Dis Nerv Syst* 36:336–339, 1975.

Sioris LJ, Krenzelok EP: Phencyclidine intoxication: A literature review. *Am J Hosp Pharm* 35:1362–1367, 1978.

Smith DE, Fischer CM: An analysis of 310 cases of acute high-dose methamphetamine toxicity in Haight-Ashbury. *Clin Toxicol* 3:117–124, 1970.

Snyder SH: Amphetamine psychosis: A "model" schizophrenia mediated by catecholamines. *Am J Psychiatry* 130:61–67, 1973.

Stern SL, Rush AJ, Mendels J: Toward a rational pharmacotherapy of depression. *Am J Psychiatry* 137:545–552, 1980.

Streltzer J, Leigh H: Amphetamine abstinence psychosis—does it exist? *Psychiat Opinion* 14:47–50, 1977.

Tennant FS, Groesbeck CJ: Psychiatric effects of hashish. *Arch Gen Psychiatry* 27:133–136, 1972.

Van Kammen DP, Murphy DL: Attenuation of the euphoriant and activating effects of d- and l-amphetamine by lithium carbonate treatment. *Psychopharmacologia* 44:215–224, 1975.

Victor M, Adams RD: Alcohol, in Isselbacher KJ, Adams RD, Braunwald E, et al (eds): *Harrison's Principles of Internal Medicine*, ed 9. New York, McGraw–Hill, 1980a, 969–977.

Victor M, Adams RD: Opiates and synthetic analgesics, in Isselbacher KJ, Adams RD, Braunwald E, et al (eds): *Harrison's Principles of Internal Medicine*, ed 9. New York, McGraw–Hill, 1980b, pp 978–982.

Weissman MM, Slobetz F, Prusoff B, et al: Clinical depression among narcotic addicts maintained on methadone in the community. *Am J Psychiatry* 133:1434–1438, 1976.

Wesson DR, Smith DE: Recognizing and treating amphetamine abuse. *Hosp Physician* 9:22–26, August 1973.

West AP: Interaction of low-dose amphetamine use with schizophrenia in outpatients: Three case reports. *Am J Psychiatry* 131:321–323, 1974.

Wharton RN, Perel JM, Dayton PG, et al: A potential clinical use for methylphenidate with tricyclic antidepressants. *Am J Psychiatry* 127:1619–1625, 1971.

Winstead DK: Coffee consumption among psychiatric inpatients. *Am J Psychiatry* 133:1447–1450, 1976.

Young D, Scoville WB: Paranoid psychosis in narcolepsy and the possible danger of benzedrine treatment. *Med Clin North Am* 22:637–646, 1938.

Index

Copper
  in Wilson disease, 206, 210–212
Cromolyn, 73, 349
Cryptotetany, 195
Cushing syndrome, see
      Hyperadrenalism
Cyanocobalamin, see Vitamin B₁₂
      deficiency
Cycloserine, 241

Death
  sudden
    antipsychotic drugs, 43
    tricyclic antidepressants, 44
Dehydration, 182
Delayed sleep phase syndrome, 339
Delirium
  anticholinergic, 11, 106–107
  due to digitalis, 11
  hallucinations, 10
Delirium tremens, 120, 347
Dementia
  cardiogenic, 17
Depression, 6–7
  due to amphetamine withdrawal,
      352
  due to amphetamines, 350
  due to arsenic, 281
  due to bromism, 284, 285
  in carcinoid syndrome, 105
  in ciliac disease, 103
  due to cimetidine, 109
  due to Cushing syndrome, 135,
      142
  differential diagnosis, 6–7
  drug induced, 7
  drug withdrawal, 7
  due to exogenous steroids,
      136–137
  due to hepatic encephalopathy,
      115, 118
  due to hypercapnia, 52–53
  due to hyperparathyroidism, 157
  due to hyperthyroidism, 146
  due to hypoadrenalism, 141, 142
  due to hypoparathyroidism, 160,
      162
  due to hypothyroidism, 149, 150
  due to infectious mononucleosis,
      267–268
  in irritable bowel syndrome, 106
  due to lupus erythematosus, 218
  due to mercury, 274, 275
  in methadone maintenance, 359
  due to methyldopa, 39
  narcolepsy
    association with, 335

Depression (cont.)
  due to oral contraceptives,
      311–313
  due to organophosphate,
      288–289
  in pancreatic carcinoma,
      111–113
  due to pellagra, 238
  due to pheochromocytoma, 21
  due to polymyalgia rheumatica-
      giant cell arteritis, 34
  postgastrectomy, 101
  in posthepatitis syndrome, 121
  due to premenstrual syndrome,
      304–305
  due to propranolol, 38
  due to reserpine, 39
  due to thiamine deficiency, 234
  viral antibodies, 265
  due to viral encephalitis, 261
  due to vitamin A toxicity, 233
  due to vitamin B₁₂ deficiency, 246
  due to vitamin B₆ deficiency,
      241–242
  due to vitamin C deficiency, 253
  due to Wilson disease, 210
Dermatologic disorders, see Skin
Dialysis
  dementia, 84–85
  disequilibrium syndrome, 83–84
  hemodialysis, 82–85
  sexual dysfunction, 86–87, 329
  subdural hematoma, 85
Diaphragmatic flutter, 67–69
  causes, 68
  clinical features, 68
  treatment, 69
Diarrhea
  in carcinoid syndrome, 104
Dicumarol
  interaction with tricyclic
      antidepressants, 45
Diethylpropion, 352
Digitalis
  cause of fatigue, 8
Diphenylhydantoin, see Phenytoin
Diphenylhydantoin (see also
Disopyramide
  neuropsychiatric symptoms, 38
  sexual dysfunction, 41
Diuretics
  interaction with lithium, 91
  potassium sparing
    interaction with lithium, 46
  thiazide
    interaction with lithium, 46, 91
    sexual dysfunction, 41